# Physical Medicine and Rehabilitation Q&A Review

# Physical Medicine and Rehabilitation Q&A Review

## Second Edition

**Lyn D. Weiss, MD**
Chairman and Program Director
Department of Physical Medicine & Rehabilitation
Nassau University Medical Center
East Meadow, New York

**Harry J. Lenaburg, MD**
Dublin Physical Medicine and Rehabilitation Associates
Dublin, Georgia

**Jay M. Weiss, MD**
Medical Director
Long Island Physical Medicine and Rehabilitation
Syosset, New York

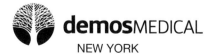
**demos**MEDICAL
NEW YORK

Visit our website at www.demosmedical.com

*ISBN:* 9781620701256
*e-book ISBN:* 9781617052989

*Acquisitions Editor:* Beth Barry
*Compositor:* Exeter Premedia Services Private Ltd.

**Library of Congress Cataloging-in-Publication Data**

Names: Weiss, Lyn D., author. | Lenaburg, Harry J., author. | Weiss, Jay M.,
   author.
Title: Physical medicine and rehabilitation Q&A review / Lyn D. Weiss, Harry
   J. Lenaburg, Jay M. Weiss.
Other titles: Physical medicine and rehabilitation Q and A review
Description: Second edition. | New York: Demos, [2017] | Includes
   bibliographical references and index.
Identifiers: LCCN 2016054245 | ISBN 9781620701256 | ISBN 9781617052989 (e-book)
Subjects: | MESH: Physical and Rehabilitation Medicine—methods | Physical
   Therapy Modalities | Rehabilitation—methods | Examination Questions
Classification: LCC RM701.6 | NLM WB 18.2 | DDC 610.76—dc23
LC record available at https://lccn.loc.gov/2016054245

Printed in the United States of America by McNaughton & Gunn.
17 18 19 20 21 / 5 4 3 2 1

*We dedicate this book to Ari, Lauren, Helene, Kyle, Stefan, Becca, and Richard. You give life meaning and inspiration.*—Jay M. Weiss and Lyn D. Weiss

*I dedicate this book to Leigh.*—Harry J. Lenaburg

# Contents

# Contributors

**Vikram Agnish, DO,** Department of Physical Medicine and Rehabilitation, Nassau University Medical Center, East Meadow, New York

**Elisa Alpert, MD,** Department of Physical Medicine and Rehabilitation, Nassau University Medical Center, East Meadow, New York

**Anu Anand, MD,** Medical Rehab Inc., Pittsburgh, Pennsylvania

**Alfred Castillo, DO,** Physical Medicine and Rehabilitation, Sports Medicine Attending, New York Methodist Hospital, Brooklyn, New York

**Rodrigo Cayme, MD,** Interventional Spine Medicine, Kansas City University of Medicine and Biosciences, Kansas City, Missouri

**Archana Chand, DO,** Cleveland Clinic, Cleveland, Ohio

**Yousaf Chowdhry, MD,** Albany Medical Center, Albany, New York

**Ricardo Cruz, MD,** Department of Physical Medicine and Rehabilitation, Nassau University Medical Center, East Meadow, New York; South Nassau Community Hospital, Oceanside, New York

**Robert Domingo, PhD,** Department of Physical Medicine and Rehabilitation, Nassau University Medical Center, East Meadow, New York

**Brian Golden, DO,** Department of Physical Medicine and Rehabilitation, Nassau University Medical Center, East Meadow, New York

**Burhan Haleem, DO,** RA Pain Services, Turnersville, New Jersey

**Sasha R. Iversen, DO,** Innovative Physical Medicine and Rehabilitation, Houston, Texas

**Navdeep Singh Jassal, MD,** Interventional Pain Attending, Florida Pain Medicine; Assistant Clinical Professor, Department of Neurology/Pain Medicine, University of South Florida, Tampa, Florida

**Sylvia John, MD,** Department of Physical Medicine and Rehabilitation, North Shore-Long Island Jewish Health System, Manhasset, New York

**Satish Kadakia, MD,** Department of Neurology, Nassau University Medical Center, East Meadow, New York

**Trishla Kanthala, DO,** Northeastern Rehabilitation Associates, Scranton, Pennsylvania

**Shilo Kramer, DO,** Physical Medicine and Rehabilitation, Complete Wellness NYC, New York, New York

**Susan Maltser, DO,** Department of Physical Medicine and Rehabilitation, North Shore-Long Island Jewish Health System, Manhasset, New York

**Yuliya Mastrovskaya, DO,** Private Practice, New York, New York

**Phillip Mendis, DO,** Department of Physical Medicine and Rehabilitation, Nassau University Medical Center, East Meadow, New York

**Kyle Menze, DO,** Fellow, Pediatric Rehabilitation Medicine, Montefiore Medical Center, Bronx, New York

**John J. Michalisin, MD,** Department of Anesthesiology, Perioperative Care and Pain Medicine, Center for the Study and Treatment of Pain, NYU Langone Medical Center, New York, New York

**Ricardo Aaron Miranda, MD,** Interventional Pain Management, St. John Medical Center, Tulsa, Oklahoma

**Matthew Moore, DO,** Department of Physical Medicine and Rehabilitation, Nassau University Medical Center, East Meadow, New York

**Kunal Oak, DO,** Rusk Institution of Rehabilitation Medicine, NYU Langone Medical Center, New York, New York

**Anup Patel, DO,** Pennsylvania State University, State College, Pennsylvania

**Arpit A. Patel, DO,** Department of Neurology and Interventional Pain Medicine, Florida Pain Medicine, Wesley Chapel; University of South Florida, Morsani School of Medicine, Tampa, Florida

**Ketan Patel, MD,** Department of Physical Medicine and Rehabilitation, Nassau University Medical Center, East Meadow, New York

**Nisha Patel, MD,** Department of Physical Medicine and Rehabilitation, North Shore-Long Island Jewish Health System, Manhasset, New York

**Craig Rosenberg, MD,** Department of Physical Medicine and Rehabilitation, Southside Hospital, Bay Shore, New York

**Rosanna Sabini, DO,** Department of Physical Medicine and Rehabilitation, North Shore-Long Island Jewish Health System, Manhasset, New York

**Lynn Schaefer, PhD,** Department of Physical Medicine and Rehabilitation, Nassau University Medical Center, East Meadow, New York

**Sameer Sharma, MD,** Attending Physician at Capitol Pain Institute, Austin, Texas

**Matthew Shatzer, DO,** Department of Physical Medicine and Rehabilitation, North Shore-Long Island Jewish Health System, Manhasset, New York

**Weibin Shi, MD,** Penn State Hershey Physical Medicine & Rehabilitation, Hummelstown, Pennsylvania

**Farah Siddiqui, MD,** Department of Physical Medicine and Rehabilitation, Nassau University Medical Center, East Meadow, New York

**Lincy Thadathil, DO,** Department of Physical Medicine and Rehabilitation, Nassau University Medical Center, East Meadow, New York

**Justin Thottam, DO,** Department of Physical Medicine and Rehabilitation, Nassau University Medical Center, East Meadow, New York

**Kevin H. Trinh, MD,** Pain Medicine, Loma Linda University Medical Center, Loma Linda, California

**Mohammad Zaidi, MD,** Department of Physical Medicine and Rehabilitation, St. Charles Hospital, Stony Brook University Medical Center, Stony Brook, New York

**Ashley Zakhary, MD,** Department of Physical Medicine and Rehabilitation, Rutgers New Jersey Medical Center, Newark, New Jersey

# *Preface*

This book is for medical students and residents who are starting to learn about the field of physical medicine and rehabilitation. It is not meant as a board review, but rather as a tool to support learning throughout training. The question and answer (Q&A) format can be utilized to teach the basics of the field and reinforce knowledge acquired. Students are encouraged to use this format to learn in a consequence-free environment and to enhance understanding in the areas they find weaknesses.

The goal of this book is not merely to get the correct answer and test knowledge, but to promote a greater understanding of this broad field of medicine. Optimal learning requires an appreciation of why the other choices are incorrect. Students are encouraged to read the answers and rationales for all of the questions to solidify and add to their understanding. If the student finds that he or she is missing questions in one particular area, further study in that area is encouraged.

We took the comments regarding the first edition very seriously. We hope that the answers are more comprehensive so that the reader's knowledge is expanded. The breadth and depth of the field has expanded. Therefore, we have expanded explanations, added questions, and included new sections.

We hope that this book stimulates learning about this ever-evolving and expanding field. If it does, our patients are the ones who will ultimately benefit.

# *Acknowledgments*

The authors would like to thank all of their students, colleagues, and mentors who encourage us to learn, grow, and teach. Thank you to the contributors for their tremendous efforts and dedication to the field. Special thank you to Beth Barry of Demos Medical Publishing for her belief in us and her support of our endeavors.

# Anatomy

## QUESTIONS

1. The gastrocnemius muscle is supplied by which nerve?
    A) Femoral nerve
    B) Obturator nerve
    C) Common peroneal nerve
    D) Tibial nerve

2. Which nerve root will most likely be affected by a posterior L3-L4 herniated disk?
    A) L2
    B) L3
    C) L4
    D) L5

3. Which meniscus is "O" shaped in the knee?
    A) Medial meniscus
    B) Anterior meniscus
    C) Lateral meniscus
    D) Posterior meniscus

4. The radial head articulates with which part of the humerus?
    A) Trochlea
    B) Capitellum
    C) Lateral epicondyle
    D) Coronoid process

5. Sensory innervation to the area of skin over the middle finger (dermatome) is subserved by afferent fibers from which dorsal root?
    A) C5
    B) C6
    C) C7
    D) C8

6. The muscles innervated by the musculocutaneous nerve includes all of the following **except**:
    A) Coracobrachialis
    B) Brachialis
    C) Biceps brachii
    D) Brachioradialis

7. What nerve innervates the levator scapulae and the rhomboids?
    A) Suprascapular nerve
    B) Subscapular nerve

ANSWERS TO THIS SECTION CAN BE FOUND ON PAGE 13

C) Dorsal scapular nerve
D) Axillary nerve

8. Which is the only carpal bone that crosses both the proximal and distal carpal rows?
   A) Hamate
   B) Scaphoid (navicular)
   C) Trapezoid
   D) Capitate

9. The intrinsic back muscles act to maintain posture and control of the spinal column and are inner-vated by the posterior rami of spinal nerves. Of these, the intermediate layer of the intrinsic back muscles include all of the following **except**:
   A) Iliocostalis
   B) Longissimus
   C) Spinalis
   D) Semispinalis

10. Which ligament of the spine resists extension?
    A) Posterior longitudinal ligament
    B) Ligamentum flavum and facet joint capsule
    C) Anterior longitudinal ligament
    D) Interspinous and supraspinous ligaments

11. All of the following are true about the anterior cruciate ligament (ACL) **except**:
    A) It originates in the medial femoral condyle and attaches to the lateral tibial eminence
    B) It draws the femoral condyles anteriorly during flexion
    C) Prevents hyperextension of the knee and backward sliding of the femur
    D) Internal rotation of the femur tightens it, and external rotation loosens it

12. Which muscle is an ankle dorsiflexor and invertor?
    A) Tibialis anterior
    B) Peroneus tertius
    C) Peroneus brevis
    D) Plantaris

13. Where is the most common location of an Achilles tendon rupture?
    A) At the attachment to the calcaneus
    B) At the aponeurosis of the gastrocnemius
    C) 2 to 5 cm proximal to tendon insertion at calcaneus
    D) Near the soleus

14. Shoulder range of motion (ROM) involves 180° of flexion, 180° of abduction, 60° of extension, and 60° of adduction. A balance exists between the glenohumeral and scapulothoracic motion during shoulder abduction. How many degrees of scapulothoracic motion is involved in shoulder abduction?
    A) 30°
    B) 60°
    C) 90°
    D) 120°

15. Nerve connective tissue includes all of the following **except**:
    A) Myelin sheath
    B) Endoneurium
    C) Perineurium
    D) Epineurium

16. What nerve innervates the subscapularis muscle?
    A) Dorsal scapular nerve
    B) Suprascapular nerve
    C) Subscapular nerve
    D) Musculocutaneous nerve

17. What is the function of the dorsal interosseous (DIO) muscles?
    A) Finger adduct and metacarpophalangeal (MCP) flexion
    B) MCP extension and wrist extension
    C) Finger abduction and MCP extension
    D) Finger abduction and MCP flexion

18. Where is the insertion of the flexor digitorum superficialis (FDS) muscle?
    A) Metacarpophalangeal (MCP) joint
    B) Proximal phalanx
    C) Middle phalanx
    D) Distal phalanx

19. What type of joint is the hip?
    A) Ball and socket
    B) Hinged
    C) Pivot
    D) Gliding

20. What part of the meniscus of the knee is poorly vascularized?
    A) Peripheral (outer) 1/3
    B) Peripheral (outer) 2/3
    C) Inner (central) 2/3
    D) Inner (central) 1/3

21. Which is **not** a compartment of the lower leg?
    A) Lateral compartment
    B) Anterior compartment
    C) Superficial posterior compartment
    D) Medial compartment

22. Where are motor axons found?
    A) Mainly in anterior (ventral) nerve roots
    B) Mainly in posterior (dorsal) nerve roots
    C) Dorsal root ganglion
    D) Proximal nerve roots

23. Finger extensors (to digits 2–5) include all of the following **except**:
    A) Extensor pollicis longus (EPL)
    B) Extensor digitorum communis

    C) Extensor indices (proprius)
    D) Extensor digiti minimi

24. Components of the neuromuscular junction include all of the following **except**:
    A) Motor nerve cell body
    B) Presynaptic region
    C) Synaptic cleft
    D) Postsynaptic region

25. What nerve innervates the teres minor muscle?
    A) Axillary nerve
    B) Musculocutaneous nerve
    C) Subscapular nerve
    D) Suprascapular nerve

26. What structures pass through the carpal tunnel?
    A) Median nerve, extensor pollicis longus (EPL), flexor digitorum superficialis (FDS), and flexor digitorum profundus (FDP) tendons
    B) Median nerve, abductor pollicis brevis (APB), FDS, and FDP tendons
    C) Median nerve, flexor pollicis longus (FPL), FDS, and FDP tendons
    D) Ulnar nerve, FPL, FDS, and FDP tendons

27. Which muscle functions to externally rotate the shoulder?
    A) Latissimus dorsi
    B) Subscapularis
    C) Infraspinatus
    D) Teres major

28. Which is **not** a hip flexor muscle?    *Per Cucc all are*
    A) Iliopsoas
    B) Gracilis
    C) Adductor magnus
    D) Rectus femoris

29. Which is **not** an anterior bursa of the knee?
    A) Prepatellar bursa
    B) Pes anserine bursa
    C) Deep infrapatellar bursa
    D) Suprapatellar bursa

30. What forms the medial malleolus?
    A) Talus and calcaneus
    B) Distal tibia
    C) Distal fibula
    D) Cuneiform bones

31. The patellar tendon reflex assesses which nerve root?
    A) L1
    B) L4
    C) L5
    D) S1

32. Finger flexors (to digits 2–4) include all of the following **except**:
    A) Dorsal and palmar interossei
    B) Flexor digitorum superficialis (FDS)
    C) Lumbricals
    D) Palmaris longus (PL)

33. The basic functional element of the neuromuscular system is a motor unit, which consists of all of the following **except**:
    A) An anterior horn cell (motor nerve cell body)
    B) The dorsal root ganglion
    C) Peripheral nerve
    D) Neuromuscular junction

34. What nerve innervates the supraspinatus muscle?
    A) Dorsal scapular nerve
    B) Suprascapular nerve
    C) Lateral pectoral nerve
    D) Axillary nerve

35. How many dorsal compartments are there in the hand?
    A) 6
    B) 5
    C) 4
    D) 3

36. Which muscle is the *main* flexor of the forearm?
    A) Anconeus
    B) Biceps brachii
    C) Brachialis
    D) Brachioradialis

37. Which is **not** a hip abductor?
    A) Gluteus medius
    B) Gluteus minimus
    C) Long head of biceps femoris
    D) Piriformis

38. What is located at the attachment of the tendons of the sartorius, gracilis, semitendinosus, and the medial collateral ligament?
    A) Baker's cyst
    B) Pes anserine bursa
    C) Posterior bursa
    D) Deep infrapatellar bursa

39. What forms the lateral malleolus?
    A) Distal tibia
    B) Distal fibula
    C) Talus
    D) Navicular

40. The Achilles reflex assesses which nerve root?
    A) L4
    B) L5
    C) S1
    D) S3

41. Ulnar deviation (also known as wrist adduction) includes paired contraction of which of the following muscle groups?
    A) Flexor carpi ulnaris (FCU) and extensor carpi ulnaris (ECU)
    B) ECU and palmaris longus (PL)
    C) ECU and extensor pollicis longus (EPL)
    D) Extensor carpi radialis (ECR) and flexor carpi radialis (FCR)

42. All of these are accessory muscles of inspiration **except**:
    A) Sternocleidomastoid
    B) Trapezius
    C) Pectoralis major
    D) Internal intercostals

43. The lumbar plexus (L1–L4) includes all of the following nerves **except**:
    A) Ilioinguinal nerve
    B) Iliohypogastric nerve
    C) Lateral cutaneous nerve of the thigh
    D) Posterior cutaneous nerve of the thigh

44. Which peripheral nerve supplies the brachialis muscle?
    A) Median
    B) Ulnar
    C) Musculocutaneous
    D) Axillary

45. Which trunk(s) of the brachial plexus contribute(s) to the radial nerve?
    A) Upper and lower trunks
    B) Upper and middle trunks
    C) Lower trunk
    D) Upper, middle, and lower trunks

46. Which muscle is an internal rotator of the hip?
    A) Obturator internus
    B) Semitendinosus
    C) Quadratus femoris
    D) Superior gemellus

47. What is the "terrible triad"?
    A) Medial/lateral meniscal injury with anterior cruciate ligament (ACL) tear
    B) ACL, medial collateral ligament (MCL), and medial meniscus injury
    C) ACL, posterior cruciate ligament (PCL), lateral meniscus injury
    D) ACL, MCL, and PCL

48. Which ligament is the weakest of the ankle ligaments?
    A) Deltoid ligament
    B) Calcaneofibular ligament

C) Anterior talofibular ligament
D) Posterior talofibular ligament

49. If someone has weak knee extension and hip flexion, what nerve is most likely injured?
    A) Obturator nerve
    B) Femoral nerve
    C) Sciatic nerve
    D) Tibial nerve

50. All of the following muscles involved in wrist and finger extension receive innervation from the radial nerve **except**:   ANSWER IS WRONG (all are Radial)
    A) Extensor carpi radialis longus
    B) Extensor carpi radialis brevis
    C) Extensor digiti minimi
    D) Extensor indicis

51. When palpating the thoracolumbar and sacral spine, which of the following statements regarding landmarks is **incorrect**?
    A) Spinous process of T3 is at the level of the spine of the scapula
    B) T8 is at the level of the inferior angle of the scapula
    C) S2 is at the level of the posterior superior iliac spine
    D) L2 is at the level of the iliac crests

52. Sacral plexus (L4–S4) includes all of the following nerves **except**:
    A) Genitofemoral nerve
    B) Superior and inferior gluteal nerves
    C) Sciatic nerve
    D) Pudendal nerve

53. Which peripheral nerve supplies the anconeus muscle?
    A) Median
    B) Ulnar
    C) Musculocutaneous
    D) Radial

54. What two tendons comprise the first dorsal compartment of the wrist?
    A) Extensor pollicis brevis (EPB) and abductor pollicis longus (APL)
    B) Extensor pollicis longus (EPL) and abductor pollicis brevis (APB)
    C) Extensor carpi radialis longus and APL
    D) Extensor carpi radialis brevis and APB

55. Which muscle is an external rotator of the hip?
    A) Tensor fasciae lata
    B) Gluteus maximus
    C) Gluteus medius
    D) Gracilis

56. Normal range of motion for the knee is:
    A) 0° to 90°
    B) 0° to 135°
    C) 10° to 150°
    D) 0° to 170°

57. Which ligament stabilizes the medial ankle?
    A) Posterior talofibular ligament
    B) Deltoid ligament
    C) Anterior talofibular ligament
    D) Calcaneofibular ligament

58. A tibial nerve injury is characterized by:
    A) Weak hip adduction
    B) Weak foot eversion and dorsiflexion
    C) Weak foot inversion and plantar flexion
    D) Weak knee extension

59. All of the following muscles involved in wrist and finger flexion receive innervation from the median nerve **except**:
    A) Flexor carpi radialis (FCR)
    B) Flexor carpi ulnaris (FCU)
    C) Palmaris longus (PL)
    D) Flexor pollicis longus (FPL)

60. When palpating the cervical spine, which of the following statements regarding landmarks is **incorrect**?
    A) Transverse process of C2 is palpated at the angle of the mandible
    B) The first palpable midline spinous process is of C2
    C) C7 has the largest cervical spinous process, also known as the *vertebra prominens*
    D) Thyroid cartilage is located at the level of C6, C7 anteriorly

61. Which one of the following is **not** a branch of the facial nerve (cranial nerve VII)?
    A) Posterior auricular nerve
    B) Temporal branches
    C) Mandibular nerve
    D) Marginal mandibular branch

62. What type of joint is the shoulder joint?
    A) Hinge
    B) Ball and socket
    C) Suture
    D) Saddle

63. What structures pass through Guyon's canal (ulnar tunnel at the wrist)?
    A) Ulnar nerve, extensor carpi ulnaris (ECU), adductor pollicis
    B) Ulnar nerve, ulnar artery, ECU
    C) Ulnar nerve, ulnar artery
    D) Ulnar nerve, adductor pollicis, ulnar artery

64. What is the function of the iliofemoral ligament?
    A) Limit extension, abduction, and external rotation of the hip
    B) Limit extension, adduction, and internal rotation of the hip
    C) Limit flexion, abduction, and external rotation of the hip
    D) Limit flexion, adduction, and internal rotation of the hip

65. Which muscle is a knee flexor?
    A) Rectus femoris
    B) Vastus lateralis
    C) Vastus medialis obliques
    D) Biceps femoris

66. What is the function of the Lisfranc ligament?
    A) Connects the distal tibia to the talus
    B) Connects the second metatarsal head to the first cuneiform
    C) Preserves the medial longitudinal arch of the foot
    D) Acts as primary ankle stabilizer

67. What is the medical term for "knock-kneed"?
    A) Genu varum
    B) Genu valgum
    C) Genu recurvatum
    D) Genu anterium

68. The proximal row of carpal bones from a radial to ulnar direction include:
    A) Scaphoid, lunate, trapezoid, pisiform
    B) Trapezium, trapezoid, capitate, hamate
    C) Scaphoid, lunate, triquetrum, pisiform
    D) Trapezium, trapezoid, triquetrum, capitate

69. Which one of the following ligaments is **not** directly attached to the spinous processes?
    A) Posterior longitudinal ligament
    B) Ligamentum nuchae
    C) Interspinous ligament
    D) Supraspinous ligament

70. Which one of the following is **not** a branch of the trigeminal nerve?
    A) Greater occipital nerve
    B) Ophthalmic nerve
    C) Maxillary nerve
    D) Mandibular nerve

71. All of the following parts of the humerus are in direct contact with the indicated nerves **except**:
    A) Surgical neck: axillary nerve
    B) Radial groove: radial nerve
    C) Distal end of humerus: musculocutaneous nerve
    D) Medial epicondyle: ulnar nerve

72. How many total articulations make up the elbow joint?
    A) 1
    B) 2
    C) 3
    D) 4

73. What is the normal range of motion for hip flexion in adults?
    A) 0° to 150°
    B) 10° to 140°

C) 0° to 100°

D) 0° to 120°

74. Which muscle is a knee extensor?
    A) Gracilis
    B) Semimembranosus
    C) Vastus intermedius
    D) Biceps femoris

75. What is the normal range of motion (ROM) for plantar flexion of the ankle?
    A) 20°
    B) 30°
    C) 50°
    D) 90°

76. Which of the following is **true** about the posterior cruciate ligament (PCL)?
    A) Primary function is to restrain posterior tibial translation
    B) Inserts on superior aspect of medial tibia
    C) Tightens in extension
    D) It attaches to the medial meniscus

77. Which bone articulates with the first metacarpal bone in the form of a saddle joint?
    A) Trapezium
    B) Trapezoid
    C) Triquetrum
    D) Scaphoid

78. The sympathetic (thoracolumbar) division of the autonomic nervous system (ANS) involves postsynaptic sympathetic fibers arising from sympathetic trunks by different means, depending on their destination. Which one of the following is **not** part of the thoracolumbar sympathetic outflow?
    A) Ciliary ganglion
    B) Celiac ganglion
    C) Aorticorenal ganglion
    D) Superior and inferior mesenteric ganglia

79. Of the following ocular muscles and cranial nerve combinations, which one is **incorrect**?
    A) Medial rectus-III
    B) Lateral rectus-VI
    C) Superior oblique-IV
    D) Inferior oblique-IV

80. Splenius capitis and splenius cervicis are part of the:
    A) Intermediate layer of the intrinsic back muscles
    B) Superficial layer of the intrinsic back muscles
    C) Deep layer of the intrinsic back muscles
    D) The minor deep layer of the intrinsic back muscles

81. Which of the following is **not** a joint of the pelvic girdle?
    A) Femoroacetabular (hip) joint
    B) The pubic symphysis

    C) Bilateral sacroiliac (SI) joints

    D) Lumbosacral joint

82. Which nerve roots innervate the quadriceps?
    A) L1, L2, L3
    B) L2, L3, L4
    C) L3, L4, L5
    D) L4, L5, S1

83. Which nerve innervates the flexor hallucis longus (FHL)?
    A) Medial plantar nerve
    B) Superficial peroneal nerve
    C) Sural nerve
    D) Tibial nerve

84. Which ligament can be mistaken for a tear of the posterior horn of the lateral meniscus on MRI?
    A) Anterior cruciate ligament (ACL)
    B) Posterior cruciate ligament (PCL)
    C) Arcuate popliteal ligament complex (APLC)
    D) Oblique popliteal ligament (OPL)

85. Structures passing through the carpal tunnel into the hand include:
    A) Five finger flexor tendons
    B) The ulnar nerve
    C) The median nerve
    D) The radial nerve

86. The parasympathetic (craniosacral) division of the autonomic nervous system (ANS) involves presynaptic parasympathetic neuron cell bodies located within two sites of the central nervous system (CNS). Which one of the following is **not** part of the cranial parasympathetic outflow?
    A) Ciliary ganglion
    B) Celiac ganglion
    C) Pterygopalatine ganglion
    D) Otic ganglion

87. An injury involving the center of the optic chiasm would result in:
    A) Homonymous hemianopsia
    B) Bitemporal hemianopsia
    C) Cortical blindness
    D) Monocular blindness

# *Anatomy*

## ANSWERS

1. **D)** The tibial nerve is a branch of the sciatic nerve. The tibial nerve innervates the gastrocnemius, popliteus, soleus, and plantaris muscles. The sural nerve is a cutaneous branch of the tibial, but also receives innervation from the peroneal nerve.

2. **C)** Posterior herniations commonly miss the nerve in the foramen, and instead tends to affect the nerve one level distal. This is because the roots from the level below are located more laterally before exiting the canal, making them more vulnerable to impingement.

3. **C)** The lateral meniscus is larger than the medial meniscus, which is shaped like a "C." There are no structures named anterior or posterior meniscus. Image source: Brown DP, Freeman ED, Cuccurullo SJ, et al. In: *Physical Medicine and Rehabilitation Board Review, Third Edition.* (Cuccurullo SJ ed.) New York, NY: Demos Medical Publishing LLC; 2015: 238.

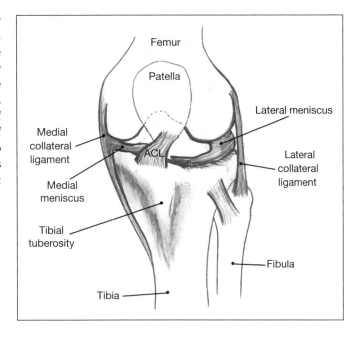

4. **B)** The distal humerus has two surfaces of articulation: the capitellum and the trochlea. The radial head articulates with the capitellum and the ulna articulates with the trochlea.

5. **C)** Although there is considerable overlap between adjacent dermatomes, the C7 dermatome supplies sensation to the area of skin over the middle finger. The C6 dermatome supplies sensation to the first digit, whereas the C8 dermatome supplies the fifth digit. The C5 dermatome supplies sensation to the lateral aspect of arm.

6. **D)** The brachioradialis muscle is innervated by the radial nerve.

7. **C)** The dorsal scapular nerve innervates both levator scapulae and the rhomboids.

8. **B)** The scaphoid bone is the only carpal bone that crosses both carpal rows. This position not only provides stability, but also places the scaphoid at the greatest risk of injury. Image source: Brown DP, Freeman ED, Cuccurullo SJ, et al. In: *Physical Medicine and Rehabilitation Board Review, Third Edition*. (Cuccurullo SJ ed.) New York, NY: Demos Medical Publishing LLC; 2015:194.

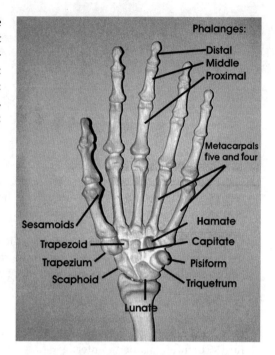

9. **D)** The semispinalis muscle is one of the deep layers of intrinsic back muscles and arises from approximately half of the spine—hence its name. It is divided into three parts: semispinalis capitis, semispinalis thoracis, and semispinalis cervices. The other muscles in the deep layer of intrinsic back muscles are the multifidus and the rotators. Collectively, the deep layer of the intrinsic back muscles is known as the *transversospinal muscle group*.

10. **C)** The anterior longitudinal ligament runs anteriorly and vertically attaching to the front of each vertebra. It traverses all of the vertebral bodies and intervertebral disks and helps resist extension.

11. **A)** The ACL originates in the lateral femoral condyle and attaches to the medial tibial eminence after traveling through the intercondylar notch. Image source: Lee SW. *Musculoskeletal Injuries and Conditions: Assessment and Management*. New York, NY: Demos Medical Publishing LLC; 2017:329.

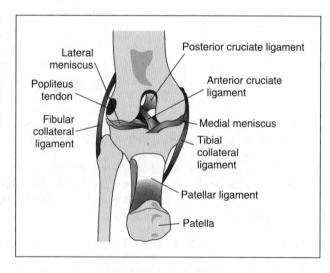

12. **A)** Tibialis anterior is an ankle dorsiflexor and inverter. Peroneus tertius dorsiflexes and everts the foot. Peroneus brevis everts and plantar flexes the foot. The plantaris is a weak plantar flexor.

13. **C)** The "watershed zone" of the Achilles is in the substance of the tendoachilles, approximately 2 to 5 cm above the calcaneal insertion of the tendon. This is an area of hypovascularity where most ruptures occur.

14. **B)** Overall, there is 2° of glenohumeral motion for every 1° of scapulothoracic motion during shoulder abduction (120° of glenohumeral motion to 60° of scapulothoracic motion). However, in a normal shoulder, the majority of the initial ROM occurs at the glenohumeral joint when the arm is supinated.

15. **A)** Endoneurium is the connective tissue that surrounds each individual axon and its myelin sheath. The perineurium surrounds the fascicles. The epineurium is the connective tissue that surrounds a peripheral nerve. The myelin sheath itself improves conductance of the electrical signal down an axon and is not part of the surrounding supportive structure.

16. **C)** The subscapular nerve innervates the subscapularis and the teres major muscles.

17. **D)** The DIO muscles are part of the intrinsic group of muscles in the hand. The DIO proximally attach at adjacent metacarpals and distally attach to proximal phalanges. Their main function is to abduct the digits and for MCP flexion.

18. **A)** The FDS inserts at the middle phalanx of the index, middle, ring, and small fingers. The FDS muscle's origins are the medial humeral epicondyle, the coronoid process of the ulna, and the upper anterior surface of the radius. Its main action is to flex the fingers at the proximal interphalangeal (PIP) joints. However, it also acts to flex the hand and wrist.

19. **A)** Hinged joints only allow a small range of motion (ROM) (eg, the humerus with the ulna and radius). Pivot joints allow a wide ROM, but not as much freedom as ball-and-socket joints (between atlas and axis). Gliding joints allow sliding motion between two bones (eg, wrist and ankle). Ball-and-socket joints have full ROM (hips, shoulders).

20. **C)** Most meniscal tissue is avascular and depends on passive diffusion and mechanical pumping to provide nutrition to the fibrocytes within the meniscal substance. The limited peripheral blood supply originates from the medial and lateral inferior and superior geniculate arteries. Repair is usually only successful in well-vascularized areas.

21. **D)** The deep posterior, superficial posterior, lateral, and anterior compartment makes up the four compartments of the lower leg.

22. **A)** The anterior nerve roots contain mostly motor nerves, whereas posterior nerve roots are mainly sensory. The dorsal root ganglion contains cell bodies of sensory nerves.

23. **A)** All of the muscles are digit 2 to 5 extensors, except the EPL, which is a thumb extensor.

24. **A)** All of the answer choices **except** the motor nerve cell body are components of the neuromuscular junction. The motor nerve cell body gives rise to motor nerve axons.

25. **A)** The axillary nerve innervates the teres minor and the deltoid muscles.

26. **C)** The carpal tunnel contains the four tendons of FDS, four tendons of FDP, FPL tendon, and median nerve. The roof of the carpal tunnel is formed by the transverse carpal ligament; the floor

is formed by the central carpal bones. The medial wall is formed by the hamate and the pisiform bones. The lateral wall is formed by the trapezius and scaphoid bones.

27. **C)** The infraspinatus muscle's proximal attachment is in the infraspinous fossa, while its distal attachment is at the greater tuberosity of the humerus. The primary action of the infraspinatus muscle is to externally rotate the arm as well as to provide stability to the rotator cuff. Image source: Miller A, DiCuccio Heckert K, Davis BA. *The 3-Minute Musculoskeletal and Peripheral Nerve Exam.* New York, NY: Demos Medical Publishing LLC; 2009:11.

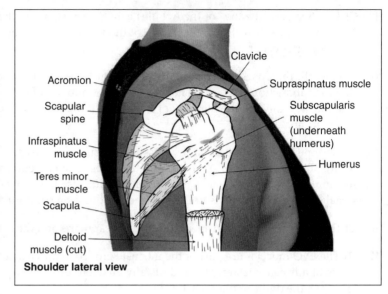

28. **C)** The adductor magnus is a hip extensor. All of the other muscles are hip flexors.

29. **B)** The pes anserine bursa is a medial bursa. There are four anterior bursae: prepatellar, suprapatellar, deep infrapatellar, and superficial (subcutaneous infrapatellar). Image source: Lee SW. *Musculoskeletal Injuries and Conditions: Assessment and Management.* New York, NY: Demos Medical Publishing LLC; 2017:333.

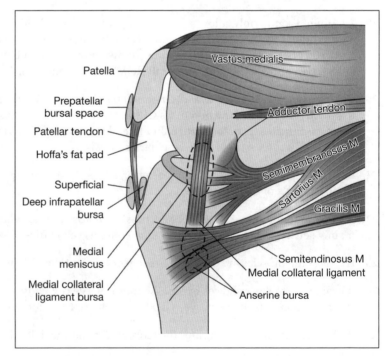

30. **B)** The medial malleolus is the prominence on the inner side of the ankle, formed by the lower end of the tibia.

31. **B)** Striking the tendon just below the patella stretches the muscle spindle in the quadriceps femoris muscle. This produces a monosynaptic reflex arc back to the spinal cord and synapses at the level of L4 in the spinal cord. From there, an alphamotor neuron conducts an efferent impulse back to the quadriceps femoris muscle, triggering contraction resulting in knee extension.

32. **D)** The palmaris longus muscle is primarily a wrist flexor. Although it is absent in about 14% of the population, its absence does not have any known effects on grip strength. All the other choices are finger flexors, including the flexor digitorum profundus (not listed).

33. **B)** The dorsal root ganglion contains cell bodies of the afferent spinal nerves responsible for relaying sensory information. A motor unit contains the following components from proximal to distal: anterior horn cell, motor nerve axons, peripheral nerve, the neuromuscular junction, muscle fibers.

34. **B)** The suprascapular nerve innervates the supraspinatus and infraspinatus muscles.

35. **A)** There are six compartments in the dorsum of the hand. The contents of each compartment are as follows: I–extensor pollicis brevis, abductor pollicis longus; II–extensor carpi radialis brevis, extensor carpi radialis longus; III–extensor pollicis longus; IV–extensor digitorum; V–extensor digiti minimi; and VI–extensor carpi ulnaris.

36. **C)** The main flexor of the forearm is the brachialis muscle. The anconeus is a relatively insignificant muscle that helps the triceps extend the forearm and it also resists ulnar abduction during pronation. The biceps brachii muscle is the major supinator of the forearm, while the brachioradialis is a forearm flexor (but not the main flexor).

37. **C)** The long head of the biceps femoris is a hip adductor. The gluteus medius and minimus muscles **ab**duct the hip. The piriformis muscle **ab**ducts, externally rotates, and extends the hip.

38. **B)** Baker's cyst is a distended bursa located between the medial head of the gastrocnemius and capsule extending under the semimembranosus. There is a second posterior bursa located between the lateral head of the gastrocnemius and the capsule. The deep infrapatellar bursa is located between the patellar tendon and the tibia.

39. **B)** The distal fibula forms the lateral malleolus of the ankle and is joined to the tibia and to the talus.

40. **C)** The ankle jerk (Achilles reflex) occurs when the Achilles tendon is tapped when the foot is slightly dorsiflexed and produces plantar flexion.

41. **A)** Paired contraction of the FCU and ECU causes ulnar deviation of the wrist.

42. **D)** The internal intercostals are accessory muscles used during expiration. In addition to the other choices, the external intercostals and scalene muscles serve as accessory muscles during inspiration. Diaphragmatic muscle contraction (innervated by the phrenic nerve) serves as the primary muscle of respiration during inspiration.

43. **D)** The posterior cutaneous nerve of the thigh (S1–S3) is part of the sacral plexus.

**44. C)** The brachialis muscle is supplied mainly by the musculocutaneous nerve. A small branch of the radial nerve may sometimes innervate the lateral portion of this muscle. The brachialis muscle originates at the lower half of the anterior humerus and inserts at the ulnar tuberosity.

**45. D)** The radial nerve originates from the C5 through T1 nerve roots and the posterior cord (originates from upper, middle, and lower trunks). Image source: Araim RJ, Aghalar MR, Weiss LD. *Neuromuscular Quick Pocket Reference.* New York, NY: Demos Medical Publishing LLC; 2012:99.

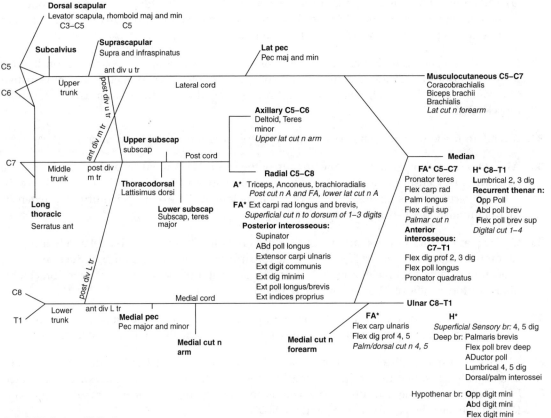

A*, Arm; FA*, Forearm; H*, Hand.

**46. B)** The semitendinosus is an internal rotator of the hip. All the other muscles are external rotators.

**47. B)** This injury usually occurs because of a lateral blow to the knee causing a rupture in the ACL, MCL, and medial meniscus. This occurs when a lateral force is applied to the knee when the foot is fixed to the ground causing a rotational force to tear all three structures.

**48. C)** Most sprains affect the anterior talofibular ligament. The ligament comes under strain and is vulnerable to injury, particularly when the foot is inverted.

**49. B)** The femoral nerve is formed from the L2 through L4 nerve roots. The main motor component innervates the iliopsoas (hip flexor) and the quadriceps (knee extensor).

LIES !!! It is PIN-Radial !

**50. C)** The extensor digiti minimi muscle is innervated by the ulnar nerve. All of the other choices are muscles that are innervated by the radial nerve. Other muscles innervated by the radial nerve include the extensor carpi ulnaris, the extensor digitorum communis, and the extensor pollicis longus.

51. **D)** L4 is at the level of the iliac crests.

52. **A)** The genitofemoral nerve is part of the lumbar plexus (L1–L4). The sacral plexus also includes the posterior cutaneous nerve of the thigh.

53. **D)** The anconeus muscle originates at the lateral epicondyle of the humerus and inserts along the lateral side of the ulna. This muscle functions in forearm extension as well as stabilization of the elbow joint against flexion or pronation-supination. The anconeus muscle is innervated by the radial nerve.

54. **A)** There are six dorsal compartments to the wrist. The first compartment houses the APL and the EPB tendons. This is the location where De Quervain's tenosynovitis can occur.

55. **B)** The gluteus maximus is an external rotator of the hip. All the other muscles are internal rotators. *+C*   *CVCC says also post fibers of glut med*

56. **B)** The normal range of motion of the knee is 0° to 135°.

57. **B)** The deltoid ligament functions to support the medial surface of the ankle. It helps to connect the tibia to the calcaneus, navicular, and talus bones.

58. **C)** The tibial nerve is comprised of L4 through S3 nerve roots. In the popliteal fossa, the nerve branches off to the gastrocnemius, popliteus, soleus, and plantaris muscles. The nerve's primary actions are foot inversion and ankle plantar flexion.

59. **B)** The FCU is innervated by the ulnar nerve. All of the other choices are muscles that are innervated by the median nerve. The median nerve also innervates the flexor digitorum superficialis. The flexor digitorum profundus is dually innervated by the median (second and third digit) and the ulnar nerves (fourth and fifth digit).

60. **D)** The thyroid cartilage is located at the level of C4, C5 anteriorly.

61. **C)** The mandibular nerve is a branch of the trigeminal nerve—cranial nerve V.

62. **B)** The shoulder joint is a ball-and-socket type joint. An example of a hinge joint is the elbow. Joints between bones of the skull are called sutures, and the base of the carpometacarpal joint of the thumb is an example of a saddle joint.

63. **C)** Guyon's canal is also known as the *ulnar tunnel*. The floor of Guyon's canal is formed by the transverse carpal ligament, the roof is the volar carpal ligament, and the medial and lateral walls are formed by the pisiform and hook of hamate. The canal houses both the ulnar nerve and the ulnar artery. Fractures or masses (eg, ganglion cyst) can compress the nerve or artery at this location.

64. **A)** The iliofemoral ligament is the strongest ligament of the body and limits extension, abduction, and external rotation of the hip.

65. **D)** The biceps femoris is part of the hamstring muscle group in the posterior thigh. The rest of the muscles are knee extensors.

66. **B)** The Lisfranc ligament connects the base of the medial cuneiform to the base of the second metatarsal. It is injured or disrupted in a Lisfranc fracture.

67. **B)** Genu valgum is excessive valgum or "knock kneed." Genu varum is "bow legged." Hyperextension or "back kneed" is genu recurvatum. Genu anterium is not a medical definition.

68. **C)** The proximal row of carpal bones (from a radial to ulnar direction) include the scaphoid, lunate, triquetrum, and pisiform. The distal row of carpal bones (from a radial to ulnar direction) include the trapezium, trapezoid, capitate, and hamate. A common acronym to remember these bones is "Some Lovers Try Positions That They Cannot Handle."

69. **A)** The posterior longitudinal ligament attaches to the posterior rim of vertebral bodies and disk from C2 to the sacrum.

70. **A)** The lesser and the greater occipital nerves arise from C2 and C3, respectively. The rest of the choices are the three main branches of the trigeminal nerve.

71. **C)** The distal end of humerus is in direct contact with the median nerve.

72. **C)** The elbow joint is comprised of three articulations: ulnohumeral, radiocapitellar, and proximal radioulnar.

73. **D)** 0° to 120°

74. **C)** The gracilis, semimembranosus, and biceps femoris are all knee flexors.

75. **C)** Normal ROM for the ankle is 50° of plantar flexion and 20° of dorsiflexion.

76. **A)** The PCL primarily restrains posterior tibial translation. It originates from the medial femoral condyle and inserts on the posterior aspect of tibial plateau. It loosens with extension and becomes tighter with flexion.

77. **A)** Synovial joints come in multiple types. Ball-and-socket joints (eg, hip joint [multiaxial], provide the most range of motion [ROM]). The saddle joint is a biaxial joint that provides the second most ROM. Other types of synovial joints include the hinge (elbow-uniaxial), pivot (atlantoaxial joint-uniaxial), condyloid joints (metacarpophalangeal joints-biaxial), and plane joints (acromioclavicular).

78. **A)** The ciliary ganglion is part of the parasympathetic (craniosacral) division of the ANS.

79. **D)** The superior oblique muscle is innervated by cranial nerve IV. The lateral rectus is innervated by cranial nerve VI. The rest of the ocular muscles, including the inferior oblique, are innervated by cranial nerve III.

80. **B)** Splenius capitis and splenius cervicis are part of the superficial layer of the intrinsic back muscles.

81. **D)** The pelvic girdle includes the hip joint, the pubic symphysis, the sacrum, and the sacroiliac joints.

82. **B)** The femoral nerve receives innervation from the L2, L3, and L4 nerve roots. The femoral nerve innervates the four heads of the quadriceps muscle as well as supplies sensation to the medial surface of the thigh.

83. **D)** The tibial nerve innervates the FHL.

84. **C)** The APLC provides attachment for the posterior lateral meniscus, and this site can be mistaken for a posterior tear of the lateral meniscus.

85. **C)** There are nine finger flexor tendons that pass into the hand through the carpal tunnel (along with the median nerve). Five of the nine tendons are deep-flexor tendons and the other four are superficial flexors. The ulnar and radial nerves do not travel through the carpal tunnel.

86. **B)** The celiac ganglion is part of the sympathetic (thoracolumbar) division of the ANS. The cranial parasympathetic outflow is via cranial nerves III, VII, and IX involving ciliary, pterygopalatine, otic, and submandibular ganglia. Cranial nerve X provides parasympathetic outflow to multiple visceral organs (heart, lungs, upper gastrointestinal system). Additionally, sacral parasympathetic outflow supplies the lower gastrointestinal and genitourinary system via pelvic splanchnic nerves arising from S2, S3, and S4 segments.

87. **B)** Homonymous hemianopsia would result from injury to the optic tract. Cortical blindness results from bilateral lesions of the primary visual cortex, as seen in Anton's syndrome. Monocular blindness would be a result of injury to the optic nerve.

# Musculoskeletal

## QUESTIONS

1. Scoliosis can be classified as structural or functional. Which one of the following is **not** characteristic of functional scoliosis?
    A) Can be due to muscle spasm
    B) Can be secondary to a herniated disc
    C) Can be due to senile changes in person's spine
    D) Can be postural

2. Which finger is commonly affected in Dupuytren's contracture?
    A) The index finger
    B) The middle finger
    C) The ring finger
    D) The pinky finger

3. Idiopathic brachial plexitis, usually preceded by a viral illness, is called:
    A) Thoracic outlet syndrome
    B) Erb's palsy
    C) Guillain-Barré syndrome
    D) Parsonage-Turner syndrome

4. Which ligament is most commonly injured in lateral ankle sprains?
    A) Calcaneofibular ligament
    B) Anterior talofibular ligament
    C) Tibionavicular ligament
    D) Posterior talofibular ligament

5. Which bone is most commonly affected in a wrist fracture?
    A) Lunate
    B) Capitate
    C) Distal radius
    D) Scaphoid

6. Which of the following statements is **not** true regarding the meniscus?
    A) Partial meniscectomy for bucket-handle tearing will still preserve most of the meniscal function as long as the peripheral rim is intact
    B) The peripheral outer 1/3 of a meniscus is well vascularized, and the inner 2/3 poorly vascularized
    C) One of the important roles the meniscus plays is in proprioception of the knee
    D) The tibial-femoral contact area is decreased by up to 25% after total meniscectomy

ANSWERS TO THIS SECTION CAN BE FOUND ON PAGE 43

7. Lateral epicondylitis most commonly affects which muscle or muscles?
   A) Extensor carpi radialis brevis and extensor digitorum communis
   B) Pronator teres, flexor carpi radialis, palmaris longus, flexor carpi ulnaris, and flexor digitorum superficialis
   C) Triceps muscle
   D) Biceps tendon

8. Which muscle is the most powerful forearm supinator?
   A) Supinator muscle
   B) Pronator teres muscle
   C) Biceps brachii muscle
   D) Brachioradialis muscle

9. The differential diagnosis of trigger finger includes all of the following **except**:
   A) Dupuytren's disease
   B) Ganglion of the tendon sheath
   C) Rheumatoid arthritis
   D) Phalange fracture

10. The true leg length should be measured between:
    A) Greater trochanter and lateral malleolus
    B) Umbilicus and lateral malleolus
    C) Anterior superior iliac spine (ASIS) and medial malleolus
    D) Anterior inferior iliac spine and medial malleolus

11. Second impact syndrome occurs when a patient:
    A) Sustains a physical injury at the same time as a concussion
    B) Sustains a brain injury before the previous concussion symptoms have resolved
    C) Sustains a second concussion after previous concussion symptoms have resolved
    D) Sustains a medical condition after a concussion

12. Adhesive capsulitis or frozen shoulder:
    A) Results from thickening and contraction of the capsule around the glenohumeral joint
    B) Is more commonly seen in middle-aged men
    C) Has risk factors including psoriasis
    D) Is more frequently noted in colder climates

13. In sports, which knee ligament is the most commonly injured?
    A) Anterior cruciate ligament (ACL)
    B) Posterior cruciate ligament (PCL)
    C) Lateral collateral ligament (LCL)
    D) Medial collateral ligament (MCL)

14. Which statement is **not** true regarding plantar fasciitis?
    A) Increased tension on the plantar fascia leads to chronic inflammation
    B) Heel spurs may contribute to its etiology
    C) A tight Achilles tendon is frequently associated with plantar fasciitis
    D) Night plantar flexion splints are not indicated

15. Heberden's nodes are found in which condition?
    A) Rheumatoid arthritis
    B) Psoriatic arthritis

C) Osteoarthritis

D) Gout

16. What radiographic finding is typical of osteoarthritis?
    A) Periarticular osteopenia
    B) "Pencil-in-cup" deformity
    C) Subchondral cysts
    D) Soft tissue swelling

17. Which joint is most commonly dislocated among pediatric patients?
    A) Shoulder
    B) Hip
    C) Elbow
    D) Proximal interphalangeal (PIP) joint

18. Which provocative test is useful in detecting rotator cuff impingement?
    A) Drop arm test
    B) O'Brien test
    C) Apley scarf test
    D) Neer's test

19. What is the most common cause of adhesive capsulitis?
    A) Diabetes
    B) Female gender
    C) Hypothyroidism
    D) Idiopathic

20. Which of the following is a static stabilizer of the shoulder joint?
    A) Biceps tendon
    B) Labrum
    C) Supraspinatus muscle
    D) Subscapularis muscle

21. The cruciate ligaments are important knee structures which lie:
    A) Inside the joint capsule, and within the synovial cavity as well
    B) Outside the synovial cavity but within the fibrous joint capsule
    C) Outside the fibrous joint capsule
    D) Outside the synovial cavity and fibrous joint capsule

22. What is a sign that the stellate ganglion was successfully blocked?
    A) Ipsilateral Horner's syndrome
    B) Increased paresthesias
    C) Anesthesia in the limb
    D) Increased pain symptoms

23. What is a Smith's fracture?
    A) Fracture of the distal radius with dorsal displacement
    B) Fracture of the distal ulna with dorsal displacement
    C) Fracture of the distal radius with volar displacement
    D) Fracture of the distal ulna with volar displacement

24. Which position should be avoided after total hip arthroplasty using an anterior approach?
    A) Bridging
    B) Adduction crossing midline
    C) Sitting on regular toilet seat
    D) Cross legs

25. Which condition/injury is not considered an absolute contraindication for return to play?
    A) Atlantoaxial instability noted on lateral flexion-extension x-rays
    B) Fused C1 to C2 segments
    C) A two- to three-level spinal fusion with normal exam
    D) An acute spinal fracture

26. What is the most common cause of nontraumatic elbow joint destruction?
    A) Osteoarthritis
    B) Rheumatoid arthritis
    C) Repetitive valgus stress injury
    D) Gout

27. Intrinsic factors contributing to the development of tendinitis include all of the following **except**:
    A) Age
    B) Genetic predisposition
    C) Poor training technique
    D) Muscle imbalance/weakness

28. The articulations of the elbow joint:
    A) Allow 3 degrees of freedom
    B) Allow 2 degrees of freedom
    C) Allow normal range of motion (ROM) of −10° extension to 120° flexion
    D) Allow 30° to 40° of pronation

29. Which of the following is **not** true regarding steroid injection for carpal tunnel syndrome (CTS)?
    A) It is indicated for mild to moderate CTS
    B) It can be used in conjunction with splinting and physical therapy
    C) Caution should be used when injecting patients with diabetes
    D) Is preferable to surgery in patients with severe CTS

30. Identify the final treatment phase of sports rehabilitation:
    A) Resolving pain and inflammation
    B) Restoring range of motion (ROM)
    C) Strengthening
    D) Sports/task-specific activities

31. What is the usual mechanism of a scaphoid fracture?
    A) Axial compression and hyperextension of the wrist
    B) Fall onto outstretched hands
    C) Direct blow to the scaphoid bone
    D) End-on blow of the fist, as in boxing

32. Hill-Sachs lesion of the shoulder:
    A) May be associated with posterior dislocations
    B) May cause shoulder instability if it accounts for 10% of the articular surface

C) Is a compression fracture of the posterolateral aspect of humeral head caused by abutment against the anterior rim of the glenoid fossa

D) Is evaluated by Speed's test

33. The diagnosis of aseptic noninflammatory olecranon bursitis:
    A) Is based on plain radiographs, demonstrating an olecranon spur in all cases
    B) Requires aspiration of bursal fluid in all cases
    C) Is usually straightforward and based on characteristic appearance on physical examination
    D) Is made only with MRI

34. What structures are found within the quadrangular space?
    A) The circumflex scapular artery
    B) The femoral nerve, artery, and vein
    C) Processus vaginalis, spermatic cord, and ilioinguinal nerve
    D) Axillary nerve, posterior circumflex artery, and humeral artery

35. **Internal** snapping hip syndrome is caused by:
    A) A tight iliopsoas tendon snapping over the lesser trochanter
    B) A tight iliotibial band snapping over the greater trochanter
    C) A tight gluteus maximus snapping over the greater trochanter
    D) An acetabular labral tear or loose body in the hip joint

36. The rotator cuff muscles include all of the following **except:**
    A) Teres minor
    B) Supraspinatus
    C) Rhomboids
    D) Infraspinatus

37. What is the Adson's test used for?
    A) To detect thoracic outlet syndrome
    B) To check for adequate blood perfusion to the hand
    C) To detect anterior instability of the shoulder joint
    D) To detect symptoms of carpal tunnel syndrome (CTS)

38. The glenohumeral joint (shoulder girdle complex) involves articulation of the humeral head with the glenoid fossa and the labrum. Approximately what percentage of the humeral head articulates with the glenoid fossa?
    A) 15
    B) 30
    C) 50
    D) 70

39. De Quervain's stenosing tenosynovitis is inflammation of the first dorsal compartment, which includes which of the following?
    A) Abductor pollicis longus and opponens pollicis
    B) Extensor pollicis brevis and opponens pollicis
    C) Abductor pollicis longus and extensor pollicis brevis
    D) Adductor pollicis longus and opponens pollicis

40. A finger locked in flexion, especially in the morning, is typical of which condition?
    A) Trigger finger
    B) Mallet finger

    C) Jersey finger

    D) Boutonnière deformity

41. What is the most common pathological "mass" to occur in the wrist joint?
    A) Madelung's deformity
    B) Ganglion cyst
    C) Heterotopic ossification
    D) Giant cell tumor of tendon sheath

42. What is the final (last) phase of sports rehabilitation?
    A) Sports/task-specific activities
    B) Immobilization
    C) Restoring range of motion (ROM)
    D) Strengthening

43. In patients younger than 20 years who have had a shoulder dislocation, what is the rate of recurrence?
    A) 10%
    B) 50%
    C) 75%
    D) 90%

44. What portion of the clavicle is most commonly fractured?
    A) Distal 1/3
    B) Middle 1/3
    C) Proximal 1/3
    D) Distal 1/3 and proximal 1/3 fractures are equally most common

45. Thomas' test is used to assess:
    A) Lumbar lordosis
    B) Hip flexion contracture
    C) Sacroiliac joint dysfunction
    D) Iliotibial band contracture

46. Rupture of the terminal extensor tendon of the distal phalanx causing loss of active extension is called:
    A) Mallet finger
    B) Jersey finger
    C) Trigger finger
    D) Coach's finger or jammed finger

47. The test of choice when looking for labral pathology is:
    A) MRI
    B) CT scan
    C) X-rays
    D) Magnetic resonance (MR) arthrogram

48. Which splint is appropriate for De Quervain's tenosynovitis?
    A) Nocturnal wrist splint
    B) Thumb spica splint
    C) Dynamic extension splint
    D) Flexor tendon splint

49. The popliteus muscle performs an important action of unlocking by:
   A) Internally rotating the femur on the tibia during an open chain movement
   B) Externally rotating the tibia on the femur during an open chain movement
   C) Externally rotating the femur on the tibia during a closed chain movement
   D) Internally rotating the tibia on the femur during a closed chain movement

50. A newborn is holding his head with his chin rotated toward the left and the ear approximating the right shoulder. Which muscle is primarily implicated?
   A) Left cervical paraspinal
   B) Right cervical paraspinal
   C) Left sternocleidomastoid
   D) Right sternocleidomastoid

51. Mechanisms proposed for superior labrum anterior to posterior (SLAP) lesions include:
   A) Falling on an outstretched arm
   B) Underhand throwing motion
   C) Repetitive overhead reaching
   D) Repetitive resistant elbow extension

52. Which portion of the humerus is most commonly affected in osteochondritis dissecans?
   A) Capitellum
   B) Medial epicondyle
   C) Lateral epicondyle
   D) Greater tubercle

53. Shoulder extension involves the use of all of the following muscles **except**:
   A) Pectoralis major, sternocostal portion
   B) Teres major
   C) Biceps brachii
   D) Posterior deltoid

54. Medial winging of the scapula is caused by which of the following nerve injuries?
   A) Weakness of serratus anterior due to spinal accessory nerve injury
   B) Trapezius weakness due to long thoracic nerve injury
   C) Serratus anterior weakness due to long thoracic nerve injury
   D) Trapezius weakness due to spinal accessory nerve injury

55. Which is the most common site for compartment syndrome?
   A) Anterior compartment of the lower leg
   B) Superficial posterior compartment of the lower leg
   C) Lateral compartment of the lower leg
   D) Deep posterior compartment of the lower leg

56. Which statement is true regarding medial tibial stress syndrome (MTSS or shin splints)?
   A) This is a type of overuse injury that results from chronic traction on the periosteum at the periosteal-fascial junction along the anterolateral border of the tibia
   B) The main predisposing factor is hypersupination
   C) Patient should continue normal activity
   D) Pain may improve with exercise but worsens afterward

57. Most patients with a grade II ankle sprain will present with:
    A) Pain in the ankle with no ligamentous injury
    B) Mild sprain of the anterior talofibular ligament and negative ankle drawer test
    C) Disruption of the anterior talofibular ligament, sprain of the calcaneofibular ligament, and positive ankle drawer test
    D) Disruption of the anterior talofibular ligament, the calcaneofibular ligament, and the lateral ligament complex, with a positive ankle drawer test

58. Which test is the most **specific** test to diagnose an anterior cruciate ligament (ACL) tear?
    A) Pivot shift
    B) Lachman test
    C) Anterior drawer sign
    D) Ege's test

59. Which ligament is affected in Gamekeeper's thumb?
    A) Tear of the ulnar collateral ligament of the thumb metacarpophalangeal (MCP)
    B) Rupture of the flexor digitorum profundus (FDP) tendon
    C) Rupture of the extensor tendon from the distal phalanx
    D) Tear of the triangular fibrocartilage complex

60. Which activity will most likely aggravate patellofemoral pain syndrome?
    A) Ambulation
    B) Climbing stairs
    C) Stationary cycling
    D) Swimming

61. A fall or blow on a hyperextended (dorsiflexed) wrist can cause osteonecrosis of which bone?
    A) Scaphoid
    B) Lunate
    C) Triquetrum
    D) Pisiform

62. The proximal tibiofibular joint:
    A) Is a source of lateral knee pain that is often overlooked
    B) Is located between the lateral tibial condyle and the fibular head, and has been construed as the "third compartment" of the knee joint
    C) Is not a synovial joint
    D) Communicates with the knee joint in approximately 90% of adults

63. O'Brien's test evaluates for:
    A) Labral abnormalities
    B) Bicipital tendinitis
    C) Stability of the glenohumeral joint
    D) Thoracic outlet syndrome

64. Gamekeeper's thumb involves an injury to the following structure:
    A) Medial collateral ligament
    B) Ulnar collateral ligament
    C) Transverse carpal ligament
    D) Triangular fibrocartilage complex

65. Test(s) to evaluate for shoulder impingement syndrome include:
    A) Finkelstein's test
    B) Speed's test
    C) Neer's sign
    D) Tinel's test

66. What is the most common cause of posterior cruciate ligament (PCL) injury?
    A) Hyperextension of the knee
    B) Rotation of femur on fixed lower leg
    C) Hyperflexion of the knee
    D) Dashboard injury

67. The Q angle is increased by:
    A) Genu varum
    B) Decreased femoral anteversion
    C) Internal tibial torsion
    D) Tight lateral retinaculum

68. What is the most common site for humeral fractures?
    A) Surgical neck
    B) Anatomical neck
    C) Midshaft
    D) Humeral head

69. Which of the following constitutes the largest tissue mass in the body (40%–45% of the total body weight)?
    A) Bone
    B) Muscle
    C) Skin
    D) Blood

70. The most sensitive imaging study to detect early changes in avascular necrosis (AVN) of the femoral head is:
    A) CT
    B) MRI
    C) Bone scan
    D) X-ray

71. A 35-year-old male plumber presents with right elbow pain. You diagnose right lateral epicondylitis. What would be expected on physical exam?
    A) Pain with passive wrist extension
    B) Pain with resisted wrist flexion and pronation
    C) Pain with resisted wrist extension and supination
    D) Pain with resisted wrist extension and pronation

72. Which statement is true regarding the anterior cruciate ligament (ACL)?
    A) It prevents backward sliding of the femur
    B) It limits external rotation of the femur when the foot is fixed
    C) It tightens in flexion and loosens with full extension
    D) Its deficiency leads to increased pressures on the anterior menisci

**73.** What provocative maneuver is used to test for lateral epicondylitis?
  A) Empty can test
  B) Valgus stress test
  C) Elbow flexion test
  D) Cozen's test

**74.** During which phase of throwing is the elbow joint placed under the most valgus stress?
  A) Follow-through
  B) Wind-up
  C) Early cocking
  D) Late cocking

**75.** Injury to the long thoracic nerve affects the function of serratus anterior, which functions primarily to:
  A) Stabilize the scapula by drawing it inferiorly and anteriorly against the thoracic wall
  B) Protract the scapula and hold it against the thoracic wall
  C) Elevate the scapula and tilt the glenoid cavity by rotating the scapula
  D) Medially rotate and adduct the arm; helps hold the humeral head in the glenoid cavity

**76.** Which radiographic view is used to visualize the humeral head for possible Hill-Sachs lesion?
  A) Scapular Y view
  B) West point view
  C) Stryker notch view
  D) Lateral view

**77.** All of the following are correct regarding the intervertebral disc **except**:
  A) The pressure obtained in the sitting position is double the pressure when the patient stands
  B) The interior of the disc has no nociceptive innervation
  C) The fibrous outer ring (annulus fibrosis) is held taut by the pressure in the central nucleus pulposus
  D) The dorsal portion of the annulus fibrosis has no nociceptive innervation

**78.** What physical exam finding will be observed in "Saturday night palsy"?
  A) Marked wrist and finger drop
  B) Atrophy of abductor pollicis brevis (APB)
  C) Weak elbow extension
  D) Painless weakness and atrophy of hand intrinsic muscle

**79.** What is Kienböck's disease?
  A) Scaphoid bone fracture
  B) Avascular necrosis (AVN) of the lunate bone
  C) Ulnar deviation of the wrist
  D) Intra-articular fracture affecting the carpometacarpal joint

**80.** Kienböck's disease involves which of the following features?
  A) Osteonecrosis of the scaphoid
  B) "Pencil-in-cup" deformities
  C) Heberden's and Bouchard's nodules
  D) Osteonecrosis of the lunate

81. Which nerve injury results in medial scapular winging?
    A) Spinal accessory nerve
    B) Axillary nerve
    C) Suprascapular nerve
    D) Long thoracic nerve

82. O'Donoghue's triad (the unhappy triad) consists of tears of which of the following?
    A) Anterior cruciate ligament (ACL), medial collateral ligament (MCL), and lateral meniscus
    B) ACL, MCL, and medial meniscus
    C) ACL, MCL, and lateral collateral ligament (LCL)
    D) ACL, MCL, and posterior collateral ligament (PCL)

83. Where is the lesion if a patient presents with isolated infraspinatus weakness and atrophy?
    A) The suprascapular notch
    B) The C5 nerve root
    C) The spinoglenoid notch of the scapula
    D) The upper trunk of the brachial plexus

84. Scapula winging is caused by an injury to which one of the following nerves?
    A) Radial nerve
    B) Suprascapular nerve
    C) Long thoracic nerve
    D) Axillary nerve

85. The primary function of tendon is to:
    A) Transmit the force generated by a muscle to bone
    B) Attach bone to bone
    C) Be primary joint stabilizers
    D) Provide nutrition to bone

86. Ankle eversion injuries often injure the:
    A) Deltoid ligament
    B) Anterior talofibular ligament
    C) Calcaneofibular ligament
    D) Posterior talofibular ligament

87. Rotator cuff tears are characterized by:
    A) Symptoms similar to rotator cuff tendinitis
    B) Pain at night with side-lying on the affected side
    C) Examination findings of supraspinatus weakness, external shoulder rotator weakness, and positive drop arm test
    D) All of the above

88. Which of the following is true regarding impact seizures after a mild head injury?
    A) Do not require treatment
    B) Occur commonly
    C) Are associated with structural brain injury
    D) Always indicates that the patient should stop participating in that sport

89. In Erb's palsy, what part of the brachial plexus is affected?
    A) The lower trunk (C8-T1)
    B) Both upper and lower trunks

C) Middle trunk (C7)

D) The upper trunk (C5-C6)

90. When is it safe for a patient to return to play after a concussion is diagnosed?

A) Patient can return to the game once they are asymptomatic

B) Neuroimaging must confirm that there is no structural damage

C) Patient must follow a stepwise approach and will be cleared once asymptomatic in all steps

D) Patient is able to play as long as there was no loss of consciousness

91. Shoulder impingement may result from:

A) C6 radiculopathy

B) Loss of competency of the biceps tendon

C) Loss of competency of scapula-stabilizing muscles

D) Thoracic outlet syndrome

92. Which of the evaluations below is the most important part of the physical evaluation of an athlete?

A) Nephrology evaluation

B) Pulmonary evaluation

C) Cardiovascular evaluation

D) Neurologic evaluation

93. A 22-year-old football player presents with right knee pain. His history reveals that he received a posteriorly directed force to his bent knee. Physical examination reveals a positive posterior drawer sign. What injury has the patient most likely sustained?

A) Patello-femoral syndrome

B) Anterior cruciate ligament (ACL) injury

C) Posterior cruciate ligament (PCL) injury

D) Medial collateral ligament (MCL) injury

94. What is a Bankart lesion?

A) Tear or avulsion of the anterior glenoid labrum

B) Compression fracture of the posterior humeral head

C) Injury to the superior glenoid labrum and biceps tendon (long head)

D) Compression of the brachial plexus and/or subclavian vessels as they exit between the superior shoulder girdle and first rib

95. A positive Froment's sign hints to which nerve being injured?

A) Median nerve

B) Radial nerve

C) Ulnar nerve

D) Musculocutaneous nerve

96. What causes Boutonnière deformity?

A) Ruptured flexor digitorum profundus (FDP) tendon

B) Thickening and nodule formation in the flexor tendon sheath

C) Median nerve entrapment

D) Rupture of the central slip and volar migration of lateral bands

97. Compression of which nerve is commonly misdiagnosed as lateral epicondylitis?

A) Posterior interosseous nerve (PIN)

B) Anterior interosseous nerve

    C) Median nerve
    D) C8/T1 nerve roots

98. Little League elbow:
    A) Involves the lateral elbow region
    B) Is an acute dislocation of the elbow
    C) Occurs most commonly between the ages of 13 and 15
    D) Occurs in athletes complaining of medial elbow pain

99. Tennis elbow typically:
    A) Is an acute lesion, lasting less than a few weeks
    B) Presents with pain and tenderness over the medial epicondyle
    C) Does not affect grip strength
    D) Can occur as a result of a poor tennis backhand stroke

100. What describes a swan neck deformity?
    A) Hyperextended metacarpophalangeal (MCP) and distal interphalangeal (DIP) joints, and flexion deformity at the proximal interphalangeal (PIP) joint
    B) Synovitis at the ulnar styloid with resultant disruption of the ulnar collateral ligament
    C) Hyperextension of the MCP and DIP joints with flexion of the PIP joint
    D) MCP and PIP joint hyperextension with flexion deformity at the DIP joint
        *disagree: mcp flexes*

101. What does FABERE (Patrick's test) test for?
    A) Hip joint dysfunction
    B) Gluteus medius weakness
    C) Femoral nerve irritation
    D) Iliotibial band tightness

102. De Quervain's is a tenosynovitis involving which two tendons?
    A) Extensor pollicis longus (EPL) and flexor digitorum superficialis (FDS)
    B) Abductor pollicis brevis (APB) and flexor digitorum profundus (FDP)
    C) Flexor carpi radialis (FCR) and palmaris longus (PL)
    D) Extensor pollicis brevis (EPB) and abductor pollicis longus (APL)

103. Which test helps determine if a patient has an anterior cruciate ligament (ACL) injury?
    A) McMurray's test
    B) Apley's grind test
    C) Lachman's test
    D) Quadriceps active test

104. In a posterior hip dislocation, how will the leg be positioned?
    A) Extended, adducted, internally rotated
    B) Flexed, adducted, internally rotated
    C) Extended, abducted, externally rotated
    D) Flexed, adducted, externally rotated

105. During which type of contraction is a hamstring injury most likely to occur?
    A) Concentric muscle contraction
    B) Eccentric muscle contraction
    C) Isometric contractions
    D) Isotonic contractions

106. An anterior superior iliac spine (ASIS) avulsion fracture can be caused by forceful contraction of:
    A) Long head of the biceps femoris
    B) Vastus intermedius muscle
    C) Sartorius muscle
    D) Iliopsoas muscle

107. Writer's cramp:
    A) Is the least common type of dystonia
    B) Is a task-specific focal dystonia
    C) Improves after attempts to perform a specific task, such as writing
    D) Has a poor prognosis

108. Which of the following statements is true regarding the use of continuous passive motion (CPM) following total knee arthroplasty (TKA)?
    A) The use of CPM has been associated with a decreased incidence of deep vein thrombosis
    B) The use of CPM has not demonstrated any difference in clinical outcomes at 1 year following surgery
    C) The use of CPM prevents the incidence of knee flexion contracture
    D) The use of CPM increases analgesic use in patients who used CPM following TKA

109. Throwing athletes, such as baseball pitchers, are most susceptible to which of the following disorders?
    A) Medial epicondylitis
    B) Lateral epicondylitis
    C) Posterior tendon tendonitis
    D) Bicipital tendonitis

110. What is the test to check for contraction of the iliotibial band?
    A) Thompson's test
    B) Painful arc test
    C) Ober's test
    D) Yergason's test

111. Which statement is **not** true regarding myositis ossificans of the hip?
    A) Ultrasound, heat, and massage are conservative treatments for new onset of myositis ossificans
    B) Prevention of contractures is important
    C) If possible, surgery should be delayed until the lesion matures at 10 to 12 months
    D) Myositis ossificans is the formation of heterotopic ossification within muscle

112. Female athletes have been shown to:
    A) Have a smaller surface area-to-mass ratio, higher bone mass, and a narrower pelvis as compared to males
    B) Have less menstrual irregularities compared to nonathletic females
    C) Have skeletal demineralization which can lead to premature osteoporosis
    D) Have less disordered eating when compared to male athletes

113. What does the anterior drawer test assess in the ankle?
    A) Integrity of calcaneofibular ligament
    B) Integrity of anterior talofibular ligament

C) Integrity of posterior talofibular ligament
D) Integrity of deltoid ligament

114. What is the pathophysiology behind avascular necrosis of the femoral head?
    A) Sepsis
    B) Crystalline deposits
    C) Interruption of the vascular supply
    D) Friction

115. All of the following are true about piriformis syndrome **except**:
    A) The sciatic nerve may be involved because in some individuals the nerve runs through the piriformis muscle fibers
    B) Pain may be in lateral buttock, posterior hip and thigh, sciatica-like pain
    C) Pain with flexion, abduction, and external rotation
    D) Pain may be exacerbated by walking up stairs or prolonged sitting

116. What diagnostic test is the "gold standard" for evaluation of the rotator cuff?
    A) Plain x-ray
    B) Physical exam of the shoulder
    C) MRI
    D) Ultrasound

117. Which test is useful in determining adequate blood supply to the hand?
    A) Hoffman's test
    B) Elson's test
    C) Phalen's test
    D) Allen's test

118. Myofascial pain syndrome is characterized by:
    A) Widespread tenderness
    B) Tender points
    C) Trigger points
    D) No change in muscle tension

119. Cervical disc disease most commonly affects which disc?
    A) C3-C4
    B) C4-C5
    C) C5-C6
    D) C6-C7

120. What are the signs of a positive Trendelenburg's test?
    A) When the pelvis on the unsupported side stays the same height
    B) When the pelvis on the unsupported side is elevated slightly
    C) When the pelvis on the unsupported side descends
    D) When the pelvis on the supported side stays level

121. The most common cause of collapse in a marathon runner after crossing the finish line is:
    A) Benign exercise–associated collapse
    B) Cardiac arrest
    C) Heat stroke
    D) Hypoglycemia

122. Boxer's fractures involve a fracture of which metacarpal bone?
    A) First metacarpal
    B) Second metacarpal
    C) Third metacarpal
    D) Fifth metacarpal

123. An Achilles tendon injury is most likely to occur with what action?
    A) Sudden pivoting
    B) Internal rotation of the ankle
    C) Abruptly starting a sprint
    D) Walking uphill

124. What is **not** true about hip fractures?
    A) Females are more likely than males to sustain a hip fracture
    B) Most common underlying cause is weakened bone from metastatic disease
    C) Approximately 25% of patients over age 50 years with hip fractures die within 1 year
    D) About 50% of hip fracture patients require some form of assistive device

125. All of the following are true about iliopsoas bursitis and tendonitis **except**:
    A) Condition may cause snapping hip syndrome with flexion
    B) Pain is elicited with hip extension
    C) Pain is usually noted deep in the groin and radiates to the front of hip
    D) Refers to a stretch, tear, or complete rupture of the iliopsoas muscle and tendon where the tendon attaches to the femur

126. When compared to paraplegic patients who were nonathletes, paraplegic patients who participated in sports had:
    A) More hospital admissions
    B) More pressure sores
    C) More susceptibility to infections
    D) More success in avoiding major medical complications

127. What physical exam maneuver is used to detect biceps tendonitis?
    A) Hawkins' test
    B) Neer's test
    C) Speed's test
    D) Empty can test

128. Which nerve is susceptible to injury with humeral shaft fractures?
    A) Radial nerve
    B) Axillary nerve
    C) Ulnar nerve
    D) Median nerve

129. Rehabilitation in patients with patellofemoral syndrome is focused on strengthening of which muscle?
    A) Vastus lateralis
    B) Rectus femoris
    C) Vastus medialis obliquus (VMO)
    D) Vastus intermedius

130. How do you measure for leg length discrepancy?
  A) Anterior superior iliac spine (ASIS) to lateral malleolus
  B) Posterior superior iliac spine (PSIS) to lateral malleolus
  C) ASIS to medial malleolus
  D) PSIS to medial malleolus

131. Weakness of which muscle would correlate with compression of the C5 nerve root?
  A) Biceps brachii
  B) Extensor carpi radialis (ECR)
  C) Triceps brachii
  D) Flexor digitorum profundus (FDP)

132. Scaphoid fractures can be ruled out if the patient:
  A) Reports falling with an outstretched hand
  B) Complains of pain over the anatomical snuff box
  C) Has negative initial x-rays
  D) Has point tenderness localized to the ulnar aspect of the wrist

133. Which is **not** a characteristic of plantar fasciitis?
  A) Affects females more than males
  B) Tenderness over lateral aspect of the heel
  C) Pain is worse in the morning
  D) Heel spurs may contribute to the etiology

134. What is the most common type of hip fracture?
  A) Femoral neck
  B) Intracapsular
  C) Intertrochanteric
  D) Subtrochanteric

135. Which of the following is false about hip dislocation?
  A) The most common type is anterior hip dislocation
  B) Sciatic nerve may be stretched or compressed during posterior hip dislocations
  C) Femoral nerve may be injured during anterior hip dislocation
  D) Motor vehicle accidents are the most common cause of hip dislocations

136. Evaluation of scoliosis involves the Adam's test (forward bending test) and measuring the Cobb angle using a posterior-anterior (PA) radiograph, which measures:
  A) The angle formed at the intersection between the horizontal line drawn along the iliac crest and a line drawn along the superior end plate of the vertebra tilted the most at the top of the curve
  B) The angle formed at the intersection between a line drawn along the superior endplate of the vertebra tilted the most at the top of the curve, and a similar line drawn along the inferior endplate of the vertebra tilted the most at the bottom of the curve
  C) The angle formed at the intersection between a line drawn along the superior endplate of the vertebra tilted the most at the top of the curve, and a similar line drawn bisecting the center of the curve
  D) The angle formed at the intersection between a line drawn along the inferior endplate of the vertebra tilted the most at the bottom of the curve, and a similar line drawn bisecting the center of the curve

137. What is the function of the flexor digitorum profundus (FDP) muscles?
    A) Flexes at the distal interphalangeal (DIP) joint
    B) Flexes at the proximal interphalangeal (PIP) joint
    C) Flexes at the metacarpophalangeal (MCP) joint
    D) Flexes at the wrist

138. Hypertrophic cardiomyopathy is an autosomal dominant hereditary condition in which the patient has a defect in:
    A) Dystrophin protein
    B) Sarcomere contractile proteins
    C) Mitochondria
    D) Tau protein

139. What is plica syndrome of the knee?
    A) Knee pain caused by a duplicated meniscus
    B) Knee pain and weakness caused by an inflamed synovial structure in rheumatoid arthritis patients
    C) Knee pain and weakness caused by a synovial fold in femorotibial joint
    D) An extension or a vestigial structure of the protective synovial capsule of the knee becomes irritated or inflamed causing anterior knee pain and weakness

140. If a patient is supine with knees flexed to 90° and feet flat on the table, how will it be determined if the right femur is longer than the left?
    A) Left knee is higher than the right
    B) Right knee is higher than the left
    C) Left knee is anterior to the right
    D) Right knee is anterior to the left

141. Mallet finger is:
    A) A rupture of the terminal extensor tendon of the distal phalanx
    B) Identified by a loss of active extension of the proximal interphalangeal (PIP) joint of the finger
    C) Caused by forced extension of the distal phalangeal joint
    D) Occurs more commonly in ice hockey than in basketball or baseball players

142. Weakness of which muscle would correlate with compression of the T1 nerve root?
    A) Abductor digiti minimi (ADM)/interossei
    B) Extensor carpi radialis (ECR)
    C) Triceps brachii
    D) Flexor digitorum profundus (FDP)

143. Scoliosis can be classified as structural or functional. Which one of the following is **not** characteristic of structural scoliosis?
    A) Most cases are idiopathic
    B) It is reversible
    C) Subtypes of structural scoliosis include idiopathic
    D) Subtypes of structural scoliosis include congenital or acquired

144. Shoulder flexion involves the use of all of the following muscles **except**:
    A) Anterior deltoid
    B) Biceps brachii

    C) Coracobrachialis
    D) Teres major

145. What diagnostic test is used to diagnose complex regional pain syndrome (CRPS) in the upper limb?
    A) Somatosensory evoked potentials (SSEP)
    B) Stellate ganglion block
    C) Lumbar vertebral ganglion block
    D) Erythrocyte sedimentation rate

146. What is the Stimson technique?
    A) A provocative maneuver to test for glenohumeral instability
    B) Gravity-assisted technique to reduce an anterior shoulder dislocation
    C) A two-person technique to reduce an anterior shoulder dislocation, using a sheet under the axilla by one person and manual traction by the other person
    D) A test for inferior shoulder laxity

147. What is Panner's disease?
    A) Osteochondritis dissecans of the trochlea
    B) Traumatic elbow dislocation
    C) Median nerve compression at the elbow by lacertus fibrosis
    D) Epiphyseal aseptic necrosis of the capitellum

148. L2 nerve root compression would cause which of the following reflex abnormalities?
    A) Patellar tendon
    B) Cremasteric
    C) Cross adductor
    D) Achilles tendon

149. Where is the most common site of injury to the spinal accessory nerve?
    A) At the foramen magnum where it passes before entering the jugular foramen
    B) At the jugular foramen
    C) At the cervical root level
    D) In the posterior cervical triangle

150. What is the physical exam to test for cervical spine radiculopathy that places the patient in passive lateral flexion and extends the neck, followed by compression of the head?
    A) Spurling's maneuver
    B) Lhermitte sign
    C) Hoffman's sign
    D) Neck distraction test

151. Motions of the hip in Patrick's test are:
    A) Flexion, adduction, and internal rotation
    B) Flexion, adduction, external rotation, and extension
    C) Flexion, abduction, internal rotation, and extension
    D) Flexion, abduction, external rotation, and extension

152. Which muscles would most commonly be affected by a nerve injury after an anterior shoulder dislocation?
    A) Deltoid and teres minor
    B) Supraspinatus and infraspinatus

C) Rhomboids

D) Biceps and Supraspinatus

153. In heat exhaustion:
    A) The patient needs to be hyperthermic to be diagnosed
    B) There are known chronic and long-lasting effects
    C) The cardiovascular system fails to respond to increased workload due to heat
    D) It is considered a medical emergency

154. A hip pointer injury is a direct blow to the pelvic brim or hip causing:
    A) Hip dislocation
    B) Contusion of soft tissues and underlying bone of the hip
    C) Hip or femur fracture
    D) Avascular necrosis of the hip

155. What is a Rockwood type II acromioclavicular (AC) joint injury?
    A) Sprain of the AC and coracoacromial (CC) ligaments
    B) Torn CC ligament and intact AC ligament
    C) Torn AC ligament and sprained CC ligament
    D) Torn AC and CC ligaments

156. All of the following muscles are involved in shoulder adduction, **except**:
    A) Pectoralis major
    B) Teres major
    C) Coracobrachialis
    D) Biceps brachii

157. Hyperextension injury of the metatarsalphalangeal joint of the great toe is called:
    A) Turf toe
    B) Lisfranc injury
    C) Plantar fasciitis
    D) Hallux rigidus

158. All the following are benefits of ice in the treatment of acute tendinitis **except**:
    A) Local vasoconstriction
    B) Decreased metabolic rate
    C) Decreased swelling
    D) Local vasodilatation

159. Most common site of Morton's neuroma is:
    A) The first intermetatarsal space
    B) The second intermetatarsal space
    C) The third intermetatarsal space
    D) The fourth intermetatarsal space

160. Among the rotator cuff muscles, a tear primarily occurs in which of the following:
    A) Supraspinatus
    B) Infraspinatus
    C) Teres minor
    D) Subscapularis

# *Musculoskeletal*

## ANSWERS

1. **C)** Senile changes in a person's spine result in the acquired type of structural scoliosis, which is not reversible. All other answer choices are characteristic of functional scoliosis and are reversible.

2. **C)** Dupuytren's contracture most commonly involves the ring finger. This condition appears in the fourth to sixth decade of life and is more severe in males of northern European descent. The pathophysiology results in collagen type III hyperproliferation affecting the palmar fascia. Treatment includes serial triamcinolone injections in early stages, collagenase injections, and surgery.

3. **D)** Parsonage-Turner syndrome commonly affects the suprascapular nerve, axillary nerve, and/ or long thoracic nerve, and can be mistakenly attributed to an athletic event because of its idiopathic nature. Its classic presentation is acute onset of pain lasting 1 to 2 weeks and a delayed onset of weakness.

4. **B)** In lateral ankle sprains, the ligaments within the lateral ligament complex are injured in a predictable sequence as forces increase: anterior talofibular ligament, calcaneofibular ligament, then posterior talofibular ligament.

5. **D)** Scaphoid fractures can be missed but should be suspected in patients with radial wrist pain after trauma. The scaphoid and triquetrum are the most common wrist fractures. Scaphoid and lunate fractures are highly susceptible to avascular necrosis.

6. **D)** The menisci appear to transmit approximately 50% of the compressive load through range of motion (ROM) of 0° to 90°. The contact area is increased, protecting articular cartilage from high concentrations of stress. The circumferential continuity of the peripheral rim of the meniscus is integral to meniscal function. Partial meniscectomy, or bucket-handle tearing, will still preserve meniscal function as long as the peripheral rim is intact. Conversely, if a radial tear extends to the periphery and interrupts the continuity of the meniscus, the load-transmitting properties of the meniscus are lost.

   The tibial femoral contact area is decreased by up to 75% in postmeniscectomy knees. This decrease results in a 235% increase in contact stresses after total meniscectomy. The peripheral outer 1/3 of a meniscus is well vascularized, and the inner 2/3 poorly vascularized. Therefore, no surgical repair is needed for the inner 2/3 of a meniscus tear. The meniscus also plays an important role in proprioception of the knee joint.

7. **A)** The pronator teres, flexor carpi radialis, palmaris longus, flexor carpi ulnaris, and flexor digitorum superficialis are affected in medial epicondylitis. The triceps muscle is affected in posterior elbow tendonitis. The biceps tendon is affected in bicipital tendonitis.

8. **C)** The most powerful forearm supinator is the biceps brachii. This muscle has two proximal attachments. The short head attaches to the coracoid process, whereas the long head attaches to the supraglenoid tubercle of the scapula. The distal attachment is at the radial tuberosity and bicipital aponeurosis into fascia of the forearm. The biceps brachii is innervated by the musculocutaneous nerve, and this muscle is best tested when the forearm is placed in flexion and supination.

9. **D)** Trigger finger is defined as the triggering, snapping, or locking of the finger as it is flexed and extended. This is due to localized inflammation or nodular swelling of the flexor tendon sheath, which inhibits the normal tendon glide. Typically, the thumb, middle, and ring fingers of the dominant hand in middle-aged women are most commonly affected.

10. **C)** The true leg length should be measured from anterior superior iliac spine to medial malleolus. Apparent leg length discrepancy should be assessed if no true leg length discrepancy exists by measuring from a nonfixed point (eg, umbilicus) to a fixed point (eg, medial malleolus), which may be associated with pelvic obliquity.

11. **B)** A second trauma can be relatively minor, but the body's response can be fatal. It is believed that the brain's autoregulation becomes impaired from the first injury leading to engorgement within the cranium. This leads to increased intracranial pressures and possible herniation of the medial temporal lobes through the tentorium or herniation of cerebellar tonsils through the foramen magnum.

12. **A)** Frozen shoulder often follows a period of prolonged shoulder immobilization and results in a decreased range of motion (ROM) of the shoulder. Thickening and contraction of the capsule occurs around the glenohumeral joint. Risk factors include diabetes. It is more commonly seen in middle-aged women.

13. **D)** The MCL is the most common knee ligament injury in sports. It is usually caused by a valgus force to the knee joint, causing stretching or tearing of the MCL. Isolated complete tears of the MCL can be treated nonoperatively.

14. **D)** Plantar fasciitis is caused by inflammation of the plantar fascia. Increased tension on the plantar fascia, such as pes cavus, pes planus, obesity, tight Achilles tendon, or bone spurs can lead to chronic inflammation. Treatment options are mostly conservative, including modalities, nonsteroidal anti-inflammatory drugs (NSAIDs), orthotics or shoe modification (heel pads, cushion, and lift), as well as Achilles tendon and plantar fascia stretching. Anesthetic/corticosteroid injection is effective. Injection from the medial side of the heel helps avoid injection into subcutaneous tissue or fascial layer, which may cause fat pad atrophy/necrosis and fascia rupture. Nighttime dorsiflexion splints may be used if other conservative measures fail.

15. **C)** Heberden's nodes are swellings of the distal interphalangeal joints seen in osteoarthritis. Contents of these swellings are gelatinous hyaluronic acid. These growths arise in the chronic phase of osteoarthritis.

16. **C)** Typical radiographic features of osteoarthritis include joint space narrowing, osteophyte formation, and subchondral cysts. Periarticular osteopenia/osteoporosis and soft tissue swelling are typically seen in rheumatoid arthritis. Pencil-in-cup deformity is a finding in psoriatic arthritis.

17. **C)** The most commonly dislocated joint in children is the elbow. The elbow is the second most commonly dislocated joint in adults.

18. **D)** Four muscles (infraspinatus, supraspinatus, subscapularis, and teres minor) form the rotator cuff. The insertion point of these four muscles is subject to repetitive microtrauma and impingement between the acromion and greater tuberosity of the humerus. *Impingement syndrome, supraspinatus syndrome,* and *bursitis* are terms commonly used. Neer's test will be positive in the setting of impingement. Hawkins' test can also be performed to further confirm impingement. Drop arm test is used to detect rotator cuff tears. O'Brien test can be used to detect superior labrum anterior to posterior (SLAP) lesions or acromioclavicular (AC) joint abnormalities. Apley scarf test is also used to detect AC joint pathology.

19. **D)** Adhesive capsulitis is usually an *idiopathic* condition resulting in the loss of both active and passive range of motion (ROM) of the shoulder. It most commonly affects middle-aged adults (40–60 years). Associated risk factors include female gender, diabetes (most common risk factor), and hypothyroidism, among other conditions. None of the aforementioned risk factors have been determined to be primary causes of this condition. Adhesive capsulitis is divided into three stages: freezing stage, frozen stage, and thawing stage.

20. **B)** Static and dynamic stabilizers contribute to shoulder joint stability. Static stabilizers are glenoid, labrum, articular congruity, glenohumeral ligaments and capsule, and negative intraarticular pressure. The dynamic stabilizers are rotator cuff muscles/tendons, biceps tendon, and periscapular muscles.

21. **B)** The cruciate ligaments lie outside the synovial cavity but within the fibrous joint capsule. Image source: Miller A, DiCuccio Heckert K, Davis BA. *The 3-Minute Musculoskeletal and Peripheral Nerve Exam.* New York, NY: Demos Medical Publishing LLC; 2009:69.

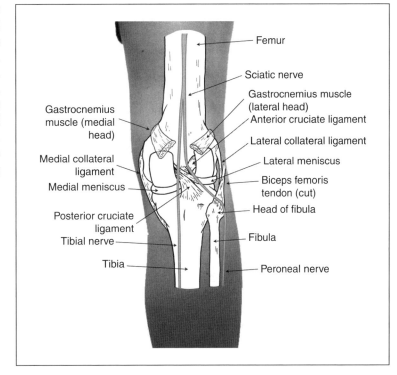

22. **A)** Ipsilateral Horner's syndrome (dropping eye, pupillary constriction, and increased skin temperature or flushing) indicates that the block was adequate.

23. **C)** Smith's fracture is when the distal radius becomes fractured and the distal fragment is displaced toward the palm (volar). It is also called a *reverse Colle's fracture* because in a Colle's fracture the distal radial fragment is displaced dorsally.

24. **A)** The anterior hip dislocation precautions are different from the posterior hip dislocation precautions: no hip extension, bridging, prone lying, or hip external rotation beyond neutral. When the patient is supine, keep the hip flexed to approximately 30° by placing a pillow under the patient's knees or by raising the head of the bed.

25. **C)** Answers A, B, and D are all absolute contraindications to return to play. A two- to three-level spinal fusion with normal exam is considered a relative contraindication. A one-level fusion with normal alignment and physical exam has no restriction whereas a fusion extending more than three levels is an absolute contraindication for return to play.

26. **B)** Rheumatoid arthritis is the most common cause of elbow joint destruction and occurs in most patients who have polyarticular involvement.

27. **C)** Age, muscle imbalance (weakness), anatomic malalignment, and genetic predisposition are all intrinsic factors that contribute to the development of tendinitis. Extrinsic variables include training errors, environmental factors, and equipment.

28. **B)** The elbow articulations allow the elbow two degrees of freedom: flexion-extension and pronation-supination. The normal elbow moves from 0° (full extension) to 135° to 150° of flexion. Pronation is approximately 70° to 90°, and supination is approximately 80° to 90°.

29. **D)** Steroid injection can be considered in patients diagnosed (by nerve conduction studies [NCV]/electromyogram [EMG]) with mild to moderate CTS. Care is taken to avoid piercing the median nerve. The needle is directed at an angle of 30°. Surgery is usually required in severe CTS, especially if abnormal spontaneous potentials are noted in the abductor pollicis brevis (APB) muscle.

30. **D)** There are five treatment phases in sports rehabilitation: the first phase is to resolve the pain and inflammation; the second phase is to restore ROM; the third phase is to strengthen; the fourth phase is proprioceptive training; and the last phase involves sports/task-specific activities.

31. **B)** Scaphoid fractures are the most common carpal bone fractures. The usual mechanism of injury (as is the case with most carpal fractures) is a fall on outstretched hands. Patients will have tenderness in the anatomical "snuffbox" area and decreased range of motion (ROM). Fracture of the middle 1/3 of the scaphoid bone (known as the waist) is most common. This bone has retrograde blood supply, making it particularly susceptible to malunion or avascular necrosis following a fracture. It is for this reason that a low threshold of suspicion is maintained for scaphoid fractures, and immobilization is usually initially prescribed if there is high clinical suspicion (despite negative x-rays).

32. **C)** Anterior glenohumeral stability is evaluated by the apprehension test. Hill-Sachs lesion accounting for greater than 30% of the articular surface may cause shoulder instability. A notch occurs in the posterior lateral aspect of humeral head owing to recurrent impingement. Image source: Brown DP, Freeman ED, Cuccurullo SJ et al. In: *Physical Medicine and Rehabilitation Board Review, Second Edition.* (Cuccurullo SJ ed.) New York, NY: Demos Medical Publishing LLC; 2010:158.

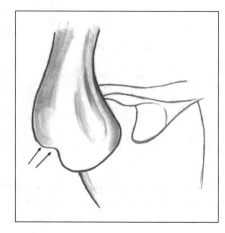

33. **C)** Additional studies are not usually necessary. If crystal-induced or septic bursitis is suspected, aspiration of the bursal fluid is usually indicated. Plain radiographs may demonstrate an olecranon spur in about 1/3 of cases.

34. **D)** The quadrangular space of the shoulder is bordered by the teres minor, teres major, long head of the triceps muscle, and medial border of the humerus. It is an area of potential compression of the posterior humeral circumflex artery or axillary nerve, especially in athletes who engage in overhead activities (throwing athletes, tennis players, swimmers). Patients will present with pain and paresthesias of the posterior lateral shoulder.

35. **D)** Internal snapping hip syndrome is caused by a tight iliopsoas tendon snapping over the iliopectineal prominence of the pelvis, or less commonly, acetabular labral tear or loose body in the hip joint. A tight iliotibial band or gluteus maximus snapping over the greater trochanter causes external snapping hip syndrome.

36. **C)** The rotator cuff muscles include the teres minor, supraspinatus, infraspinatus, and subscapularis muscles. These muscles are dynamic stabilizers of the shoulder.

37. **A)** Adson's test is performed by locating the radial pulse of the affected arm and asking the patient to turn their head toward the affected shoulder. The arm may be abducted and externally rotated as part of the maneuver. If the radial pulse diminishes on the affected side, this is positive for possible thoracic outlet syndrome. Thoracic outlet syndrome is the compression of the neurovascular structures in the neck, usually by a cervical rib or first rib and scalene muscles. Image source: Araim RJ, Aghalar MR, Weiss LD. *Neuromuscular Quick Pocket Reference.* New York, NY: Demos Medical Publishing LLC; 2012:4.

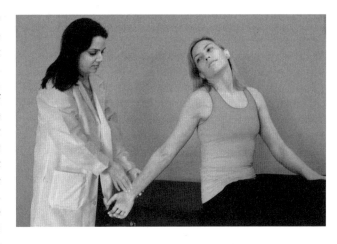

38. **B)** Approximately 30% of the humeral head articulates directly with the glenoid fossa. A fibrocartilaginous complex called the *labrum* surrounds the glenoid fossa, effectively increasing the total contact of the humeral head with the glenoid to 70%. This allows for the stabilization of the glenohumeral joint and prevents anterior and posterior humeral head dislocation.

39. **C)** De Quervain's affects the abductor pollicis longus and extensor pollicis brevis tendons. It can be seen with overuse in sports with gripped equipment such as golf and racquet sports. The patient usually has pain with resisted thumb extension. Finkelstein's test can be positive.

40. **A)** Individual flexor tendons for each digit of the hand are housed within a flexor tendon sheath. The tendon sheath has areas of thickening called annular and cruciate pulleys that function to stabilize the tendon. In stenosing tenosynovitis (trigger finger), the proximal pulley becomes inflamed and thickened with concurrent nodular enlargement of the tendon itself. As the inflamed tendon passes through the thickened pulley, it occasionally becomes stuck, locking the finger in flexion. This condition usually affects the middle or ring fingers. Therapy includes local steroid injection or surgery.

41. **B)** The most common "mass" to occur in the wrist is a ganglion cyst. It is essentially a "ballooning-out" of the joint lining and the fluid inside is synovial fluid. Ganglion cysts most commonly occur on the dorsal aspect of the wrist (usually from the scapholunate joint). On physical examination, the cyst may transilluminate. They can be evaluated by MRI, while x-rays will often be normal. Observational management is indicated for asymptomatic cases. If the cysts interfere with activity, aspiration may be warranted. Ganglion cysts tend to recur at a rate of 20%, while recurrence rate drops to less than 10% following excision.

42. **A)** Sports rehabilitation can be categorized into five phases: (1) resolving the pain and inflammation, (2) restoring range of motion, (3) strengthening, (4) proprioceptive training, and (5) sports/task-specific activities. Immobilization is generally avoided as it can limit range of motion (which can cause contractures and atrophy).

43. **D)** Approximately 90% of patients under 20 years of age will dislocate their shoulder again after a prior dislocation. Individuals age 20 to 40 years old carry a moderate risk of dislocation and there is an approximate 10% rate for dislocation in patients over 40 years.

44. **B)** Clavicle fractures are one of the most common bony injuries. The most common location is the middle 1/3 (80%), 15% occur in the distal 1/3, and 5% occur in the proximal 1/3.

45. **B)** Thomas' test is used to assess for a hip flexion contracture. With the patient supine, flex one hip to obliterate the lumbar lordosis. The angle between the affected thigh and the table reveals the fixed flexion contracture of the hip. Ober's test is used to assess for an iliotibial band contracture. Image source: Araim RJ, Aghalar MR, Weiss LD. *Neuromuscular Quick Pocket Reference*. New York, NY: Demos Medical Publishing LLC; 2012:32.

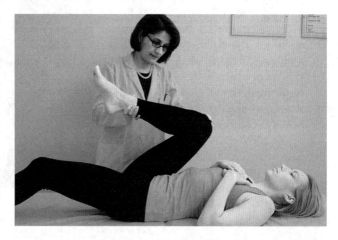

46. **A)** Mallet finger is usually caused by forced flexion of the distal phalangeal joint. Jersey finger is avulsion of the flexor digitorum profundus from the distal phalanx. It usually occurs in the fourth finger. Trigger finger is thickening of the proximal portion of the flexor tendon sheath which may cause the finger to get "stuck" in flexion. Coach's finger is an interphalangeal dislocation that usually dislocates dorsally.

47. **D)** MR arthrogram is the test of choice when evaluating for labral pathology.

48. **B)** De Quervain's tenosynovitis is a condition in which inflammation causes thickening and stenosis of the synovial sheath surrounding the first dorsal compartment of the wrist. This produces pain with tendon movement. On examination, there may be appreciable thickening of the fibrous sheath and Finkelstein's test will be positive. Nonoperative management is indicated in most cases. Splinting with a thumb spica splint is applied such that pinching is possible. Steroid injection can help for symptomatic relief, and surgery may be indicated for decompression in refractory cases.

49. **C)** During the last 20° of extension of the knee, the femur slightly internally rotates on the tibia to lock the knee joint in place in the closed chain, or the tibia slightly externally rotates on femur in

the open chain, which is also called the *screw-home mechanism*. In the closed chain, the popliteus can externally rotate the femur to unlock the knee for flexion.

50. **D)** Congenital torticollis occurs in approximately 1 per 250 live births, with 75% involving the right side. The most common cause is fibrosis of the sternocleidomastoid. The presence of a cervical hemivertebra is less common. On physical examination, a nontender enlargement in the sternocleidomastoid is noted.

51. **A)** SLAP lesions occur as a result of falling on an outstretched arm causing a traction and compression injury related to the fall. Overhead throwing motion in the deceleration phase can also cause a SLAP lesion by causing traction on the superior labrum by the biceps muscle. The cocking phase of the overhead throw causes a torsional peeling-back stress to the glenoid labrum leading to a SLAP lesion.

52. **A)** Osteochondritis dissecans is characterized by fragmentation of the bone and cartilage overlying the capitellum in the elbow. This condition often occurs in teenage boys involved in throwing sports because of the valgus stress on the elbow. It is often mistakenly confused with Panner's disease, which has more to do with a circulatory problem affecting the bone in the elbow and occurs in children 5 to 12 years of age.

53. *C* **D)** Shoulder extension involves the use of the posterior deltoid, latissimus dorsi, teres major, long head of triceps, and sternocostal portion of the pectoralis major.

54. **C)** Choices (A) and (B) are paired with the incorrect nerves. Choice (D) is responsible for lateral winging of the scapula.

55. **A)** The most common site of compartment syndrome is the lower leg. The anterior compartment is the most frequently affected, followed by the lateral compartment and the deep posterior compartment.

56. **D)** MTSS, also known as shin splints, is a common type of overuse injury that results from chronic traction on the periosteum at the periosteal-fascial junction along the posteromedial border of the tibia. The main predisposing factor is hyperpronation. Pain may improve with exercise but may worsen afterward. Rest is the first priority in management of MTSS. Return to activity should be gradual.

57. **C)** It is important to rule out a fracture of the fibula and/or the fifth metatarsal. Mild sprain of the anterior talofibular ligament and negative ankle drawer test is considered a grade I ankle sprain. Disruption of the anterior talofibular ligament, the calcaneofibular ligament, and the lateral ligament complex with positive ankle drawer test is considered a grade III ankle sprain.

58. **A)** The pivot shift test is the most **specific** test to diagnose an ACL tear. Under anesthesia, the specificity approaches 100%. Lachman's test is usually considered the most **sensitive** test for an ACL tear. Ege's test is used for diagnosis of a meniscal injury.

59. **A)** Gamekeeper's thumb is an injury to the ulnar collateral ligament of the thumb-MCP joint resulting in joint instability. Usually, the mechanism of injury is a forced radial deviation of the thumb or from a ski pole injury. Patients may describe pain and decreased grip strength at this location. There may be appreciable laxity of the MCP. A palpable mass at the location of the ulnar collateral ligament is called a Stener lesion, where the adductor pollicis aponeurosis falls under the torn collateral ligament.

60. **B)** The patellofemoral joint is under high levels of compression during stair climbing owing to significantly increased quadriceps activity.

61. **A)** The scaphoid is the most commonly fractured carpal bone (70%). It is subject to osteonecrosis because of its poor blood supply. Clinical features of a scaphoid fracture include tenderness in the anatomical snuff box. Complications include collapse of carpal bones, especially scapholunate instability.

62. **A)** The proximal tibiofibular joint is located between the lateral tibial condyle and the fibular head and has been construed as the "fourth compartment" of the knee joint. It is a synovial joint and communicates with the knee joint in approximately 10% of adults. It is a source of lateral knee pain that is often overlooked.

63. **A)** O'Brien's test evaluates for labral abnormalities. The shoulder is flexed to 90° with the elbow fully extended. The arm is then adducted 15° and the shoulder is internally rotated with the patient's thumb pointing down. Downward force is applied to the arm against resistance. The shoulder is then externally rotated with the palm facing up and the examiner applies downward force on the patient's arm, which the patient is instructed to resist. A positive test is indicated by pain during the first part of the maneuver with the patient's thumb pointing down. The pain is lessened when the patient resists a downward force with the palm facing up. Image source: Araim RJ, Aghalar MR, Weiss LD. *Neuromuscular Quick Pocket Reference*. New York, NY: Demos Medical Publishing LLC; 2012:15.

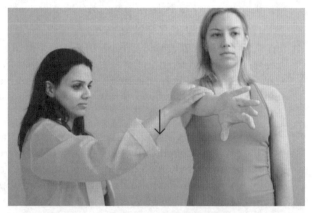
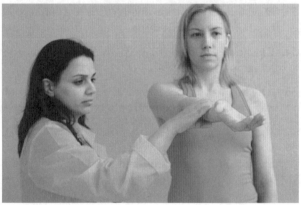

64. **B)** Injuries caused by forcible abduction of the thumb are associated with injury to the ulnar collateral ligament of the first metacarpophalangeal joint (MCP). Skiers are at risk owing to falling while holding a ski pole.

65. **C)** Neer's impingement sign is performed by bringing the arm in extreme forward flexion with the humerus externally rotated. Hawkins' test is also used to assess for impingement sign. The arm is forward flexed to 90° and medially rotated. A positive sign elicits pain during movement. Speed's test is used to assess for bicipital tendonitis. Finkelstein's test is used to assess for De Quervain's, and Tinel's test is used to evaluate for nerve irritability. Image source: Araim RJ, Aghalar MR, Weiss LD. *Neuromuscular Quick Pocket Reference*. New York, NY: Demos Medical Publishing LLC; 2012:8.

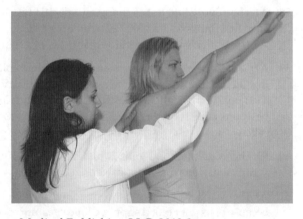

66. **D)** Sudden impact to the front of the tibia with the knee flexed (as in a motor vehicle accident) is the most frequent cause of a PCL injury. Hyperflexion is the most common cause of PCL injuries in athletes.

67. **D)** Q angle is the angle formed by a line drawn from the anterior superior iliac spine (ASIS) to the central patella, and a second line drawn from the central patella to the tibial tubercle. Normally, Q angle is 14° for males and 17° for females. An increased Q angle is a risk factor for patellar sub-luxation. The Q angle is increased by genu valgum, increased femoral anteversion, external tibial torsion, a laterally positioned tibial tuberosity, or a tight lateral retinaculum.

68. **A)** The surgical neck is called so because of frequent fractures which occur here. This area lies below the head and tubercle and is narrow. The anatomical neck is located at the junction point of the head with the shaft, and is between the head and tubercles.

69. **B)** Muscle comprises 40% to 45% of the total body weight.

70. **B)** MRI of both hips is indicated to assess for a diagnosis of AVN of the femoral head. MRI is most sensitive to early changes with a low signal intensity noted on T1 imaging.

71. **C)** Pain with resisted wrist extension and supination as well as pain with passive wrist flexion are seen in lateral epicondylitis. Once diagnosed, it is important to identify the behavior causing the problem, and to modify it. Pain with wrist flexion and pronation, as well as pain with passive wrist extension, is seen in medial epicondylitis

72. **A)** The ACL originates at the lateral femoral condyle, travels through the intercondylar notch, and attaches to the medial tibial eminence. Its primary function is to limit anterior tibial transla-tion, or prevent backward sliding of the femur. It limits internal rotation of the femur when the foot is fixed. The ACL loosens in flexion and tightens in full extension. ACL pathology leads to increased pressures on the posterior menisci.

73. **D)** Cozen's test is performed with the examiner stabilizing the patient's elbow and his or her thumb over the extensor tendon origin along the lat-eral epicondyle. With the opposite hand, the examiner provides resis-tance as the patient tries to extend and radially deviate the wrist. Pain over the lateral epicondyle indi-cates a positive test. Image source: Araim RJ, Aghalar MR, Weiss LD. *Neuromuscular Quick Pocket Reference.* New York, NY: Demos Medical Publishing LLC; 2012:20.

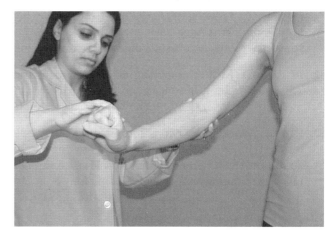

74. **D)** The phases of throwing in order are: wind up, early cocking, late cocking, acceleration, and follow-through. During late cocking there is significant valgus stress on the elbow joint, with maximal stress on the medial collateral ligament (MCL). The elbow also experiences a significant degree of valgus stress during acceleration, but not as much as late cocking.

75. **B)** The serratus anterior protracts the scapula and holds it against the thoracic wall. The other choices refer to the pectoralis minor (A), levator scapulae (C), and subscapularis (D).

76. **C)** Recurrent anterior shoulder dislocations can lead to a compression fracture of the posterolateral humeral head known as a Hill-Sachs deformity. Radiographic evaluation with anterior-posterior views and Stryker notch view are used. In the Stryker notch view, the patient is supine with a cassette placed under the involved shoulder. The palm of the affected arm is placed on top of the head with the fingers pointing posteriorly, and the elbow pointing upward toward the ceiling. The x-ray beam is centered over the coracoid process with the beam directed 10° towards the head.

77. **D)** The dorsal portion of the annulus fibrosis is innervated by the medial branch of the segmental spinal nerves.

78. **A)** Saturday night palsy, honeymooner's palsy, or radial nerve mononeuropathy usually presents with wrist and finger drop. It may present with numbness and paresthesias of the forearm and wrist as well. Acute compression of the radial nerve typically occurs at the spiral groove.

79. **B)** Kienböck's disease is a consequence of traumatic or repetitive microtrauma to the lunate leading to osteonecrosis. Patients present with pain, stiffness, and wrist dysfunction. Physical examination reveals local tenderness over the lunate, limited range of motion (ROM), and decreased grip strength. Radiographs may show lunate sclerosis and degeneration of adjacent joints in later stages. In later stages, wrist fusion may be indicated.

80. **D)** Clinical features of Kienböck's disease include pain over the dorsal aspect of the wrist, directly over the lunate. The mechanism is hypothesized to be an idiopathic loss of blood supply to the lunate, causing avascular necrosis. The disease is correlated with repetitive stress or fracture. Risk factors include short ulnar variance and poor vascular supply. In later stages, the collapse of the lunate results in multiple degenerative changes at the wrist.

81. **D)** Long thoracic nerve injury or palsy will result in serratus anterior weakness. The long thoracic nerve originates from the C5-C7 nerve roots, and travels below the brachial plexus and clavicle before ultimately innervating the serratus anterior muscle. The serratus anterior muscle works to protract the scapula and cause its upward rotation, pulling it forward against the rib cage. In medial scapular winging, the scapula comes away from the chest wall medially. Forward flexion of the shoulder is often weaker and limited to 90° relative to the unaffected side. Injury to the spinal accessory nerve results in lateral scapular winging.

82. **B)** The ACL, MCL, and medial meniscus are structures that are damaged in the unhappy triad. This usually occurs in contact sports, usually with valgus stress and rotation of the knee. Lateral meniscus tears can also be seen with ACL and MCL injuries.

83. **C)** The suprascapular nerve is commonly compressed at the level of the suprascapular notch, resulting in deep, boring shoulder pain along the superior scapula and weakness of shoulder abduction and external rotation. If nerve entrapment occurs at the level of the spinoglenoid notch, then the only appreciable finding may be isolated atrophy and weakness of the infraspinatus muscle. Pain is not so prominent at this level because the sensory fibers have already exited.

84. **C)** Injury to the long thoracic and spinal accessory nerves causes weakness of the serratus anterior and trapezius muscles, respectively, and are most commonly associated with scapular winging. Patients present with symptoms of pain in the upper back or shoulder, muscle fatigue, and weakness with the use of the shoulder. Initial management includes immobilization to prevent overstretching of the weakened muscle.

85. **A)** Tendons consist of dense, regularly arranged collagen fibers meshed with elastin and a proteoglycan/glycosaminoglycan ground substance. The primary function of the tendon is to transmit the force generated in muscle to the bone allowing for the generation of movement of the extremities.

86. **A)** Eversion injuries are not as common as inversion injuries but can cause damage to the deltoid ligament. The anterior talofibular ligament, calcaneofibular ligament, and posterior talofibular ligament can be injured in inversion injuries.

87. **D)** A full thickness tear can cause immediate functional impairments. The pain quality can be described as dull and achy, and symptoms are similar to those of rotator cuff tendinitis. The greatest limitation is difficulty performing overhead activities.

88. **A)** Seizures can occur within seconds of the insult and do not warrant treatment. They are uncommon and are not associated with structural brain injury or long-term risks. The athlete should not necessarily be eliminated from the sport.

89. **D)** In Erb's palsy, the upper trunk of the brachial plexus is affected (C5-C6) resulting in shoulder abduction, elbow flexion, and forearm supination weakness. It is the most common brachial plexopathy seen in newborns.

90. **C)** Patients must be asymptomatic before starting the stepwise approach, which goes from light aerobic activity to sport-specific training to non–contact drills to full contact practice to game play. The patient is able to progress as long as they are asymptomatic in all steps.

91. **C)** Impingement can result from extrinsic compression or as a result of loss of competency of the rotator cuff and/or scapula-stabilizing muscles. The biceps tendon also passes within the space. The impingement interval, which is the space between the undersurface of the acromion and the superior aspect of the humeral head, is maximally narrowed when the arm is abducted.

92. **C)** It is important to identify and prevent sudden cardiac death during physical activity. Conditions such as hypertrophic cardiomyopathy, arrhythmias, coronary artery anomalies, ruptured aortic aneurysms, and commotio cordis are some examples of dangerous and life-threatening conditions.

93. **C)** This injury can occur when there is a force to a flexed knee. PCL injuries can also be seen in motor vehicle collisions. Isolated PCL injury rehabilitation is focused on quadriceps strengthening and closed kinetic training.

94. **A)** When there is shoulder instability, there are recurrent episodes of subluxation where the humeral head partially comes out of the socket. Anterior instability is more commonly seen than posterior instability, hence dislocations also more commonly occur anteriorly. With recurrent anterior dislocations (where the humeral head remains fully out of socket), the anterior glenoid labrum may become torn or even avulsed off of the glenoid rim (called a *Bankart lesion*). Choice (B) describes a Hill-Sachs lesion; choice (C) is a SLAP lesion; and choice (D) describes the setting of thoracic outlet syndrome. Image source: Brown DP, Freeman ED, Cuccurullo SJ, et al. In: *Physical Medicine and Rehabilitation Board Review, Third Edition.* (Cuccurullo SJ ed.) New York, NY: Demos Medical Publishing LLC; 2015:160.

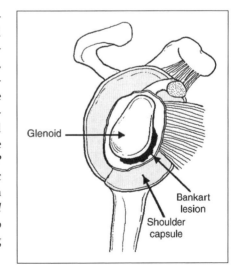

95. **C)** Froment's sign is performed by asking the patient to pinch a piece of paper between his or her index finger and thumb while the examiner tries to pull the paper away. If the patient flexes the first interphalangeal joint, suggesting adductor pollicis weakness, the test is considered a positive Froment's sign and indicates possible ulnar nerve palsy. Image source: Friedrich J, Akuthota V. In: *Sports Medicine: Study Guide and Review for Boards, Second Edition.* (Harrast MA, Finnoff JT, eds.) New York, NY: Demos Medical Publishing LLC; 2017:510.

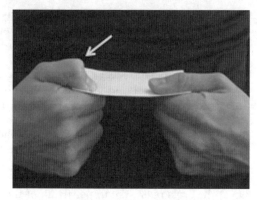

96. **D)** Boutonnière deformity is seen in patients with rheumatoid arthritis and is a consequence of disruption of the central slip of the extensor tendons with volar migration of the lateral bands. This results in hyperflexion of the proximal interphalangeal (PIP) joint. Treatment in early stages includes splinting of the PIP joint in extension.

97. **A)** The PIN is a deep branch of the radial nerve, which if compressed may present with lateral elbow pain. The PIN usually gets compressed by a fibrous band located between two heads of the supinator muscle (the radial tunnel). Patients may present with symptoms similar to lateral epicondylitis, but remain refractory to treatment. In such situations, an electromyogram (EMG)/nerve conduction study (NCS) should be sought to evaluate for PIN compression.

98. **D)** Little League elbow is suspected in a throwing athlete between the ages of 9 and 12 with medial elbow pain and a recent history of throwing. There is tenderness over the medial epicondyle and pain with resisted flexion of the wrist and valgus stress testing of the elbow. There may also be a slight elbow flexion contracture. The pathology is irritation and inflammation of the growth plate on the medial epicondyle.

99. **D)** Tennis elbow is commonly known as lateral epicondylitis. Patients present with pain and tenderness over the lateral epicondyle as well as over the extensor tendon. There is pain with resistance to wrist and third digit extension. Occasionally, grip strength testing elicits pain. Acutely, there will be inflammatory responses to tension overload placed in the tendon-bone junction. Lateral epicondylitis typically lasts longer than a few weeks. It is caused by a poor backhand stroke in tennis, although this is not always the cause.

100. **D)** Swan neck deformity is characteristic of rheumatoid arthritis. The deformity may start at the MCP, PIP, or DIP joint. If the flexor tendon at the MCP joint tightens, this may result in hyperextension at the PIP joint. Alternatively, if the PIP volar capsule becomes lax secondary to tenosynovitis, the PIP joint will hyperextend causing swan necking of the remaining joints. More commonly, however, stretching or disruption of the distal extensor mechanism results in a mallet finger deformity, which leads to eventual PIP hyperextension.

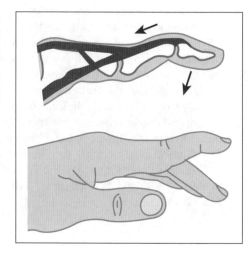

101. **A)** Flex, **ab**duct, **e**xternally **r**otate the hip, with downward force causing **e**xtension is the FABERE test. Anterior hip/groin pain is suggestive of hip joint pathology. Image source: Araim RJ, Aghalar MR, Weiss LD. *Neuromuscular Quick Pocket Reference*. New York, NY: Demos Medical Publishing LLC; 2012:31.

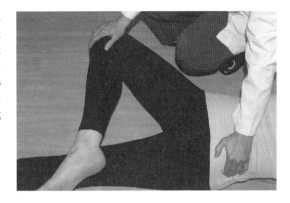

102. **D)** De Quervain's is a tenosynovitis of the first dorsal compartment of the hand/wrist. The APL and EPB tendons are involved. Finkelstein's test is usually positive (pain is elicited along the radial aspect of the wrist when the wrist is forced into ulnar deviation with the thumb in a closed fist).

103. **C)** Lachman's test is the most sensitive test for ACL injury or laxity. McMurray's and Apley's grind tests assess injury to the lateral meniscus and medial meniscus. The quadriceps active test assesses posterior collateral ligament disruption. Image source: Araim RJ, Aghalar MR, Weiss LD. *Neuromuscular Quick Pocket Reference*. New York, NY: Demos Medical Publishing LLC, 2012:41

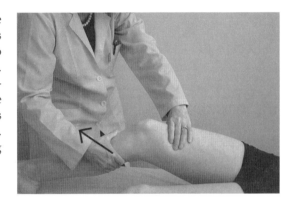

104. **B)** The hip will be flexed, adducted, and internally rotated. The affected leg is shorter because the dislocated femoral head is higher than on the normal side, and the patient will be unable to abduct the affected side.

105. **B)** During concentric contractions, muscles shorten. In eccentric contractions, muscles lengthen. This usually occurs under tension, and the muscles are more prone to injury. Isometric contractions are static where muscle fibers do not change length. Isotonic contractions involve muscle length changes and encompass both concentric and eccentric contraction.

106. **C)** An avulsion fracture of the ASIS, especially in an adolescent athlete, often occurs from forceful eccentric contraction of the sartorius or tensor fascia lata muscle with hip extension and knee flexion, as in sprinting or swinging a baseball bat. Surgery may be needed for a displaced apophysis. The rectus femoris muscle is involved in an anterior inferior iliac spine avulsion fracture.

107. **B)** Writer's cramp is the most common type of dystonia. Patients with dystonia have simultaneous contraction of agonist and antagonist muscle groups. Initial complaints present as poor coordination, cramping, and aching of the hand with task-specific movements. Prognosis for recovery is good.

108. **B)** No differences have been found in knee range of motion (ROM), pain scores, or analgesic use in patients who used CPM following TKA. One study did reveal some evidence suggesting that CPM can shorten the length of hospital stay and improve knee flexion at early time points, but does not affect other functional outcomes. The postoperative use of a continuous passive motion machine does not improve outcomes after anterior cruciate ligament tear surgical repair either.

109. **A)** Medial epicondylitis is associated with pitchers and golfers. Medial epicondylitis is felt to occur from microtears of the common flexor tendon origin or failed healing response that alters normal biomechanics. Lateral epicondylitis is seen in tennis players.

110. **C)** Ober's test is used to assess for tensor fascia lata/iliotibial band tightness. Thomson's test is used to assess for Achilles tendon injury or rupture. Image source: Araim RJ, Aghalar MR, Weiss LD. *Neuromuscular Quick Pocket Reference.* New York, NY: Demos Medical Publishing LLC; 2012:30.

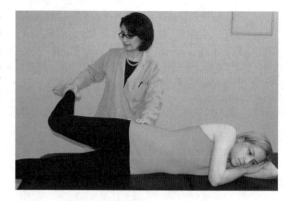

111. **A)** Myositis ossificans is the formation of heterotopic ossification within muscle. Prevention of contractures is a priority and can be accomplished by gentle range of motion (ROM). Surgery may be needed if the myositis ossificans causes nerve entrapment, decreased ROM, or loss of function. However, surgery should be delayed until heterotopic ossification matures at 10 to 12 months.

112. **C)** Female athletes were seen to have more skeletal demineralization, inadequate eating, and menstrual abnormalities. On average, women have a larger surface area–to-mass ratio, lower bone mass, and a wider, shallower pelvis than men.

113. **B)** Anterior talofibular ligament. To perform this test, stabilize the distal part of the leg with one hand and apply anterior force to the heel with the other hand. This attempts to sublux the talus anteriorly from beneath the tibia when performing the test. Image source: Araim RJ, Aghalar MR, Weiss LD. *Neuromuscular Quick Pocket Reference.* New York, NY: Demos Medical Publishing LLC; 2012:47.

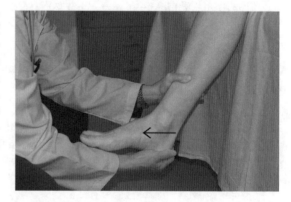

114. **C)** Also known as osteonecrosis of the hip or aseptic necrosis of the hip, this condition is characterized by destruction of the femoral head without sepsis. Interruption of the vascular supply is the defining common pathway of the disease process. The most common causes in adults are steroid use or alcohol abuse.

115. **C)** The provocative test for piriformis syndrome is flexion, adduction, and internal rotation (FAIR), which helps reproduce the symptoms.

116. **C)** MRI has replaced arthrography as the gold standard test for rotator cuff injuries. It offers high sensitivity and specificity that can be used to identify size, location, and quality of injury. It is relatively expensive and requires lack of motion by the patient in order to avoid artifact.

117. **D)** Allen's test is used to check for patent ulnar and/or radial artery circulation to the hand. To perform the test, the examiner manually occludes the patient's ulnar and radial arteries while the patient makes a fist. As the examiner releases pressure one by one, visible reperfusion of the palm indicates patency of the arteries. This test is usually performed prior to doing a radial artery arterial blood gas to ensure that collateral circulation will be possible should the radial artery become occluded.

118. **C)** Trigger points can develop owing to a variety of factors, including direct or indirect trauma, overuse, or stress. A trigger point is an area of tautness, which on compression can cause local or referred manifestations. Trigger points can refer symptoms to more remote regions. In contrast, palpation of a tender point causes local discomfort without referred pain.

119. **C)** C5-C6 is the most common cervical disc disease followed by C6-C7 and then C4-C5.

120. **C)** The Trendelenburg's sign indicates gluteus medius weakness. The strength of the gluteus medius (which acts as an abductor) is assessed. If the unsupported side descends, this is a positive test. For example, pelvic drop on the right side in a patient standing on left leg indicates left gluteus medius weakness.

121. **A)** Benign exercise–associated collapse is due to a form of orthostatic hypotension. When the patient stops running, venous blood pools to the lower extremities and the patient becomes hypotensive, which can cause them to collapse. It can be prevented by having the athlete continue to walk/jog to maintain the muscular venous pumping after the marathon.

122. **D)** Boxer's fractures involve a fracture of the fifth metacarpal and are the most common fractures occurring in the metacarpals. They usually occur after the patient strikes a hard object with a closed fist. Treatment typically involves closed reduction and casting.

123. **C)** The Achilles tendon attaches the gastrocnemius to the heel. As the muscle shortens, the tendon plantarflexes the foot. An acute injury occurs when a healthy tendon is subjected to a sudden, unexpected force, such as pushing off for a sprint or landing from a jump.

124. **B)** The most common cause of hip fractures is osteoporosis. In the vast majority of cases, a hip fracture is a fragility fracture owing to a fall or minor trauma in someone with weakened, osteoporotic bone. They are classified as intracapsular, which includes femoral head and neck fractures, or extracapsular, which includes trochanteric, intertrochanteric, and subtrochanteric fractures. The location of the fracture and the amount of angulation and comminution play integral roles in the overall morbidity of the patient, as does the preexisting physical condition of the individual. The other options are all true.

125. **B)** Pain is elicited with hip flexion. The acute injury often involves eccentric contraction of the iliopsoas muscle or rapid flexion against extension force/resistance, but may less commonly result from direct trauma. The overuse phenomenon may occur in any activity resulting in repeated hip flexion or external rotation of the femur.

126. **D)** Paraplegic athletes were shown to have fewer hospitalizations, fewer pressure sores, and were less susceptible to infections. There is an increase in athletic opportunities for patients with impairments—there has been a rise in participants in the Paralympic games.

127. **C)** Speed's test is performed by asking the patient to anteriorly flex the shoulder against resistance while the elbow is extended. Hawkins' and Neer's both test for rotator cuff impingement. Empty can test is used to detect supraspinatus tendinopathy. Image source: Araim RJ, Aghalar MR, Weiss LD. *Neuromuscular Quick Pocket Reference*. New York, NY: Demos Medical Publishing LLC; 2012:16.

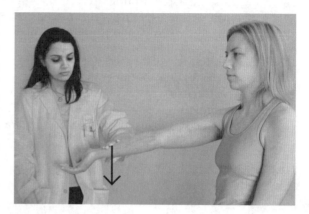

128. **A)** Up to 18% of humeral shaft fractures are associated with radial nerve injury, particularly if the fracture occurs at the junction between the middle and distal 1/3 of the shaft. The axillary nerve is the most commonly injured nerve with more proximal humerus fractures (ie, surgical neck fractures).

129. **C)** The VMO is a dynamic medial stabilizer which helps maintain proper patellar tracking during extension of the knee.

130. **C)** To assess for a leg length discrepancy, measure from the anterior superior iliac spine to the medial malleolus. Leg length discrepancies of less than 1/2 in. do not need correction.

131. **A)** Compression of the C5 nerve root will result in weakness of the biceps brachii. Compression of C6 and C7 nerve roots would result in weakness of the extensor carpi radialis and triceps, respectively. Compression of C8 and T1 nerve roots would result in weakness of flexor digitorum profundus and abductor digiti minimi (ADM)/interossei, respectively.

132. **D)** Scaphoid fractures are the most common carpal bone fractures. They often occur due to a fall on an outstretched hand. Snuff box tenderness may be noted. If initial plain films are negative, then wrist should be immobilized and films repeated in approximately 2 weeks. There is a high incidence of nonunion and avascular necrosis.

133. **B)** Tenderness usually occurs over the medial aspect of the heel in plantar fasciitis.

134. **C)** An intertrochanteric hip fracture occurs three to four inches from the hip joint. This type of fracture does not interrupt the blood supply to the bone and may be easier to repair.

135. **A)** The most common type of hip dislocation is posterior (90%).

136. **B)** If the Cobb angle exceeds 50° to 60°, abnormalities in pulmonary function tests may appear. Treatments are based on the degree of curvature: 1° to 20°—observation; 20° to 40°—bracing; greater than 40°—evaluation for surgery.

137. **A)** The FDP muscle's origin is at the anterior ulna and interosseous membrane. The insertion is the distal phalanx of the index, middle, ring, and small fingers. Its main action is flexion of the DIP joint of the fingers. The FDP is innervated by the anterior interosseous nerve from the median nerve (index and middle fingers) as well as the ulnar nerve (ring and small finger).

138. **B)** This defect leads to increased ventricular muscle mass but not an increase in ventricular cavity size. Hypertrophic cardiomyopathy leads to a net reduction in inner ventricular cavity size because of the hypertrophied muscle. Dystrophin abnormalities are seen in Duchenne muscular dystrophy. Tau proteins are affected in Alzheimer's disease.

139. **D)** The knee plica is considered a vestigial structure because of remnant embryological tissue that compartmentalizes the knee during fetal development. This horseshoe-shaped structure can become irritated or inflamed, which causes anterior knee pain and weakness, known as the *plica syndrome.*

140. **D)** If one knee projects further anteriorly in the position described, then that femur is longer. In this case, the right knee will be anterior to the left. If one knee is higher than the other, that tibia is longer.

141. **A)** Mallet finger is a rupture of the terminal extensor tendon of the distal phalanx causing loss of active extension of the distal interphalangeal joint. It is usually caused by forced flexion of the distal phalangeal joint as can occur when a ball hits the end of the finger. It occurs most commonly in sports like basketball or baseball.

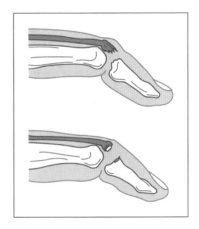

142. **A)** Compression of the T1 nerve root would result in weakness of the ADM/interossei. Compression of C6 and C7 nerve roots would result in weakness of the extensor carpi radialis and triceps, respectively. Compression of the C8 nerve roots would result in weakness of the flexor digitorum profundus.

143. **B)** Structural scoliosis is not reversible. Subtypes include idiopathic, congenital, or acquired. Idiopathic scoliosis accounts for 80% of structural scoliosis.

144. **D)** Shoulder flexion involves the use of the anterior deltoid, pectoralis major, biceps brachii, and coracobrachialis.

145. **B)** CRPS is a condition characterized as a chronic pain syndrome due to dysfunction in the central and peripheral nervous systems. It presents with changes in skin color and temperature and is accompanied by intense burning pain symptoms and sensitivity. The stellate ganglion block is a sympathetic block used primarily to diagnose and treat symptoms of CRPS. Such blocks are usually performed by a pain specialist and may result in complete or partial pain relief. An adequate block may result in a temporary Horner's syndrome. Sympathetic blocks performed for the lower extremities are called lumbar sympathetic blocks.

146. **B)** In the Stimson's technique, the patient with an anterior shoulder dislocation is placed prone on the stretcher with the dislocated arm hanging off the edge of the bed. A 5- to 15-lb. weight is attached to the distal arm so that it is not touching the floor. The physician places their thumb on the patient's acromion and using fingers of the same hand places them over the humeral head. As the patient's muscles gradually relax, the provider gently pushes the humeral head caudally until it reduces. Choice (C) describes another type of technique different from Stimson's.

147. **D)** Panner's disease is usually seen in young boys aged 5 to 12 years. It is felt to be due to an interruption in the blood supply to the epiphysis resulting in initial resorption followed by eventual remodeling of the epiphysis. This condition most commonly occurs in the dominant arm and is found to be due to chronic repetitive trauma, hereditary factors, and certain endocrine disorders.

148. **B)** L2 nerve root compression would result in cremasteric reflex abnormalities. The cremaster muscle receives innervation via the genitofemoral nerve (L1 and L2). Patellar tendon and Achilles tendon reflexes would be present in L3/L4 and S1 nerve root compressions, respectively. Cross-adductor reflex is a withdrawal reflex on one side, with an inhibitory response on the contralateral side to maintain balance—for example, stepping on a nail would result in flexion of the affected limb and extension of the contralateral limb.

149. **D)** The spinal accessory nerve is most commonly injured in the posterior cervical triangle. This will result in isolated trapezius muscle weakness. The mechanism of injury may be stretch or external compression or after surgical procedure (ie, cervical lymph node biopsy). A lesion in this region will spare the sternocleidomastoid of the affected side. Mild scapular winging may also be observed with shoulder abduction (lateral winging).

150. **A)** Spurling's maneuver is a highly specific, but not a sensitive test for cervical radiculopathy. Lhermitte's sign is rapid passive cervical flexion while the patient is seated, which causes a shock sensation. Hoffman's sign signifies an upper motor neuron insult.

151. **D)** Patrick's test is a provocative maneuver to assess for sacroiliac joint dysfunction as well as hip joint pathology by **f**lexion, **ab**duction, **e**xternal **r**otation, and **e**xtension of the hip joint (hence it is also called the FABERE test). FAIR test (**f**lexion, **a**dduction, and **i**nternal **r**otation) is a provocative test for piriformis syndrome.

152. **A)** The axillary nerve is most commonly injured in an anterior shoulder dislocation. The axillary nerve innervates the deltoid and teres minor. Supraspinatus and infraspinatus are innervated by suprascapular nerve. The suprascapular nerve is rarely associated with glenohumeral dislocation, but can be injured from repetitive traction trauma. The rhomboids are innervated by the dorsal scapular nerve.

153. **C)** Heat exhaustion is due to failure of the cardiovascular system to respond to an increased workload secondary to heat. Heat **stroke** is considered a medical emergency (when the rectal core temperature is greater than 39°C). Heat stroke can cause organ damage. Heat stroke can occur because of endogenous heat production, and does not necessarily occur only in warm environments. The treatment is immediate cooling.

154. **B)** Hip pointers are seen in contact sports such as football and hockey, and are usually seen at the greater trochanter and iliac crest. There can be hematoma formation but there is usually focal tenderness. Patients should have full range of motion of the hip. X-rays should be considered if there is severe pain with passive range of motion.

155. **C)** The Rockwood classification system is used to describe AC joint injuries. Type I is mild injury with intact AC and CC ligaments. Type II is a complete tear of the AC ligament and intact CC ligament. Type III to VI each describe complete disruption of both AC and CC ligaments with varying degrees of dislocation of the clavicle. In type III injuries, the clavicle is displaced superiorly, whereas in type IV the clavicle is displaced superiorly and posteriorly into the trapezius. In type V injuries, the clavicle is displaced superiorly with more than 100% increase in the coracoclavicular interspace. In type VI, the clavicle is displaced inferiorly below the acromion or coracoid process.

156. **D)** The biceps brachii is not involved in shoulder adduction. In addition to the pectoralis major, teres major, and coracobrachialis, shoulder adduction involves the latissimus dorsi, infraspinatus, anterior and posterior deltoid, and the long head of the triceps.

157. **A)** Turf toe is associated with metatarsophalangeal joint pain that worsens with weight bearing. It can be exacerbated by turf fields which have stiff surfaces.

158. **D)** Ice is used more frequently in the acute stages of inflammation, particularly during the first 24 to 48 hours. It is a very effective anti-inflammatory modality. Benefits of ice include vasoconstriction, decreased swelling, and relief of pain and muscle spasm.

159. **C)** Morton's neuroma is a benign neuroma of an intermetatarsal plantar nerve, and most commonly affects the third intermetatarsal space (between the third and fourth metatarsal bones).

160. **A)** The supraspinatus is the primary muscle implicated in rotator cuff tears. The supraspinatus tendon has a poor blood supply and is susceptible to chronic subacromial impingement—a mechanism which is rarely seen in people younger than 40 years of age.

# *Electrodiagnostics*

## QUESTIONS

1. What is the clinical manifestation of conduction block?
   A) Weakness
   B) There is no clinical manifestation
   C) Rash
   D) Atrophy

2. In myopathies, the motor unit action potentials (MUAPs) may demonstrate all of the following **except**:
   A) Low amplitude
   B) Long duration
   C) Polyphasicity
   D) Early recruitment

3. As opposed to acquired neuropathies, congenital neuropathies usually:
   A) Have proximal more than distal slowing
   B) Have uniform slowing throughout the nerve
   C) Have segmental slowing throughout the nerve
   D) Are distal

4. In electrodiagnostic testing, a cold limb (less than 32°C in the arms or 30°C in the legs) could lead to:
   A) Decreased latency of compound motor action potentials (CMAPs)
   B) Increased amplitude of sensory nerve action potentials (SNAPs)
   C) Increased conduction velocity of SNAPs
   D) Decreased amplitude of CMAPs

5. On needle electromyographic (EMG) testing, normal muscles at rest:
   A) Are electrically silent
   B) Will spontaneously discharge potentials with an initial negative deflection
   C) Will spontaneously discharge potentials with an initial positive deflection
   D) Will discharge potentials only if the muscle belly is tapped

6. Miniature end-plate potentials are:
   A) A postsynaptic response
   B) A prerequisite for depolarization
   C) The result of single muscle fiber depolarizations
   D) The release of one quantum of acetylcholine from the presynaptic terminal

7. All of the following are possible reasons why a compound motor action potential (CMAP) would have an initial positive deflection **except**:
   A) Not over the muscle you are trying to stimulate
   B) Not stimulating the nerve that innervates that muscle

    C) With proximal stimulation of the median nerve in a Martin-Gruber anastomosis

    D) With distal stimulation of the median nerve in a Martin-Gruber anastomosis

8. While performing a motor nerve study, the reference electrode (G2) is placed:
   A) Distally over an electrically neutral area (tendon or bone)
   B) Proximally over an electrically neutral area (tendon or bone)
   C) Distally over an electrically active area (muscle)
   D) Proximally over an electrically active area (muscle)

9. All of the following muscles include innervation from the L4 nerve root **except**:
   A) Tibialis anterior
   B) Gluteus maximus
   C) Sartorius
   D) Adductor magnus

10. To diagnose a conduction block with electrodiagnostic testing, what percentage decrease in compound motor action potential amplitude should be noted from the proximal to the distal segment?
    A) 20%
    B) 50%
    C) 75%
    D) 10%

11. What muscle does the long thoracic nerve innervate?
    A) Supraspinatus
    B) Trapezius
    C) Infraspinatus
    D) Serratus anterior

12. Which of these statements regarding the H-reflex is **not** true?
    A) This reflex is elicited with submaximal stimulation
    B) As the intensity of the stimulation is subtly increased from the peak H-reflex amplitude, there is a gradual drop in H-reflex amplitude with a concomitant increase in M-wave amplitude
    C) The H-reflex is often used to assess for S1 radiculopathy (with pickup over the gastrocnemius-soleus group), but can also be used to assess for C6/C7 radiculopathy with pickup over the flexor carpi radialis
    D) Side-to-side differences in H-reflex latencies of greater than 1.0 msec are suggestive of S1 radiculopathies

13. In patients with myasthenia gravis, repetitive nerve stimulation will usually result in:
    A) At least a 20% increment in amplitude between the first and fifth stimulation
    B) No response
    C) At least a 10% decrement in amplitude between the first and fifth stimulation
    D) A decrease in the amplitude of the sensory response

14. Axonal damage (with Wallerian degeneration) would present with:
    A) Decreased compound motor action potential (CMAP) amplitude with proximal stimulation and distal stimulation
    B) Decreased CMAP amplitude with proximal stimulation but not distal stimulation
    C) Decreased CMAP amplitude distally but not proximally
    D) Slowing of conduction velocity across the lesion
    E) Slowing of conduction velocity distal to the lesion

**15.** In amyotrophic lateral sclerosis (ALS), the sensory nerve action potential (SNAP) will be:
  A) Normal
  B) Decreased amplitude distally and proximally
  C) Decreased amplitude distally
  D) Increased

**16.** To definitively state that a patient who presents for electrodiagnostic (EMG) testing has a radicu-lopathy, the following must all be present **except**:
  A) Denervation in two different muscles innervated by different peripheral nerves but the same nerve root
  B) Normal sensory nerve action potentials (SNAPs)
  C) An abnormal F-wave
  D) Denervation in the corresponding paraspinal muscles

**17.** If it can be avoided, why should short distances not be used when measuring conduction veloci-ties in electrodiagnostic testing?
  A) They are not reproducible
  B) They may not include the area of injury
  C) You cannot use the measuring tape
  D) The margin of error is larger

**18.** If a patient has tarsal tunnel syndrome, one would likely find which of the following on nerve conduction studies?
  A) Increased latency of the sural nerve at the ankle
  B) Increased latency of the tibial nerve at the ankle
  C) Decreased conduction velocity of the tibial nerve
  D) Decreased conduction velocity of the peroneal (fibular) nerve

**19.** On needle electromyographic (EMG) testing, myotonic discharges:
  A) May have an initial positive deflection
  B) Are stable and do not change
  C) Sound like marching soldiers
  D) Are not seen in chronic radiculopathies

**20.** When the electromyographic (EMG) needle is inserted into the muscle, there is not a crisp sound and the feel of the needle is "gritty." This may be a result of all of the following **except**:
  A) The needle has passed through the muscle and is touching periosteum
  B) The needle is in an adjacent muscle
  C) The needle is in fat
  D) The muscle is atrophied

**21.** Which is the worst nerve injury, according to the Seddon classification of nerve injuries?
  A) Neurapraxia
  B) Neurotmesis
  C) Axonotmesis
  D) Conduction block

**22.** All of the following muscles usually receive at least some innervation from the C7 nerve root **except**:
  A) Extensor carpi radialis
  B) Opponens pollicis

C) Pronator teres

D) Flexor carpi radialis

23. During nerve conduction testing, dispersion of the compound motor action potential (CMAP) is noted in which of the following:
    A) Axonal injury
    B) Focal nerve slowing
    C) Conduction block
    D) Segmental demyelination

24. What are the clinical symptoms of a patient with anterior interosseous nerve (AIN) syndrome?
    A) Impairment of all median nerve–innervated muscles
    B) A dull, achy sensation in the distal forearm along with weakness in grip strength and wrist flexion
    C) Numbness and paresthesias radiating to the first, second, third, and fourth lateral digits of the hand
    D) Abnormal "okay" sign, difficulty forming a fist, inability to approximate the thumb and index finger

25. Which one of the following muscles is **not** dually innervated?
    A) Flexor pollicis brevis
    B) Gracilis
    C) Biceps femoris
    D) Lumbricals of the hand

26. Myokymic discharges are usually seen in:
    A) Radiation plexopathy
    B) Acute carpal tunnel syndrome
    C) Myasthenia gravis
    D) Myotonic dystrophy

27. Conduction block in the forearm would present with:
    A) Decreased compound motor action potential (CMAP) amplitude with proximal stimulation and distal stimulation
    B) Decreased CMAP amplitude with proximal stimulation but not distal stimulation
    C) Decreased CMAP amplitude distally but not proximally
    D) Slowing of conduction velocity across the lesion

28. In a healthy adult, from what muscle can an H-reflex be obtained?
    A) Hamstring
    B) Flexor carpi radialis
    C) Biceps
    D) Extensor digitorum

29. A lumbar plexopathy affecting the posterior division will affect all of the following muscles **except**:
    A) Sartorius
    B) Rectus femoris
    C) Adductor longus
    D) Pectineus

30. The best way to localize whether a lesion is in the plexus or a radiculopathy is:
    A) Assess sensory nerve action potential (SNAP) amplitude
    B) Look for denervation in the extremity muscles
    C) Assess compound motor action potential (CMAP) amplitude
    D) F-waves

31. The anterior interosseous nerve innervates all of the following muscles **except**:
    A) Flexor digitorum profundus to digits 2 and 3
    B) Pronator quadratus
    C) Flexor digitorum superficialis to digits 1 and 2
    D) Flexor pollicis longus

32. When performing an electromyography (EMG), 60-cycle interference can be reduced by:
    A) Turning on the notch filter
    B) Moving the reference electrode closer to the active electrode during nerve conduction studies
    C) Moving the ground to the opposite limb
    D) Changing to a sensory setting (from a motor setting)

33. Hereditary neuropathies are usually:
    A) Segmental demyelinating
    B) Uniform demyelinating
    C) Axonal
    D) Mixed sensory and motor axonal and demyelinating

34. The connective tissue that surrounds bundles or fascicles of nerve fibers is called the:
    A) Epineurium
    B) Endoneurium
    C) Perineurium
    D) Paraneurium

35. All of the following muscles are innervated by the posterior cord of the brachial plexus **except**:
    A) Triceps
    B) Deltoid
    C) Biceps
    D) Brachioradialis

36. What is the best way to ensure that the biceps muscle is electrically silent during electrodiagnostic testing?
    A) Extend the elbow
    B) Supinate the forearm
    C) Extend the elbow and pronate the forearm
    D) Flex the elbow and supinate the forearm

37. What are the areas of median nerve entrapment?
    A) Ligament of Struthers (LOS), bicipital aponeurosis, cubital tunnel, anterior interosseous nerve, carpal tunnel
    B) Arcade of Struthers, bicipital aponeurosis, pronator teres syndrome, Guyon's canal, carpal tunnel
    C) LOS, cubital tunnel, carpal tunnel
    D) LOS, bicipital aponeurosis, pronator teres, anterior interosseous nerve, carpal tunnel

38. A patient who underwent a pelvic surgery is noted to have an impingement of the obturator nerve. Which muscle would you **least** suspect to show signs of denervation on electrodiagnostic testing?
    A) Gracilis
    B) Adductor longus
    C) Adductor brevis
    D) Adductor magnus

39. Electrodiagnostic findings in patients with critical illness myopathy (CIM) most commonly include:
    A) Low amplitude sensory nerve action potentials (SNAPs)
    B) Denervation potentials (fibrillations and positive sharp waves) in proximal muscles
    C) Low amplitude compound motor action potentials (CMAPs)
    D) Decreased motor conduction velocities

40. To determine whether an ulnar nerve lesion is at the wrist or the elbow, it is important to:
    A) Test conduction velocity across the elbow
    B) Needle test the first dorsal interosseous muscle
    C) Test the dorsal ulnar cutaneous nerve
    D) Test the ulnar motor response to the first dorsal interosseous muscle

41. Which muscles are innervated, at least partially, by the L5 nerve root?
    A) Peroneus longus, semimembranosus, vastus medialis
    B) Adductor longus, gluteus medius, extensor digitorum longus
    C) Tibialis anterior, adductor magnus, biceps femoris
    D) Tibialis anterior, gluteus maximus, peroneus longus

42. In an axonal injury, all of the following may be noted **except**:
    A) Denervation in all muscles innervated by that nerve
    B) Decreased compound motor action potential (CMAP) amplitude with distal stimulation
    C) Decreased CMAP amplitude with proximal stimulation
    D) Decreased sensory nerve action potential (SNAP) amplitude

43. During electrodiagnostic testing, motor unit analysis should be done:
    A) With the muscle at rest
    B) With a surface electrode
    C) With minimal contraction
    D) With maximum contraction

44. Your patient has a distal median sensory conduction velocity of 65 m/sec and a proximal (across the carpal tunnel) median sensory conduction velocity of 50 m/sec. This indicates:
    A) Carpal tunnel syndrome
    B) Normal findings
    C) Peripheral neuropathy
    D) Sensory carpal tunnel syndrome

45. What is the difference in findings on electromyography (EMG)/nerve conduction studies (NCS) between someone with a conduction block and someone with an axonotmetic lesion distal to the point of stimulation?
    A) The axonotmetic lesion will have decreased compound motor action potential (CMAP) amplitude, whereas the conduction block will not
    B) They will have the same findings

C) Both will have decreased CMAP amplitudes, but only the axonotmetic lesion will have evidence of denervation on needle study

D) Both will have normal CMAP amplitudes, but only the sensory nerve action potential (SNAP) will be affected with an axonotmetic lesion

46. The waveform below is most likely:
    A) An end-plate potential
    B) A fibrillation (fib) potential
    C) A positive sharp wave
    D) A motor unit

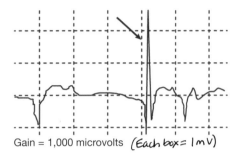

Gain = 1,000 microvolts  (Each box = 1 mV)

47. Needle electrodiagnostic studies evaluate what types of fiber?
    A) Only Ib (large, myelinated)
    B) Only Ia (large, myelinated)
    C) All A-alpha
    D) Ia and Ib, myelinated

48. To minimize electrical noise in the electrodiagnostics (EMG) lab, you should do all of the following **except**:
    A) Place the ground between the recording and the reference electrode
    B) Make sure that the skin is cleaned appropriately (usually with alcohol)
    C) Unplug equipment that is not being used
    D) Turn off fluorescent lights

49. In needle electromyographic (EMG) testing, insertional activity:
    A) Is the result of discrete quanta of ACh
    B) Is considered abnormal
    C) Is the electrical activity generated as a result of disruption of the muscle membrane by a needle
    D) Is performed with muscle activation

50. Axonotmesis refers to:
    A) An injury of the axon of a nerve but not the supporting connective tissue and results in Wallerian degeneration
    B) Complete injury of a nerve involving the myelin, axon, and all supporting structures
    C) A lesion where conduction block is present but the axon remains intact
    D) A nerve injury that results in degeneration of the axon starting distally and ascending proximally

51. A patient presents to your office with complaints of right arm weakness. On examination, you appreciate a positive Spurling's test and notice mild weakness of the wrist extensors. With deep tendon reflex (DTR) testing, you notice a diminished brachioradialis reflex, but normal biceps and triceps DTR. At what root level do you suspect a radiculopathy?
    A) C5
    B) C6
    C) C7
    D) C8

52. The combined sensory index (CSI) is used to assess:
    A) Sensory axonal neuropathy
    B) Sensory demyelinating neuropathy
    C) Ulnar neuropathy at the elbow
    D) Carpal tunnel syndrome (CTS)

53. What is the most proximal muscle innervated by the common peroneal nerve?
    A) Anterior tibialis
    B) Short head of biceps femoris
    C) Hamstring
    D) Peroneus longus

54. Why should the elbow be bent to about 90° when performing and measuring ulnar nerve stimulation across the elbow?
    A) The ulnar nerve is not slack in that position and its length is more accurately estimated, so the conduction velocity will not be falsely slowed
    B) The ulnar nerve is not taught in that position, so the conduction velocity will not be falsely slowed
    C) The ulnar nerve is not slack in that position, so the conduction velocity will not be falsely increased
    D) The ulnar nerve is not taught in that position, so the conduction velocity will not be falsely increased

55. When calculating a "normal" H-reflex, all of the following should be taken into consideration **except**:
    A) Age
    B) Height
    C) Temperature
    D) Latency on the opposite side

56. What type of neuropathy is usually seen on electrodiagnostic testing in paraneoplastic syndrome?
    A) Axonal sensory neuropathy
    B) Demyelinating sensory motor neuropathy
    C) Axonal and demyelinating sensory motor neuropathy
    D) Axonal sensory motor neuropathy

57. When performing a needle electromyographic (EMG) study, rise time of a motor unit action potential (MUAP) refers to:
    A) Time for a motor unit to fire
    B) Time from baseline to initial negative peak
    C) Time lag from the peak of the initial negative deflection to the subsequent positive (downward) peak
    D) Time from the baseline takeoff to when the waveform returns to baseline

58. Somatosensory evoked potentials (SSEPs) may have utility in the diagnosis of:
    A) Radiculopathy
    B) Meralgia paresthetica
    C) Anterior interosseous nerve injury
    D) Sacral plexopathy

59. What will happen if a compound motor action potential (CMAP) waveform is viewed at a gain of 100 mV?
   A) It would appear truncated
   B) It would appear as a small blip on the baseline
   C) It would appear normal
   D) It would appear half its size

60. What would be considered orthodromic conduction for a sensory nerve?
   A) Stimulating the wrist with a pickup over the finger
   B) Stimulating the wrist with a pickup over the muscle
   C) Stimulating the distal aspect of a finger and picking up more proximally over the wrist
   D) Stimulating the distal aspect of a finger and picking up more proximally over the muscle

61. The accessory peroneal nerve:
   A) Is noted when the amplitude at the fibular head is larger than at the ankle
   B) Innervates the extensor digitorum hallucis muscle
   C) Is a branch of the deep peroneal nerve
   D) All of the above

62. You are performing an electromyography (EMG) on a patient and notice that the sensory and motor amplitudes are low throughout, latencies are prolonged throughout, and conduction velocities are slow throughout. The most likely conclusion is:
   A) Alcoholic neuropathy
   B) Paraneoplastic syndrome
   C) Diabetic neuropathy
   D) Guillain-Barré syndrome

63. On needle electromyographic (EMG) testing, myotonic discharges are characterized by:
   A) Involuntary group repetitive discharge of the same motor unit action potential with a high-frequency pattern within the burst and a slow-frequency between the burst
   B) Spontaneous discharge of a single motor unit potential at very high frequencies, with a notable decrementing response
   C) Action potentials of muscle fibers firing in a prolonged fashion that wax and wane in both amplitude and frequency
   D) Spontaneous action potentials of single muscle fibers that are firing autonomously in a regular fashion

64. Which muscle is innervated solely by the C5 root?
   A) Serratus anterior
   B) Rhomboids
   C) Supraspinatus
   D) Biceps brachii

65. What type of neuropathy is critical illness neuropathy?
   A) Sensorimotor demyelinating
   B) Sensorimotor axonal
   C) Motor axonal
   D) Sensory demyelinating

66. Which of the following has the poorest prognosis of nerve recovery?
    A) Axonotmesis
    B) Conduction block
    C) Demyelination
    D) Neurapraxia
    E) Neurotmesis

67. What is the difference between an unmyelinated nerve and a demyelinated nerve?
    A) The location of the sodium channels
    B) The resting transmembrane potential
    C) The way the sodium-potassium pump operates
    D) The ions that are required

68. In a brachial plexopathy, the sensory nerve action potentials (SNAPs):
    A) Would be affected as the lesion is distal to the dorsal root ganglion
    B) Would not be affected as the lesion is distal to the dorsal root ganglion
    C) Would be affected as the lesion is proximal to the dorsal root ganglion
    D) Would not be affected as the lesion is proximal to the dorsal root ganglion

69. What type of neuropathy is usually seen on electrodiagnostic testing in diabetic neuropathy?
    A) Axonal sensory neuropathy
    B) Demyelinating sensory motor neuropathy
    C) Axonal and demyelinating sensory motor neuropathy
    D) Axonal sensory motor neuropathy

70. In electrodiagnostic testing, the ideal minimal distance between the active and the reference electrode in a sensory nerve study is:
    A) 1 cm
    B) 4 cm
    C) 1 in.
    D) 2 cm

71. In a sensory nerve (as opposed to a motor nerve), the conduction velocity can be calculated from the distance from the stimulator to the active electrode because:
    A) The sensory nerve pickup is more distal than a motor nerve pickup
    B) The sensory nerve has no myoneural junction
    C) Sensory nerves are more superficial
    D) This is not true; a conduction velocity can be calculated in a motor nerve by knowing the distance from the stimulator to the active electrode

72. What gain would you typically use for a sensory nerve conduction study?
    A) 10 mcV
    B) 100 mcV
    C) 1 mV
    D) 10 mV

73. A good way to differentiate between an upper trunk and a lateral cord brachial plexopathy is the finding of decreased amplitude in the:
    A) Musculocutaneous nerve compound motor action potential (CMAP) to the biceps muscle
    B) Axillary nerve CMAP to the deltoid muscle
    C) Lateral antebrachial nerve sensory nerve action potential (SNAP)
    D) Median nerve SNAP

74. The Riche-Cannieu anastomosis:
    A) Is a communication between the deep branch of the ulnar nerve and the recurrent branch of the median nerve in the hand
    B) Can result in an all ulnar hand
    C) May have denervation in the abductor pollicis brevis (APB) with an ulnar nerve lesion at the elbow
    D) All of the above

75. You are performing an electromyography (EMG)/nerve conduction study (NCS) of the upper extremities to evaluate for carpal tunnel syndrome and notice that the sensory and motor, median, and ulnar latencies are delayed. One possible mistake that you may have made that could have resulted in this finding would be:
    A) Your anode and cathode were reversed on the stimulator
    B) You did not use maximal stimulation
    C) You did not stimulate over the nerve
    D) There was too much electrical interference

76. One of the common findings in ulnar neuropathy is the Froment's sign, which is demonstrated by:
    A) Difficulty in abducting the fourth and fifth digits
    B) Pain and numbness in dorsal aspect of the hand
    C) Weakness of the flexor digitorum profundus muscle to the fourth and fifth digits
    D) Substitution of the flexor pollicis longus muscle for a weakened adductor pollicis

77. How does limb temperature cooling affect electrodiagnostic findings?
    A) No change in conduction velocity, decreased amplitude
    B) No change in conduction velocity, no change in amplitude
    C) Decreased conduction velocity, increased amplitude
    D) Increased conduction velocity, decreased amplitude

78. A typical amplitude of a compound muscle action potential (CMAP) is:
    A) 10 msec
    B) 10 mcV
    C) 10 mV
    D) 10 mcsec

79. Which of the following does the nerve conduction component of the neurodiagnostic study fail to assess or give information about?
    A) Autonomic nerve
    B) Integrity of myelin
    C) Motor nerve
    D) Sensory nerve
    E) Speed of transmission

80. When is it most appropriate to perform F-waves?
    A) For the evaluation of radiculopathy
    B) For the evaluation of peroneal neuropathy at the fibular head
    C) For the evaluation of possible acute inflammatory demyelinating polyneuropathy (AIDP)
    D) For the evaluation of peripheral neuropathy

81. When determining the location and extent of a peroneal nerve lesion, an important nerve to include in the electrodiagnostic test is:
    A) The lateral femoral cutaneous nerve
    B) The superficial peroneal nerve
    C) The lateral peroneal nerve
    D) The medial peroneal nerve

82. What type of neuropathy is usually seen on electrodiagnostic testing in alcoholic neuropathy?
    A) Axonal sensory neuropathy
    B) Demyelinating sensory motor neuropathy
    C) Axonal and demyelinating sensory motor neuropathy
    D) Axonal sensory motor neuropathy

83. All of the following can affect H-reflex latency on electrodiagnostic testing **except**:
    A) Demyelinating sensory neuropathy
    B) Demyelinating motor neuropathy
    C) Height
    D) Weight

84. Certain medical conditions predispose a patient to an entrapment neuropathy, such as carpal tunnel syndrome. These include all of the following **except**:
    A) Diabetes
    B) Pregnancy
    C) Thyroid disorders
    D) Psoriasis

85. During electrodiagnostic (EMG) testing, if the patient requests termination of the test:
    A) The test should be continued
    B) The test should be stopped
    C) The test should be paused, and then continued when the patient is more relaxed
    D) The patient should be given a sedative to calm him or her down

86. A patient presents with weakness in the right hand. Electromyography (EMG)/nerve conduction study (NCS) findings are as follows:
    - Right median motor latency = 4.3 msec
    - Right ulnar motor latency = 2.2 msec
    - Left median motor latency = 3.2 msec
    - Right median sensory conduction velocity across the wrist = 36 m/sec
    - Right median sensory conduction velocity distally = 44 m/sec
    - Needle EMG of the right abductor pollicis brevis (APB) muscle = +3 fibrillation potentials

    What would be an appropriate next step?
    A) No more testing is indicated
    B) Test the left ulnar motor nerve
    C) Needle evaluation of the right pronator teres muscle
    D) Test the right ulnar sensory nerve

87. What would be seen on a needle study in a patient with steroid myopathy?
    A) Normal motor units
    B) Small amplitude, short duration polyphasic motor units
    C) Large amplitude, long duration motor units
    D) Small amplitude, long duration polyphasic potentials

88. You are performing an electromyography (EMG)/nerve conduction study (NCS) of the upper extremities to evaluate for carpal tunnel syndrome and notice that the sensory and motor, median and ulnar latencies are delayed. Your next steps should be:
    A) Test radial sensory nerve
    B) Needle testing of bilateral abductor pollicis brevis (APB) muscles
    C) Test tibial motor nerve
    D) Test the peroneal and sural nerves

89. In a patient with an accessory peroneal nerve, stimulation proximally at the fibular head with pickup over the extensor digitorum brevis (EDB) muscle will lead to:
    A) Larger compound motor action potential (CMAP) amplitude than distally at the ankle
    B) Increased CMAP conduction velocity proximally
    C) Positive deflection of the CMAP
    D) No changes from that of an individual without an accessory peroneal nerve

90. Electrodiagnostic findings in a classic radiculopathy will include which of the following?
    A) Decreased sensory nerve action potential (SNAP) and compound motor action potential (CMAP) amplitudes, with spontaneous potentials seen in the paraspinal muscles
    B) Normal SNAP and CMAP amplitudes, with spontaneous potentials from two muscles innervated by the same peripheral nerve
    C) Normal SNAP and CMAP amplitudes, with spontaneous potentials in the paraspinal muscles and two muscles from different peripheral nerves innervated by the same affected root
    D) Decreased SNAP and CMAP amplitudes, with spontaneous potentials seen in paraspinal muscles and two muscles from different peripheral nerves innervated by the same affected root

91. What findings would you expect to see on electrodiagnostic testing in a patient with spinal stenosis?
    A) Increased sensory nerve action potential (SNAP) and compound motor action potential (CMAP) amplitudes with normal conduction velocities
    B) Decreased SNAP and CMAP amplitudes with decreased conduction velocities
    C) Normal SNAP and CMAP findings with normal needle electromyography (EMG) findings
    D) Normal SNAP and CMAP findings with possible abnormal spontaneous potentials at multiple levels

92. The most common error in the realm of neurodiagnostic testing is typically related to which of the following?
    A) Computer analysis failure
    B) Excessive ambient temperature/room temperature
    C) Lack of repeat calibration of the testing probe with each measurement
    D) Operator error
    E) Patient's inability to fully relax

93. What is the only muscle that is innervated exclusively by the C5 nerve root?
    A) Supraspinatus
    B) Levator scapulae
    C) Trapezius
    D) Rhomboid (major and minor)

94. The X-axis on the oscilloscope (screen) represents:
    A) Time in microseconds
    B) Time in milliseconds
    C) Distance in centimeters
    D) Distance in millimeters

95. What muscles would be affected in a C6 radiculopathy?
    A) Extensor carpi radialis
    B) Flexor digitorum superficialis
    C) Extensor indicis
    D) Rhomboid major

96. In the newborn, nerve conduction velocities are approximately what percentage of adult values?
    A) 50%
    B) 25%
    C) 100%
    D) 75%

97. On needle electromyographic (EMG) testing, muscles that would be affected in a lesion to the posterior cord include all of the following **except**:
    A) Extensor indicis proprius
    B) Deltoid
    C) Pronator teres
    D) Triceps

98. During the needle portion of the examination, when assessing motor unit action potential (MUAP) recruitment:
    A) Full recruitment should be attempted
    B) Minimal recruitment should be used
    C) The muscle should be relaxed
    D) Any of the above can be used

99. Which of the following can result in a prolongation of the H-reflex?
    A) S1 radiculopathy
    B) Sacral plexopathy
    C) Polyneuropathy
    D) All of the above

100. In what condition might you see a potential such as this one?

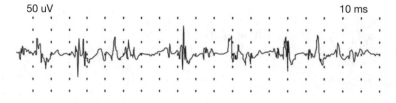

50 uV                                                    10 ms

    A) Normal muscle
    B) Myopathy
    C) Neuropathy
    D) Disorder of the neuromuscular junction

101. The only muscle that is innervated by the common peroneal (fibular) nerve is:
    A) Tibialis anterior
    B) Short head of the biceps femoris
    C) Peroneus longus
    D) Long head of the biceps femoris

102. The sartorius muscle is innervated by which nerve?
    A) Superior gluteal nerve
    B) Inferior gluteal nerve
    C) Sciatic nerve
    D) Femoral nerve

103. The common peroneal nerve splits at the fibular head into the superficial and deep peroneal nerve. Which muscle is innervated by the superficial peroneal nerve?
    A) Tibialis anterior
    B) Extensor digitorum brevis
    C) Extensor hallucis longus
    D) Peroneus brevis

104. During repetitive nerve stimulation in a patient with myasthenia gravis, what should be seen?
    A) Incremental increase in amplitude of the compound motor action potential (CMAP) from the first to the fifth stimulation
    B) Greater than 10% decrease in amplitude of the CMAPs from the first to the fifth stimulation
    C) Greater than 10% decrease in latency of the CMAPs from the first to the fifth stimulation
    D) None of the above

105. The amplitude of the compound motor action potential (CMAP) you have obtained is very small, and you are unable to assess where the takeoff is. In order to see the takeoff more clearly, you should:
    A) Increase the sweep speed
    B) Decrease the sweep speed
    C) Increase the gain
    D) Decrease the gain

106. During electrodiagnostic testing, how can you tell if an accessory peroneal nerve is present?
    A) There is decreased compound motor action potential (CMAP) amplitude when the peroneal nerve is stimulated at the ankle, and normal CMAP amplitude with stimulation at the fibular head
    B) There is decreased CMAP amplitude when the peroneal nerve is stimulated at the fibular head, and normal CMAP amplitude with stimulation at the ankle
    C) There is unusually slowed conduction velocity in the peroneal nerve
    D) There is unusually fast conduction velocity in the peroneal nerve

107. The normal gain for a sensory nerve study is:
    A) 100 mcV/division
    B) 1,000 mcV (1 mV)/division
    C) 10 mV/division
    D) 20 mcV/division

**108.** In electrodiagnostic testing, increased firing frequency refers to:
   A) A firing rate of more than 10 Hz before the next motor unit is recruited
   B) Increased recruitment
   C) A myopathic process
   D) Fibrillations and positive sharp waves (PSWs)

**109.** When performing needle electromyography (EMG) with a monopolar needle, the best location for the reference electrode is:
   A) Over nonmuscle distal to the needle
   B) Over nonmuscle but close to the needle
   C) Over a muscle innervated by the same nerve as the muscle you are testing
   D) Over the same muscle and close to the needle

**110.** When noted during electrodiagnostic testing, all of the following indicate a chronic (more than 6 months) process **except**:
   A) Polyphasicity
   B) Complex repetitive discharges
   C) Fibrillations and positive sharp waves
   D) Large amplitude motor units

**111.** When performing the needle portion of an electrodiagnostic test examination, it is important for the muscle to be at rest. This is best accomplished by:
   A) Putting a pillow under the muscle
   B) Activating the antagonist muscle
   C) Having the patient use imagery
   D) Activating the agonist muscle

**112.** A patient presents for electrodiagnostic testing for left-sided low-back pain. The study is normal **except** for a prolonged left H-reflex. What is your diagnosis?
   A) Left S1 radiculopathy
   B) Polyneuropathy
   C) Lumbar plexopathy
   D) None of the above

**113.** The motor unit action potential below was taken using a monopolar needle in the quadriceps muscle.

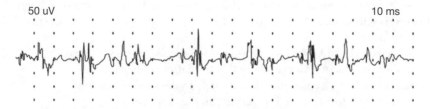

50 uV                                                                                          10 ms

   What can you determine about the amplitude of the motor unit?
   A) Normal
   B) Decreased amplitude
   C) Increased amplitude
   D) Mixed increased and decreased amplitude

114. The sural nerve is made up of sensory fibers from:
    A) Femoral nerve
    B) Peroneal nerve
    C) Tibial nerve
    D) Tibial and peroneal nerves

115. Which of the following muscles has dual innervation?
    A) Pronator quadratus
    B) Flexor carpi ulnaris (FCU)
    C) Flexor digitorum profundus (FDP)
    D) Rhomboids

116. In alcohol-induced polyneuropathy, what kind of findings would you expect to see on nerve conduction studies (NCS)?
    A) Increased compound motor action potential (CMAP) amplitude, increased sensory nerve action potential (SNAP) amplitude, decreased conduction velocity
    B) Increased CMAP amplitude, decreased SNAP amplitude, decreased conduction velocity
    C) Decreased CMAP amplitude, decreased SNAP amplitude, decreased conduction velocity
    D) Decreased CMAP amplitude, decreased SNAP amplitude, normal conduction velocity

117. All the following are true regarding F-wave studies **except**:
    A) F-waves are obtained using supramaximal stimulation, initiating an antidromic motor response to the anterior horn cells in the spinal cord
    B) The F-wave is a pure motor response that does not represent a true reflex
    C) The latency of the F-wave is constant
    D) In some chronically injured nerves, an A-wave may be seen

118. Assuming correct timing of performing the complete neurodiagnostic study, which of the following conditions would most likely result in a normal electromyographic (EMG)/nerve conduction studies (NCS) test?
    A) Bell's palsy
    B) Brachial plexopathy (eg, medial cord)
    C) Botulism
    D) Myofascial pain
    E) Ulnar nerve impingement at elbow

119. Which of the following is **not** an indication that a Martin-Gruber anastomosis is present?
    A) An initial positive deflection of the median compound motor action potential (CMAP) when stimulating the median nerve at the antecubital fossa
    B) Slowed median nerve conduction velocity in the forearm
    C) Decreased amplitude of the median CMAP with distal stimulation as compared with proximal stimulation
    D) An excessively fast median nerve forearm conduction velocity when carpal tunnel is present

120. Complex repetitive discharges (CRDs) are most likely seen in:
    A) Radiculopathy of 4 weeks duration
    B) Carpal tunnel syndrome of 1 year duration
    C) Lumbar radiculopathy of 1 week duration
    D) Sensory axonal peripheral neuropathy of 2 years duration

121. Electrodiagnostic findings common in myopathies include:
     A) Low amplitude sensory nerve action potentials (SNAP)
     B) Long duration motor units
     C) Abnormal spontaneous potentials (denervation) on needle electromyography (EMG)
     D) Increased firing frequency of motor units

122. Monopolar needles generally have higher amplitude motor unit action potentials (MUAPs) than concentric needles because:
     A) Monopolar needles are longer than concentric needles
     B) The needle samples from 360° rather than 180°
     C) The tip of a concentric needle is smaller
     D) Concentric needles have the ground electrode as part of the needle

123. On needle electromyography (EMG), normal motor units have a duration of:
     A) 20 to 30 msec
     B) 5 to 15 mcsec
     C) 20 to 30 mcsec
     D) 5 to 15 msec

124. A motor point is:
     A) The thickest part of the muscle
     B) The tip of the needle
     C) The point where the nerve enters the muscle
     D) Not seen in all muscles

125. In nerve conduction studies, temporal dispersion is a result of:
     A) A large variance in conduction velocities in the fibers that make up the compound motor action potential (CMAP)
     B) Slowed conduction velocity in all fibers
     C) Axonal loss
     D) Different velocities in different segments of the nerve

126. While performing a needle electromyography (EMG) study, the reference electrode (G2) is placed:
     A) Distally over an electrically neutral area (tendon or bone)
     B) Proximally over an electrically neutral area (tendon or bone)
     C) Distally over a muscle
     D) Over the same muscle that the needle is in

127. The sensory continuation of the femoral nerve is the:
     A) Lateral femoral cutaneous nerve
     B) Obturator nerve
     C) Sural nerve
     D) Saphenous nerve

128. Which muscle is innervated by the sciatic nerve?
     A) Tensor fascia lata
     B) Iliopsoas
     C) Gracilis
     D) Adductor magnus

**129.** The classic finding on electrodiagnostic testing in a patient with diabetic neuropathy indicates what type of polyneuropathy?
A) Axonal motor polyneuropathy
B) Uniform-demyelinating mixed sensorimotor polyneuropathy
C) Segmental-demyelinating motor polyneuropathy
D) Mixed axonal demyelinating sensorimotor polyneuropathy

**130.** Limitations of the H-reflex include all the following **except**:
A) Abnormal H-reflex is not truly indicative of radiculopathy, as the lesion may involve other parts of the long pathway (such as the plexus or spinal cord)
B) H-reflex is often absent in otherwise normal individuals older than 60 years
C) Patients with an S1 radiculopathy can have a normal H-reflex
D) All of the above are limitations

# *Electrodiagnostics*

## ANSWERS

1. **A)** Conduction block is an area of focal demyelination that is so severe that the action potential cannot propagate. This leads to a decreased number of motor units available to contribute to the strength of a contraction. The prognosis is excellent once the offending mechanism (usually pressure on the nerve) has been removed. (For sensory fibers, the clinical manifestation would be sensory loss.)

2. **B)** In myopathies, motor units usually have low amplitude (less than 1 mV when using a monopolar needle), short duration, polyphasicity, and early recruitment.

3. **B)** Congenital (hereditary) neuropathies usually have slowing throughout the entire course of the nerve. Acquired neuropathies are usually more distal or segmental. Temporal dispersion is a feature of an acquired neuropathy.

4. **B)** It is better to warm a limb than use correction formulas. A limb that is cold may demonstrate increased latency, decreased conduction velocity, and increased amplitude of SNAPs and CMAPs. With cooling, the latency is prolonged about 0.2 msec/°C, amplitude increases (sensory more than motor), conduction velocity decreases 1.8 to 2.4 m/s/°C, and duration increases. This is presumed to be due to sodium channels taking longer to open, but staying open longer, with cooling.

5. **A)** Normal muscles at rest are electrically silent. Sticking a needle in a muscle will damage it, and a potential with an initial positive deflection may be noted. However, this potential does not persist. A muscle that has been damaged or denervated will spontaneously discharge potentials that have an initial positive (downward) deflection and persist when the needle is not moving. Fibers with an initial negative (upward) potential most likely indicate incomplete relaxation. Tapping over the muscle belly is not recommended as it serves no purpose, except perhaps to occasionally confuse the electromyographer when a waveform is seen as the needle is moved in the muscle.

6. **D)** Miniature end-plate potentials are produced spontaneously by the release of one quantum of acetylcholine from the presynaptic terminal. End-plate spikes are believed to be the result of single muscle fiber depolarizations. With needle electromyographic (EMG) testing, there is usually increased pain when the needle is in the end-plate region.

7. **D)** If the muscle that you are recording from is not innervated by the nerve you are stimulating, the recording electrode will pick up the electrical activity from a distant muscle that is being stimulated. However, this will result in an initial positive deflection. With a Martin-Gruber anastomosis, proximal stimulation of the median nerve will stimulate both the median nerve destined for the abductor pollicis brevis (APB) muscle and the ulnar nerve that is traveling with the median nerve (until the forearm where it crosses over). These ulnar nerve fibers innervate the nearby adductor pollicis muscle. Because the ulnar nerve does not have to traverse the carpal tunnel, the adductor pollicis muscle is stimulated before the APB muscle via the median nerve. Therefore, the recording electrode first picks up the distant action potential from the adductor pollicis, and a positive deflection is seen. This is especially evident when there is carpal tunnel syndrome and the median nerve is especially slow.

8. **A)** The reference (G2) electrode is always placed distally over an electrically neutral area (ie, tendon or bone). The electromyography (EMG) machine will "subtract" the electrical signal of the reference from the active electrode signal. Therefore, whenever possible, it is important that for motor studies, the reference be placed over an electrically neutral area.

9. **B)** The tibialis anterior is innervated by the peroneal (fibular) nerve (L4, L5, and some S1). The sartorius is innervated by the femoral nerve (L2, L3, L4). The adductor magnus is innervated by the obturator nerve (L2, L3, L4). However, the gluteus maximus is innervated by the inferior gluteal nerve (L5, S1, S2).

10. **A)** A more than 20% decrease in amplitude of the proximal segment (compared with the distal segment) usually indicates a conduction block. One must be careful to compare the affected with the nonaffected side. Sometimes if there is obesity or fluid accumulation proximally, the amplitude may be decreased because the stimulation is not close enough to the nerve. A 50% decrease in amplitude side to side usually indicates an axonal lesion.

11. **D)** The supraspinatus and infraspinatus are innervated by the suprascapular nerve, which originates from C5 and C6 roots. The trapezius is innervated by the spinal accessory nerve. Injury to this nerve can cause lateral winging of the scapula. The serratus anterior is innervated by the long thoracic nerve (C5, C6, and C7 roots), and injury to it can cause medial winging of the scapula. Remember SALT (serratus anterior long thoracic).

12. **D)** All the statements about the H-reflex are true except for choice (D). The H-reflex is a monosynaptic spinal reflex involving both motor and sensory fibers. As it is a reflex and involves the Ia fibers, very little intensity is required (hence the submaximal stimulation, unlike the F-wave test). Increasing the intensity past the H-reflex peak amplitude will result in a drop in H-reflex amplitude and an increase in M-wave amplitude. The H-reflex tests for the same fibers involved in the ankle reflex (S1) and can help in differentiating an L5 from an S1 radiculopathy. An H-reflex side-to-side difference of more than 1.5 msec is considered significant.

13. **C)** Myasthenia gravis is a disorder of the neuromuscular junction. Antibodies to the acetylcholine receptor affect the postsynaptic membrane. Repetitive nerve stimulation usually results in at least a 10% decrement in the amplitude between the first and fifth stimulation. Proximal muscles are affected more than distal muscles, so proximal muscles should be included in the testing. Sensory responses should be normal, as this disorder affects the neuromuscular junction. Testing should be performed with the muscle warm, and the patient should be off medication for myasthenia gravis. The test should be repeated after exercise of the muscle, and after 1-minute intervals to assess for postexercise exhaustion. Patients with myasthenia gravis have a 15% association with thymomas.

14. **A)** Wallerian degeneration occurs distal to the level of an axonal injury. As with CMAP stimulation the pickup is always over a distal muscle, and both proximal and distal stimulation would result in decreased CMAP amplitude.

15. **A)** ALS is a disorder of the motor nerves. As such, the motor fibers, but not the sensory fibers, would be affected. Therefore, the SNAPs should be normal, whereas the compound motor action potentials might show decreased amplitudes.

16. **C)** To definitively state that the patient has a radiculopathy, the findings must include denervation in the paraspinal muscles as well as denervation in two different muscles innervated by different peripheral nerves but the same nerve root. Because the lesion is preganglionic, the SNAPs should be normal. Abnormal F-waves are nonspecific and not helpful in the evaluation of a radiculopathy.

17. **D)** A 1-cm error in measurement over a 10-cm segment will lead to a 10% margin of error. If a 5-cm segment is used, the margin of error becomes 20%.

18. **B)** Tarsal tunnel syndrome is an entrapment neuropathy of the tibial nerve below the flexor retinaculum behind the medial malleolus. The most sensitive test is the mixed medial and lateral plantar nerves.

19. **A)** Myotonic discharges wax and wane in frequency and amplitude. They may have an initial positive deflection and look like a positive sharp wave (PSW), or they may appear as biphasic or triphasic potentials. They fire at variable rates (20–100 Hz) and sound like a "dive bomber." Myokymic discharges sound like marching soldiers. Myotonic discharges may be found in myotonic dystrophy, myotonia congenita, paramyotonia, hyperkalemic periodic paralysis, polymyositis, acid maltase deficiency, and chronic radiculopathies and neuropathies.

20. **B)** If the needle is in fat, atrophied tissue, periosteum, or subcutaneous tissue, the sound on the amplifier will not be crisp. If the needle is an adjacent muscle, the sound will be crisp with needle insertion (you are in a muscle). However, the rise time will be decreased when the muscle is activated, as you are not recording from the muscle that is being activated.

21. **B)** Neurotmesis is complete transection of the nerve and involves the axon, the myelin, and all supporting tissue (connective tissue including the epineurium). There is complete disruption of any pathway, and nerve action potentials cannot propagate. There is little chance for regeneration (collateral sprouting or axonal regrowth) because of the loss of a pathway of connective tissue for the axon to follow. Neurapraxia is the same thing as conduction block. This is a focal area of severe demyelination. The demyelination is so severe that the action potential cannot propagate. As remyelination takes place, the myelin is immature. Therefore, with remyelination, there will be slowing of the segment where the conduction block occurred. Axonotmesis is damage to the axon itself. However, the connective tissues and Schwann cells are intact, so recovery can take place.

22. **B)** The extensor carpi radialis is innervated by the radial nerve (C6/C7). The pronator teres is innervated by the median nerve (C6/C7). The flexor carpi radialis is innervated by the median nerve (C6/C7). However, the opponens pollicis is innervated by the median nerve (C8/T1).

23. **D)** Dispersion is noted when the various components of the action potential travel at different speeds. Uneven degrees of demyelination and remyelination in the different nerve fibers make the entire CMAP waveform of lower amplitude and longer duration. This is frequently seen in segmental demyelination. The area under the entire waveform is not decreased. The sum of all of the nerve fibers contributes to the shape of the CMAP. If some of the fibers are traveling at 30 m/sec, some at 40 m/sec, and some at 50 m/sec, the duration of the waveform will be prolonged (and the amplitude decreased). This can be confused with an axonal injury if the clinician only assesses amplitude, and not duration. In axonal injury, the amplitude is decreased, but the duration of the waveform is normal. Focal nerve slowing will present with a normal CMAP amplitude, but with conduction velocity slowing across the involved area. With conduction block, the CMAP amplitude distal to the lesion will be normal, but the CMAP amplitude will be decreased with stimulation across the lesion.

24. **D)** The AIN is a motor nerve branch of the median nerve. An injury to this nerve results in a pure motor syndrome with no sensory deficits. The muscles innervated by the AIN are the flexor pollicis longus (FPL), pronator quadratus, and the flexor digitorum profundus (FDP) to digits 2 and 3. The FPL is usually the first muscle to be affected. As a result of the muscle impairments, patients are unable to approximate the thumb and index finger or give an "OK" sign.

25. **B)** All the muscles listed are dually innervated except for the gracilis. The flexor pollicis brevis is innervated by the median and ulnar nerves. The lumbricals are supplied by the median and ulnar nerves. The long head of the biceps femoris is innervated by the sciatic tibial division, whereas the short head of the biceps femoris is innervated by the common peroneal nerve. Only the gracilis is innervated by one nerve—the obturator nerve.

26. **A)** Myokymic discharges are spontaneous motor unit action potentials that fire repetitively and have the sound of "marching soldiers." They have a regular rate and rhythm. These single or paired discharges fire at a rate of 5 to 10 Hz. They may be seen in chronic nerve lesions, radiation plexopathy, facial muscles in Bell's palsy, multiple sclerosis, and chronic polyradiculopathy.

27. **B)** Conduction block is an area of **focal** demyelination that is so severe that the action potential cannot propagate. If the conduction block were located in the forearm, stimulation distal to the conduction block would be normal. When stimulation occurred **across** the area of conduction block, some of the action potentials could not propagate. This would lead to a drop in CMAP amplitude (with proximal stimulation). Choice (D) is incorrect because slowing of conduction velocity is actually the result of a conduction block with subsequent remyelination. The immature myelin conducts slower than normal myelin, leading to a slowing of conduction velocity.

28. **B)** In healthy adults, an H-reflex can be obtained in the flexor carpi radialis muscle and can therefore be useful in the assessment of C6/C7 radiculopathies. In the healthy adult, an H-reflex elicited in any muscle besides the gastrocnemius-soleus or the flexor carpi radialis is considered pathological and may indicate an upper motor neuron lesion.

29. **C)** The adductor longus muscle is innervated by the obturator nerve, which comes off of the anterior division. The other muscles are innervated by the femoral nerve, which comes off of the posterior division.

30. **A)** If a lesion is in the plexus, it will be postganglionic (ie, distal) to the dorsal root ganglion. Therefore, the SNAP amplitudes will be affected. If a lesion is at the root level, it will be preganglionic (ie, proximal to the dorsal root ganglion). Therefore, the SNAP amplitudes will not be affected. In both cases, there may be denervation in the extremity muscles. In a radiculopathy, there may be denervation in the paraspinal muscles as well. F-wave abnormalities are nonspecific and may indicate that the problem is between the stimulation point and the spinal cord. This would include both plexopathy and radiculopathy, and so does not distinguish between the two.

31. **C)** The anterior interosseous nerve is a motor branch of the median nerve that innervates the flexor digitorum profundus to digits 2 and 3, the flexor pollicis longus, and the pronator quadratus. Its function can be tested by asking the patient to make the "okay" sign, which uses these muscles. When testing for anterior interosseous nerve injury, the nerve conduction studies are usually normal, as the active electrode is over the abductor pollicis brevis muscle. Needle electromyography (EMG) findings of denervation limited to the three muscles listed would be diagnostic of an anterior interosseous nerve (AIN) lesion.

32. **A)** A 60-cycle (60-Hz) interference happens frequently and is usually caused by electrical sources near the EMG machine. Turning on the notch filter will get rid of all components of the waveform that have 60-cycle components. Although this is usually a good thing (making the baseline flatter), the electromyographer must remember that just like all filters, you may be removing parts of the waveform that you want to see. Turning on the notch filter will remove part of the waveform, which may affect amplitude, latency, and conduction velocity as well as motor unit action potential (MUAP) morphology. Eliminating extraneous electrical currents and ensuring better electrical contacts may be a better solution.

33. **B)** Hereditary neuropathies are usually uniform-demyelinating neuropathies. They will therefore show uniformly slowed conduction velocity without temporal dispersion. Temporal dispersion would be seen in segmental demyelination, where some fibers are conducting much slower than others.

34. **C)** The perineurium is a protective connective tissue that surrounds fascicles of myelinated and unmyelinated nerve fibers. The endoneurium is connective tissue that surrounds each individual axon and its myelin sheath. The epineurium is the loose connective tissue that surrounds the entire nerve.

35. **C)** The triceps and brachioradialis are innervated by the posterior cord via the radial nerve. The deltoid is innervated by the posterior cord via the axillary nerve. The biceps is innervated by the lateral cord via the musculocutaneous nerve.

36. **C)** The biceps is an elbow flexor, but it is also a strong supinator. To relax the biceps muscle, it is important to extend the elbow and pronate the forearm.

37. **D)** The median nerve is known to have five classic areas of possible impingement. The LOS is a rudimentary ligament seen in only 1% of the population. It connects the medial epicondyle to a 2-cm bone spur that is a few centimeters proximal to the epicondyle. The median nerve, along with the brachial artery, can become entrapped under this ligament. The bicipital aponeurosis is a thickening of the antebrachial fascia, which attaches the biceps to the ulna and spreads over the median nerve in the forearm. The median nerve then travels between the two heads of the pronator teres muscle (where it can become entrapped) and runs below the flexor digitorum superficialis. In pronator teres syndrome, the pronator teres muscle is usually not affected as the muscle receives its nerve innervation proximal to the nerve entering the two heads of the muscle. The anterior interosseous nerve, a motor branch of the median nerve, can be injured by a fracture of the forearm, compression, or laceration. Finally, the carpal tunnel syndrome is the most common site of median nerve compression.

38. **D)** The only muscle listed here that is not solely innervated by the obturator nerve is the adductor magnus. This muscle has dual innervation from both the obturator nerve and the tibial division of the sciatic nerve.

39. **B)** CIM affects predominantly proximal muscles. Sensory responses should not be affected. Although CMAP amplitudes may be affected, they are usually normal to borderline normal as the pickup is over a distal muscle (and proximal muscles are affected in CIM). Electrodiagnostic findings include denervation potentials (fibrillations and positive sharp waves) in proximal muscles as well as low amplitude, short duration, polyphasic motor units with early recruitment.

40. **C)** The dorsal ulnar cutaneous nerve is a sensory branch of the ulnar nerve that supplies the dorsum of the hand. It can easily be obtained (and compared with the nonaffected hand). The dorsal ulnar cutaneous nerve branches above the wrist. Therefore, in lesions at the wrist, the dorsal ulnar cutaneous nerve will be spared. Decreased amplitude of the dorsal ulnar cutaneous nerve indicates that the ulnar nerve lesion is above the wrist.

41. **D)** All three of these muscles contain innervation from the L5 nerve root, although through different peripheral nerves. The tibialis anterior is from the deep peroneal nerve, the gluteus maximus from the inferior gluteal nerve, and the peroneus longus from the superficial peroneal nerve.

42. **A)** In an axonal injury, Wallerian degeneration occurs *distal* to the nerve lesion, and therefore, denervation may be noted in all muscles *distal* to the area of injury. Muscles innervated by a particular nerve, but proximal to the level of the axonal injury, should not be affected. With nerve conduction studies, the pickup is over a distal muscle (which would have been innervated by a nerve that has undergone Wallerian degeneration). Therefore, with both distal and proximal stimulation, the CMAP amplitude may be decreased.

43. **C)** The patient should be asked to contract the muscle minimally so that only one or two motor units are noted on the screen. If there is maximal contraction, individual motor units will not be able to be evaluated (as they will "run into" each other). In addition, it is important to note the recruitment frequency (ie, how fast one motor unit is firing when another motor unit is recruited).

44. **D)** Although 50 m/sec is considered a "normal" conduction velocity, you must interpret the results in relation to the patient's other nerves. If the distal sensory conduction velocity is greater than 10 m/sec more than the conduction velocity across the carpal tunnel, then a sensory carpal tunnel is presumed to exist. Note that sensory carpal tunnel is the correct answer and not carpal tunnel syndrome. It is important to be as descriptive as possible. Here, we do not know what the median motor latency is, so sensory carpal tunnel is more descriptive. In addition, nerves usually conduct slower the more distal they are. This is because they are thinner with less myelin and are more superficial (and therefore cooler—cooling slows down nerves). Findings in a peripheral neuropathy would be slower conduction in the distal segment rather than the proximal (across the carpal tunnel).

45. **C)** Conduction block is a focal area of demyelination that is so severe that the action potential cannot propagate. Axonotmesis is damage to the axon. Decreased amplitude will be noted if conduction block occurs between stimulator and recording electrodes (in both motor and sensory studies). If the conduction block occurs in the forearm, the distal amplitude will be normal, whereas conduction across the lesion will be affected. However, if the conduction block is distal, the distal CMAP and SNAP amplitudes would be affected (the lesion is in between the active electrode and the stimulator). This can easily be confused with an axonotmetic lesion. However, on needle testing, the axonotmetic lesion will show denervation or changes to the motor unit action potential (MUAP). Because conduction block is a focal problem with the myelin, no denervation should be noted on needle study.

46. **D)** Although this waveform has an initial positive deflection, it is a motor unit. The gain is set at 1,000 mcV (ie, each box represents 1 mV). The waveform is much too large to be a fib, a positive sharp wave (PSW), or an end-plate potential (which are usually seen when the gain is set at 100 mcV/division). If it were a fib or PSW, it would appear as a very small blip on the baseline.

47. **B)** Needle electrodiagnostic studies evaluate only large myelinated Ia fibers. This is the reason that in steroid myopathies (which usually affect type II fibers) the electromyography will usually be negative.

48. **A)** The ground electrode should be between the recording and the stimulating electrodes. All of the other measures should help to decrease extraneous electrical noise.

49. **C)** Insertional activity is a result of actual damage to the muscle membrane by the needle. It is normal if it lasts less than a few hundred milliseconds (just barely longer than the needle movement itself). The muscle should be at rest during this part of the testing.

50. **A)** Choice (A) describes axonotmesis, an injury to the axon that results in axonal interruption with the connective tissue and Schwann cell remaining intact. Wallerian degeneration proceeds in a proximal to distal manner. Choice (B) refers to neurotmesis, or nerve transection injury. This injury involves the axon and connective tissue disruption. This leads to conduction failure. Choice (C) refers to neurapraxia, which is a nerve injury that results in focal myelin injury with an intact axon; conduction block is present.

51. **B)** Although most radiculopathies are not clearly delineated by focal muscle weakness (as most are innervated by more than one root), this scenario clearly depicts a presentation consistent with a C6 radiculopathy. Wrist extensor weakness and brachioradialis weakness are consistent with a C6-level lesion. C5 radiculopathy would involve some weakness of the biceps, C7 weakness of the triceps, and C8 weakness of finger flexors.

52. **D)** The CSI uses three parameters to increase the sensitivity for evaluating CTS using electrodiagnostic testing. Three parameters are tested: difference in the latency of the ulnar and median sensory response from digit 4 (at 14 cm), difference in the radial and median sensory response from the thumb (at 10 cm), and median and ulnar midpalm orthodromic stimulation (at 8 cm). If the added differences total more than 0.9 msec, CTS is confirmed.

53. **B)** The short head of the biceps femoris is the first (and only) muscle innervated by the common peroneal nerve. The sciatic nerve divides into the tibial and peroneal (also called the fibular) nerves in the posterior thigh. The only muscle innervated by the peroneal nerve proximal to the knee is the short head of the biceps femoris. Testing this muscle is important when a patient presents with foot drop or suspected peroneal nerve injury to localize the lesion. Abnormal spontaneous potentials (fibrillations and positive sharp waves) in the short head of the biceps femoris place the lesion at the common peroneal nerve in the thigh or more proximal. The tibial innervated muscles must also be examined, as the lesion may involve the sciatic nerve. The peroneal division of the sciatic nerve is often more affected than the tibial division.

54. **A)** The ulnar nerve is slack when the arm is extended. When the arm is bent, the ulnar nerve is no longer slack. The measurement should also be done in this position, following the path of the nerve. As speed = distance/unit of time, a falsely low distance will falsely slow the conduction velocity.

55. **C)** H-reflex represents the time in milliseconds for a stimulation from the popliteal fossa to travel orthodromically in afferent sensory fibers, synapse in the spinal cord, and then travel orthodromically in efferent motor fibers to a pickup over the gastrocnemius-soleus muscle. Of course, the taller the individual, the longer this pathway will take. In addition, nerves conduct slower as a person ages, so an older individual will likely have a longer latency. There are nomograms to correct for the H-reflex given a person's age and height. Comparing the affected side with the nonaffected side is important. A side-to-side latency difference of more than 1.5 msec is usually considered significant. Although temperature usually plays a role in latency and amplitude when testing peripheral nerves with a distal pickup, with an H-reflex the pickup is over a more proximal (and therefore warmer) muscle. Therefore, the temperature is not usually a significant factor.

56. **A)** A patient who has low-amplitude sensory nerve action potentials with preserved compound motor action potential amplitudes (and relatively normal conduction velocities and latencies) should be suspected of having a paraneoplastic syndrome.

57. **B)** The rise time is measured as the time from the peak of the initial positive deflection to the subsequent negative upward peak. The rise time is used to estimate the distance between the recording tip and the discharging motor unit. If the needle is far from the muscle that is being activated, the rise time will be prolonged (more than 0.5 msec) and the motor unit will sound duller or "thuddier." If this occurs, the needle should be repositioned. A distant motor unit will have a longer rise time because of the resistance and capacitance of the tissues that separate the needle from the activated muscle. This will act as a high-frequency filter.

58. **B)** SSEPs may be helpful in diagnosing problems in sensory nerves (such as in meralgia pares-thetica, also known as *lateral femoral cutaneous nerve injury*) that are not accessible to routine elec-trodiagnostic testing. SSEPs are not the test of choice in assessing for a radiculopathy, as only the sensory pathway is tested and the pathway is very long. Problems anywhere along the pathway may affect latency and amplitude. They are not at all useful in assessing motor nerves (anterior interosseous nerve injury). The pathway is too long to be of use in a sacral plexopathy.

59. **B)** As each "box" is 100 mV and as a CMAP amplitude is typically 5 to 10 mV in amplitude, the waveform would appear as a blip on the baseline. To adequately view the waveform, one would have to *increase* the gain by changing it from 100 mV to 1 mV.

60. **C)** Orthodromic conduction means conduction in the same direction as physiologic conduction. For a sensory nerve, this would be an electrical impulse that is transmitted from the distal aspect of the sensory nerve (ie, the finger or the toe) to the more proximal pickup. Sensory studies are usually performed antidromically (stimulating at the wrist or ankle and picking up more distally over the sensory area of the nerve).

61. **A)** The accessory peroneal nerve is a branch from the superficial peroneal nerve. It travels pos-terior to the lateral malleolus and innervates the lateral portion of the extensor digitorum brevis (EDB) muscle. The anomaly is usually noted when the amplitude of the compound motor action potential (CMAP) at the fibular head is larger than the CMAP amplitude at the ankle. With stimu-lation behind the lateral malleolus, a CMAP is produced. Usually, the amplitude of the CMAP at the ankle combined with the amplitude of the CMAP posterior to the lateral malleolus equals the amplitude of the CMAP obtained at the fibular head.

62. **C)** Diabetic neuropathy usually presents as sensory and motor, axonal and demyelinating peripheral polyneuropathy. Alcoholic neuropathy is usually a sensory motor axonal neuropathy. Paraneoplastic syndrome is usually a sensory axonal neuropathy. Guillain-Barré syndrome usu-ally presents with segmental demyelination.

63. **C)** Choice (A) describes myokymic discharges. It is often noted to sound like "soldiers marching" and is often seen in conditions such as multiple sclerosis, Bell's palsy, and polyradiculopathy. Choice (B) refers to neuromyotonic discharges. Generalized neuromyotonia is usually an autoim-mune disease characterized by widespread muscle stiffness and delayed muscle relaxation after voluntary movement. Choice (D) refers to fibrillation potentials, which are usually triphasic in nature. Myotonia is clinically seen as delayed relaxation of a muscle after contraction. Potentials tend to fire at a variable rate, waxing and waning in appearance, and its variation causes a char-acteristic "dive bomber" sound.

64. **B)** The serratus anterior is innervated by the long thoracic nerve (roots C5, C6, and C7), which helps to protract the scapula and rotate the glenoid upward. The supraspinatus is innervated by the suprascapular nerve (roots C5, C6), which helps in shoulder abduction and external rota-tion. The biceps brachii is innervated by the musculocutaneous nerve (roots C5, C6) and assists in

elbow flexion and forearm supination. The rhomboids are innervated by the dorsal scapular nerve (solely C5 root) and help to elevate and retract the scapula as well as rotate the glenoid downward.

65. **B)** Critical illness neuropathy is a sensorimotor axonal neuropathy. On nerve conduction studies, sensory and motor amplitudes are low. Three extremities should be tested and temperature should be maintained at 32°C in the upper extremities and 30°C in the lower extremities. Latencies and conduction velocities remain normal to borderline normal. (If the fastest axons are affected, latency may be mildly increased, and conduction velocities mildly decreased. However, the axonal loss (amplitude) is out of proportion to the slowing.) Critical illness neuropathy is seen in the critical care setting and is most commonly associated with sepsis, systemic inflammatory response syndrome (SIRS) and multiorgan failure. Patients who have abnormal weakness (out of proportion to their disease) should be considered for electrodiagnostic testing.

66. **E)** Neurotmesis is a complete disruption of the axon, myelin, and all supporting connective tissues. Complete nerve regeneration is unlikely, as there is no path for the nerve to follow when trying to connect to the distal muscles.

67. **A)** A myelinated nerve has sodium channels located only at the nodes of Ranvier. An unmyelinated nerve has sodium channels throughout the length of the nerve. Therefore, if a myelinated nerve loses its myelin (becomes demyelinated), the sodium channels are still located at distinct intervals throughout the nerve. If saltatory conduction cannot occur (because the myelin has been lost), the action potential cannot propagate along the nerve. Therefore, conduction block will occur. Conduction block does not occur in an unmyelinated nerve because the lesion in a conduction block is myelin.

68. **A)** In a brachial plexopathy, the lesion is distal to the sensory nerve body (the dorsal root ganglion). As such, the continuity between the cell body and the end organ has been affected. Therefore, the SNAP would be affected. Conversely, in a radicular lesion, there is continuity between the dorsal root ganglion and the end organ (the sensation over the hand or foot), so the SNAP is not affected.

69. **C)** The peripheral neuropathy seen in diabetic neuropathy is usually axonal and demyelinating sensory motor neuropathy. This means that low-amplitude sensory nerve action potentials (SNAPs) and compound motor action potentials (CMAPs) would be noted with slowing of nerve conduction velocities (both sensory and motor) and increased latencies.

70. **B)** There should be at least 4 cm between the active and the reference electrodes. If the electrodes are placed too close together, the sensory nerve action potential (SNAP) amplitude could falsely decrease (resembling an axonal lesion). This has to do with the rise time of the SNAP. The electrodiagnosis (EMG) machine will "subtract" the recorded action potential of the reference electrode from the recorded action potential of the active electrode. If the action potential reaches the reference electrode during the rise time of the action potential seen by the active electrode, the EMG machine will subtract one from the other, resulting in a decreased SNAP amplitude.

71. **B)** Because the sensory nerve has no myoneural junction, the speed ($V = D/T$) can be directly calculated if the distance and the time (latency) is known. Motor nerves, on the other hand, have a myoneural junction. As it is not known how long it takes for the action potential to cross the myoneural junction and for conduction in the muscle, the conduction velocity in a motor nerve must be calculated using the formula $V$ = change in distance/change in time. Therefore, two stimulations must be performed (one proximal and one distal) to assess velocity. The difference in distance is divided by the difference in latency.

72. **A)** Sensory amplitudes are generally about 10 to 20 mcV. These are much smaller than compound motor action potential (CMAP) amplitudes, where the gain is usually 1,000 mcV. Remember that the gain is the Y-axis and is also called the *sensitivity*. Therefore, a lower number (10 mcV) represents a higher sensitivity than a higher number (1 mV). The waveform is the same. What differs is how much the waveform is "blown up" so that it can be visualized.

73. **B)** The axillary nerve comes off at the trunk level. With either an upper trunk or a lateral cord lesion, the musculocutaneous CMAP to the biceps, the lateral antebrachial SNAP, and the median SNAP will all be affected.

74. **D)** The Riche-Cannieu anastomosis is a communication between the deep branch of the ulnar nerve and the recurrent branch of the median nerve in the hand. It can produce an all-ulnar hand. Therefore, if the ulnar nerve is injured proximally, the muscles normally innervated by the median nerve (but now innervated via the ulnar nerve anastomosis) may show signs of injury. Conversely, if the patient has a complete laceration of the median nerve at the wrist, he or she may still retain thenar function via the anastomosis.

75. **A)** If the anode and cathode were reversed on the stimulator, there would be an extra 3 to 4 cm in length between the stimulator and the active electrode. The longer the distance that the stimulation has to travel, the longer the latency. If maximal stimulation were not used, the sensory and motor amplitudes may be decreased. If you did not stimulate over the nerve, the sensory and motor amplitudes may be decreased as well. If there was too much electrical interference, the baseline would not be flat.

76. **D)** Froment's sign is often found in ulnar neuropathy. It is demonstrated by having the patient grasp a piece of paper between the thumb and the radial side of the second digit. As the examiner tries to pull the paper out of the patient's hand, the patient will try to substitute his or her median-innervated flexor pollicis longus muscle for a weakened ulnarly innervated adductor pollicis muscle.

77. **C)** Cooling results in a longer time for the action potential to proceed down the axon. This is in part due to a change in protein configuration of the Na+ channels as its structure is changed by temperature change. Cooling can cause slow opening and even slower closing of Na+ channels, which slows the propagation of action potentials in axons. For every 1°C drop in temperature, there is an approximate 5% decrease in conduction velocity. Amplitude is increased along with the duration of the action potential because of prolonged opening times of the sodium channels.

78. **C)** The typical amplitude of a compound muscle action potential (CMAP) is above 4 mV. A millivolt is one thousandth of a volt. A microvolt is a thousandth of a millivolt (or a millionth of a volt)—this is a typical amplitude of a sensory nerve action potential (SNAP). The other choices are measures of time, not amplitude. Amplitude is on the Y-axis, whereas time is on the X-axis of the electromyography (EMG) screen.

79. **A)** Except for somatosensory-evoked potentials, electrodiagnostic testing only assesses the peripheral nervous system. Testing is possible of both the motor and the sensory fibers. Assessment can be made about the integrity of the myoneural junction, the axon, and the myelin. However, the autonomic nervous system is not evaluated by conventional nerve studies and electrodiagnosis (EMG).

80. **C)** F-waves are low-amplitude late responses thought to be due to antidromic activation of motor neurons. They have variable latency and configuration with variable responses. They are indicated to assess proximal conduction in conditions such as AIDP (also known as Guillain-Barré

syndrome). F-waves are reported to be among the earliest electrodiagnostic findings in AIDP. F-waves should not be used routinely to assess for radiculopathy. The most commonly assessed parameter of F-waves is the shortest F latency. F-waves evaluate a very long neural pathway, are nonspecific, and can be affected by anything that would slow the pathway (ie, peripheral neuropathy and focal slowing). The exact location of the slowing cannot be assessed, so to use an F-wave to say the slowing is at the root level is faulty. In addition, because the active electrode is over a muscle that would have multiple root innervations and because the F-wave only assesses the fastest fibers, in theory the F-wave should be normal in a radiculopathy. Radiculopathies may affect the axon, and the F-wave is a test of latency. If there is slowing of the neural path in a radiculopathy, the area of slowing is small compared with the length of the pathway assessed with an F-wave. Finally, as the F-wave latency is extremely variable, multiple stimulations must be performed to find the shortest latency. The number of stimulations, therefore, has to be high (more than 10) and even then, the electromyographer is never sure that the shortest latency has been recorded.

81. **B)** Below the knee, the common peroneal nerve branches into the superficial and deep peroneal nerves. The superficial nerve innervates the peroneus longus and brevis and provides innervation to the lateral aspect of the lower leg as well as the dorsum of the foot (except for the first dorsal web space, which is innervated by the deep peroneal nerve). Nerve conduction study of the superficial peroneal sensory nerve is easy to perform, but often omitted. Just like the dorsal ulnar cutaneous nerve, it can be helpful in determining location and severity of a lesion. It should be noted that the peroneal nerve is also known as the fibular nerve.

82. **D)** The peripheral neuropathy usually seen in alcoholic neuropathy is axonal sensory motor neuropathy. This means that low amplitudes would be seen in the sensory nerve action potentials (SNAPs) and compound motor action potentials (CMAPs) with relative preservation of the velocities (up to 20% decrease in velocity can be seen, as the fastest fibers may be affected).

83. **D)** A demyelinating neuropathy will slow nerves and therefore increase the latency of the H-reflex. Because the pathway of the H-reflex involves both sensory and motor fibers, either type of neuropathy will affect the H-reflex. The height of the person will affect the H-reflex latency because the pathway is longer (it takes a longer time to travel a longer distance).

84. **D)** Diabetes, pregnancy, and thyroid disorders (as well as rheumatoid arthritis, edema, gout, and peripheral neuropathy) can predispose patients to entrapment neuropathies. Psoriasis has not been related to an increase in entrapment neuropathies.

85. **B)** The patient has the right to terminate the test at any point. It is best to explain the benefits of continuing the test and ask the patient whether they are sure that this is what they want. If the patient insists, this should be documented in the EMG report.

86. **C)** Although this appears to be a simple right carpal tunnel syndrome, it is important (especially considering the denervation in the APB muscle) to rule out a median neuropathy more proximally, a double-crush syndrome with cervical radiculopathy, or even an anterior horn cell disorder. Any of these can occur with a carpal tunnel syndrome. It is important to test a more proximal median-innervated muscle (pronator teres) as well as another ulnarly innervated hand muscle. If these are positive, it behooves the electromyographer to continue the needle evaluation.

87. **A)** The motor units in a patient with steroid myopathy would typically have normal-appearing motor units. That is because steroid myopathies typically affect type II fibers. Electromyographic (EMG) testing evaluates type I fibers.

88. **D)** To assess whether a patient has a peripheral neuropathy, it is necessary to test sensory and motor nerves in three limbs. Therefore, the peroneal and sural (or any other sensory and motor nerve in the lower extremity) should be performed.

89. **A)** The accessory peroneal nerve is a branch of the superficial peroneal nerve that innervates the lateral aspect of the EDB. The nerve runs deep to the peroneus brevis and behind the lateral malleolus. The best way to test for this anomalous innervation is to stimulate the peroneal nerve posterior to the lateral malleolus (with pickup over the EDB). The amplitude of the CMAP obtained posterior to the malleolus plus (+) that of the normal ankle peroneal amplitude should summate and equal that of the amplitude proximally at the fibular head.

90. **C)** Radiculopathy is a lesion of a nerve root. Clinically, it may present as sensory, motor, or mixed sensory/motor findings. In radiculopathy, the injury is proximal to the area being stimulated and therefore conduction block or slowing of conduction velocity will not be noted on electrodiagnostic testing. Any damage to the sensory fibers is generally proximal to the dorsal root ganglion (DRG). As there is physical continuity between the sensory nerve cell and the end unit, nerve conduction studies (NCS) will show normal sensory findings. Motor nerve conduction studies will generally be normal too because peripheral nerves contain multiple nerve roots. The classic needle electromyography (EMG) findings in a radiculopathy are abnormal spontaneous potentials (fibs and positive sharp waves) in the paraspinal muscles of the suspected root level as well as two muscles innervated by different peripheral nerves but the same root level.

91. **D)** In spinal stenosis, there is narrowing of the vertebral canal, which is usually exacerbated by extending the spine (standing) and relieved with flexion of the spine (sitting). Pain may radiate from the back down to the extremities, especially with extension of the spine. SNAPs are normal as the dorsal root ganglion (DRG) is located outside the spinal canal. CMAPs should not be affected as the distal portion of the nerve is not affected. There may be abnormal spontaneous potentials at rest (positive sharp waves [PSW] or fibrillations) or chronic motor unit action potential (MUAP) changes (polyphasic potentials) that are often bilateral. Bilateral paraspinals and extremities should be tested for EMG abnormalities.

92. **D)** Of all of the possible mistakes that can lead to false-positive or false-negative electrodiagnostic results, the most common one is due to the person performing the test. These include not performing the test correctly, not interpreting the test correctly, not testing the appropriate nerves or muscles, failing to account for anomalous innervation, improper technique, or performing the test too early (before findings would be apparent on neurodiagnostic testing).

93. **D)** The dorsal scapular nerve (which innervates the rhomboid muscle) is the first branch of the upper trunk and is usually composed of C5 fibers only.

94. **B)** The X-axis (sweep) represents time, which is usually in milliseconds per division.

95. **A)** The extensor carpi radialis is innervated by the radial nerve C6/7. The flexor digitorum superficialis is via the median nerve C7-T1. The extensor indicis is via the radial nerve C7/8. The rhomboid is innervated by the dorsal scapular nerve, C5.

96. **A)** At birth, most of the myelination is incomplete. Conduction velocities are about half of adult values. By 1 year of age, the velocity is about 75%. Myelination is usually complete by age 3 to 5 years.

97. **C)** The posterior cord includes the axillary nerve (to the deltoid) and the radial nerve (to the triceps and extensor indicis proprius). The pronator teres is innervated through the lateral cord and the median nerve.

98. **B)** When evaluating the recruitment pattern of MUAPs, it is important to use minimal recruitment. Ideally, you would like to see the firing rate of one motor unit when a second motor unit is recruited. If maximal recruitment is attempted, individual motor units cannot be assessed and the recruitment frequency cannot be assessed. In addition, there is a risk of the needle breaking in the muscle if the contraction is too strong.

99. **D)** Although the H-reflex is very sensitive, it is not specific. Any of the conditions listed can result in a prolongation of the H-reflex.

100. **B)** Small-amplitude, short-duration polyphasic motor units are often seen in myopathies. In chronic neuropathies, the motor units may be of large amplitude, long duration, and polyphasic.

101. **B)** The short head of the biceps femoris is the only nerve that is innervated by the common peroneal (fibular) nerve. It is also the only muscle innervated by the peroneal nerve that is above the popliteal fossa. Therefore, it is a very important muscle to test to determine the location of a lesion. The tibialis anterior muscle is innervated by the deep peroneal (fibular) nerve. The peroneus longus is innervated by the superficial peroneal (fibular) nerve, and the long head of the biceps femoris is innervated by the tibial nerve.

102. **D)** The sartorius is innervated by the femoral nerve. The femoral nerve also innervates the pectineus, iliopsoas, and quadriceps muscles.

103. **D)** The superficial peroneal nerve innervates the peroneus brevis and peroneus longus muscles. These muscles help to plantarflex and evert the foot. This nerve provides cutaneous sensation to the lower lateral aspect of the leg and dorsum of the foot with the exception of the first web space between the great and the second toes (innervated by the deep peroneal nerve). Choices (A), (B), and (C) are all innervated by the deep peroneal nerve along with the peroneus tertius and the extensor digitorum longus.

104. **B)** In repetitive nerve stimulation, a greater than 10% decrease in CMAP amplitude from the first to the fifth stimulation is considered significant for pathology at the neuromuscular junction.

105. **C)** Increasing the gain is equal to increasing the sensitivity. By **increasing** the gain from 1,000 mcV (1 mV)/division to 500 mcV/division, each "box" on the Y-axis will portray a smaller percentage of the waveform. If the CMAP amplitude is 2,000 mcV in amplitude, and if the gain is 1,000 mcV (1 mV)/division, the waveform will be two boxes high. If the gain is increased to 500 mcV/division, the waveform will be four boxes tall (hence amplified). The sweep speed is represented on the X-axis and is measured in milliseconds per division.

106. **A)** An accessory peroneal nerve is a branch from the superficial peroneal nerve that travels posterior to the lateral malleolus and can innervate the lateral portion of the extensor digitorum brevis (EDB) muscle. The fibers from the accessory branch are not activated with ankle stimulation and therefore cannot contribute to the distal CMAP amplitude. These fibers are activated with proximal stimulation. If the accessory branch is stimulated posterior to the lateral malleolus (with pickup on the EDB), a waveform will be obtained. Usually, this CMAP amplitude, when added to the CMAP amplitude of the ankle stimulation, will equal the CMAP amplitude of stimulation at the fibular head.

107. **D)** The gain is the Y-axis on the screen. Normal sensory nerve amplitudes are between 10 and 20 mcV/division. If the gain is set too low, the sensory nerve action potential (SNAP) will be merely a blip on the screen (oscilloscope). (Remember that gain means sensitivity. A **low** gain would be 1,000 mcV/division or 1 mV/division.) Compound motor action potentials, which have an amplitude of about 5 mV, can be visualized on a gain of 1 mV/division.

108. **A)** An increased firing frequency is frequently reported as "decreased recruitment." Both mean that a single motor unit fires faster than normal before a second motor unit is recruited. Muscles can increase their strength in one of two ways: they can recruit more motor units, or the motor units that are there can fire faster. In a neuropathic process, there are not more motor units that can be recruited. Therefore, the remaining motor units have to fire faster to increase the strength of the contraction. One motor unit may fire at 20 Hz (cycles per second) or faster. If the sweep is set at 10 msec/division, and there are 10 divisions per screen, then the screen represents 1/10 of a second. Therefore, if a motor unit fires twice in a screen, it is firing at about 20 Hz.

109. **D)** To decrease interference and make the baseline as quiet as possible, the reference electrode should be placed over the same muscle that is being tested. The EMG machine will "subtract" the electrical activity of the reference electrode, therefore getting rid of any excess noise.

110. **C)** Fibrillations and positive sharp waves are seen in acute processes (either neuropathic or myopathic). Polyphasicity and long duration motor units are noted with reinnervation and asynchronous firing of the individual muscle fibers that make up a motor unit. Complex repetitive discharges are noted in chronic processes as well.

111. **B)** It is very difficult to have the patient relax a muscle during needle testing. The best way to do this is to have the patient activate the antagonist muscle. This will automatically relax the muscle that you are testing. For example, if the needle is in the biceps muscle (which flexes the elbow and supinates), have the patient extend the elbow and pronate. It is important to know the function of each muscle. As described, simply extending the elbow will often not be enough to relax the biceps, as it also functions as a supinator.

112. **D)** You cannot state that the patient has an S1 radiculopathy based solely on a prolonged H-reflex. Many conditions can lead to a prolonged H-reflex. To definitively state that the patient has a radiculopathy, there must be findings of denervation in the corresponding paraspinal muscle as well as two limb muscles innervated by the same root level, but different peripheral nerves.

113. **B)** The gain is set at 50 mcV. Therefore, the largest motor unit is 200 mcV in amplitude. This is considered a small-amplitude potential, as normal amplitude of a motor unit using a monopolar needle is about 1 to 7 mV in amplitude.

114. **D)** The sural nerve receives sensory branches from both the tibial and the peroneal (fibular) nerves.

115. **C)** The FDP is innervated by the median nerve (anterior interosseous branch) and the ulnar nerve. The median nerve innervates the FDP to digits 2 and 3, whereas the ulnar nerve innervates the FDP to digits 4 and 5. The pronator quadratus is innervated by the anterior interosseous nerve via the median nerve. The ulnar nerve innervates the flexor carpi ulnaris. The dorsal scapular nerve innervates the rhomboids.

116. **D)** Alcohol abuse can lead to axonal injury to the nerves, involving both sensory and motor nerves. Thus, both CMAP and SNAP amplitudes would be expected to be decreased. As the myelin is usually not affected, the conduction velocity and latency should not be affected.

117. **C)** F-waves are a delayed pure motor response. They are triggered by antidromic activation of motor neurons from peripheral stimulation of a nerve. This stimulation travels antidromically to the anterior horn cell. From there, it proceeds orthodromically to the muscle fiber. This backfiring of the axon is thought to represent a small portion (about 5%) of the orthodromically

generated motor response (M-wave) that first occurs with stimulation. F-waves vary in their waveforms and latency and thus are averaged over multiple trials (usually 10). A-waves are seen in chronically injured nerves and represent regeneration or collateral sprouting of a nerve, as the orthodromic response is diverted along a collateral neural branch to circumvent the conventional path. This alternative path has a constant latency and is seen between the M- and the F-wave, with submaximal stimulation.

118. **D)** Myofascial pain does not lead to changes in the nerves or muscles that are quantifiable by electrodiagnostic testing. In general, changes to the sensory or motor nerve (axonal, demyelinating, or both), the neuromuscular junction, or the muscle itself can lead to electrophysiological changes that can be quantifiable by electrodiagnostic testing.

119. **B)** Martin-Gruber anastomosis is a median to ulnar nerve anastomosis in the forearm. Most commonly these are ulnar fibers that are destined for the ulnarly innervated hand muscles that travel with the median nerve proximally and then cross over to the ulnar nerve in the forearm (usually from the anterior interosseous nerve). When the active electrode is placed over the abductor pollicis brevis (APB) muscle (median nerve study), and the median nerve is stimulated at the antecubital fossa, the ulnarly innervated adductor pollicis muscle is stimulated as well (from the ulnar fibers that travel with the median nerve). Remember, in the forearm, these fibers switch over to again travel with the ulnar nerve. Because these fibers do not have to go through the carpal tunnel, the action potential reaches the adductor pollicis muscle before the median fibers get to the APB muscle. Therefore, there is an initial positive (downward) deflection with stimulation of the median nerve in the antecubital fossa (this occurs because the active electrode is not over the motor point of the muscle being activated, the active electrode is over the APB muscle, not the adductor motor point). There is decreased amplitude of the median CMAP with distal stimulation as compared with proximal stimulation, because distal stimulation only activates the median-innervated APB muscle. Proximal stimulation activates the median-innervated APB muscle as well as the nearby ulnar-innervated adductor pollicis muscle. The excessively fast median forearm conduction velocity noted with a Martin-Gruber anastomosis when carpal tunnel is present is due to the proximal stimulation of ulnar fibers (which do not have to travel through the carpal tunnel). This leads to a spuriously decreased latency with proximal stimulation compared with the increased latency of the distally stimulated median nerve.

120. **B)** CRDs are usually noted in longstanding disorders (of more than 6 months). They represent groups of spontaneously firing action potentials with an affected area of muscle electrically stimulating an adjacent muscle fiber. This produces a local muscular arrhythmia. The patterns repeat regularly with a frequency of 10 to 100 Hz. They have the sound of a motorboat misfiring. They can be seen in chronic neurogenic or myopathic disorders. As the needle study would be normal in a sensory neuropathy (only the motor fibers are tested with needle testing), CRDs would not be noted in a sensory peripheral neuropathy.

121. **C)** Denervation can be found in neuropathic or myopathic processes. As myopathies only affect the muscle, SNAPs should be preserved. The motor units are usually short-duration, small-amplitude, polyphasic potentials with early recruitment.

122. **B)** Concentric needles are beveled and therefore only pick up from 180° around the needle tip. Monopolar needles pick up electrical activity from 360°. Therefore, the MUAP amplitudes from a monopolar needle are usually larger than those from a concentric needle. It is important to include information about the type of needle in the report so that the amplitude can be interpreted correctly. Concentric needles have the reference electrode as part of the needle and require a separate ground.

123. **D)** Duration is the time from the initial baseline departure to the final return to baseline. Normal duration is about 5 to 15 msec or approximately one horizontal division with a commonly used sweep speed of 10 msec/division. It represents the degree of synchrony in the firing of the individual motor fibers that contribute to the motor unit. With reinnervation, there is asynchrony of firing of individual muscle fibers due to immature myelin. Therefore, duration of a motor unit increases with reinnervation and can be seen in chronic neuropathic processes. Decreased duration may be seen in myopathic disorders.

124. **C)** The motor point is the area where the nerve enters the muscle. This is usually located near the middle of the muscle belly. It is also known as the end-plate zone.

125. **A)** When many of the fibers that make up the CMAP have different velocities, the resulting waveform will be more dispersed. Remember that the latency reflects the fastest fibers. Those at the end of the CMAP reflect the slowest fibers. Even though this slowing is a result of a demyelinating lesion, the CMAP amplitude may be decreased with temporal dispersion. Again, this is because there is a wider variation of conduction velocities and the CMAP has a longer duration. However, the area under the CMAP curve will be the same. Therefore, if a decreased amplitude is noted, do not automatically assume it is due to an axonal lesion. Assess the duration of the waveform. If it is prolonged, the decreased amplitude may be due to dispersion.

126. **D)** Placing the surface reference electrode over the same muscle that the needle is in will decrease the baseline noise. The EMG machine will "subtract" the electrical signal of the reference from the active electrode signal. Therefore, any surface "noise" will be eliminated.

127. **D)** The saphenous nerve is the sensory continuation of the femoral nerve. It supplies sensation to the medial leg and foot.

128. **D)** The adductor magnus is innervated by both the obturator and the sciatic nerves. The superior gluteal nerve innervates the tensor fascia lata, the femoral nerve innervates the iliopsoas, and the obturator nerve innervates the gracilis.

129. **D)** Diabetes (along with uremia) usually involves both the axon and the myelin with findings in motor and sensory fibers. Conditions associated with axonal motor polyneuropathy include porphyria and axonal type Guillain-Barré syndrome. Hereditary neuropathies usually present with uniform-demyelinating mixed sensorimotor polyneuropathy. Conditions that may present with segmental-demyelinating motor polyneuropathy include Guillain-Barré syndrome (acute inflammatory demyelinating polyneuropathy) and hypothyroidism.

130. **D)** All the choices are valid limitations of the clinical utility of the H-reflex. As this reflex assesses a long neural pathway (including the orthodromic Ia afferents, the dorsal root ganglion to the spinal cord, interneurons, and then orthodromically to the muscle), a delay may not be specific to a radiculopathy. The lesion can be anywhere along the pathway.

# 4

# Speech

## QUESTIONS

1. A patient demonstrates paraphasic speech with semantic substitutions. Most striking is the patient's echolalia, or repetition of phrases that are heard. Comprehension is poor in this patient, whereas verbal repetition is considered good. Reading and writing skills are also poor. This individual may be diagnosed as having:
   A) Wernicke's aphasia
   B) Transcortical sensory aphasia
   C) Broca's aphasia
   D) Conduction aphasia

2. Sustained, rhythmic, jerky motions that are elicited when a muscle or tendon is held in extension are called:
   A) Tremors
   B) Athetosis
   C) Clonus
   D) Fasciculations

3. Dysphagia may be due to:
   A) Neurological dysfunction
   B) Cancer
   C) Aging
   D) All of the above

4. Apraxia of swallowing:
   A) May follow a left anterior stroke
   B) Results in delayed initiation of the oral stage of swallowing
   C) Has accompanying limited tongue movement for bolus preparation
   D) Is all of the above

5. Proximal escape occurs when:
   A) Stomach acid flows up the esophagus
   B) A bolus escapes through the nasal cavity
   C) A bolus enters the pyriform sinuses
   D) A bolus moves back up the esophagus before entering the stomach

6. Techniques for a delayed swallow reflex include all of the following **except**:
   A) Chin tuck
   B) Supraglottic swallow
   C) Head rotation to the weaker side
   D) Thinned liquids

ANSWERS TO THIS SECTION CAN BE FOUND ON PAGE 111

7. Which imaging modality is best to capture tongue movements and swallowing motion?
   A) Ultrasound
   B) Scintigraphy
   C) MRI
   D) Fast low-angle shot MRI (FLASH-MRI)

8. Which of the choices below describes a fluent aphasia?
   A) Transcortical motor
   B) Mixed transcortical
   C) Transcortical sensory
   D) All of the above

9. A 78-year-old male who presented with clinical signs and symptoms of an acute cerebrovascular accident (CVA) is admitted to the stroke service. He undergoes an MRI of the brain, which shows abnormal signal around the area of the arcuate fasciculus. During rehabilitation, the patient regains his speech but seems to have trouble with repetition and naming. His fluency and comprehension are intact. Which type of aphasia does this patient most likely have?
   A) Wernicke's aphasia
   B) Broca's aphasia
   C) Global aphasia
   D) Conduction aphasia
   E) Anomic aphasia

10. A patient's signs and symptoms include effortful speech and difficulties with verbal expression, difficulty in organizing verbal responses, phonemic and global paraphasias, and verbal perseverations. The patient can be diagnosed as having:
    A) Wernicke's aphasia
    B) Global aphasia
    C) Transcortical motor aphasia
    D) Conduction aphasia

11. A patient who has been diagnosed with Huntington's disease is likely to experience:
    A) Hypokinetic dysarthria
    B) Hyperkinetic dysarthria
    C) Ataxic dysarthria
    D) Apraxia of speech

12. What happens during the pharyngeal stage of swallowing?
    A) Vocal folds adduct
    B) Epiglottis folds over
    C) Larynx elevates and moves anteriorly
    D) All of the above

13. When a patient does not cough after material has passed into the trachea because of a lack of sensation, this is called:
    A) Vallecular pooling
    B) Pyriform sinus pooling
    C) Silent aspiration
    D) Poor bolus transport

14. Disordered swallowing may result from lesions in the basal ganglia and is likely associated with:
    A) Postural instability
    B) Prolonged oral phase of swallowing
    C) Tongue rigidity
    D) All of the above

15. The most common type of dysphagia is:
    A) Oral-phase dysphagia
    B) Pharyngeal-phase dysphagia
    C) Supraglottal-phase dysphagia
    D) Esophageal-phase dysphagia

16. In patients with swallowing disorders, water-soluble agents with high osmolality should not be used because of the risk of aspiration-induced pulmonary edema.
    A) True
    B) False

17. Which vessel is often involved in patients with global aphasia?
    A) Anterior cerebral artery (ACA)
    B) Middle cerebral artery (MCA)
    C) Posterior cerebral artery (PCA)
    D) Basilar artery

18. A 35-year-old male with no past medical history was struck by a car and admitted to the surgical ICU. He had positive loss of consciousness and was found to have a subarachnoid hemorrhage on CT scan. After being stabilized, he was transferred to the surgical floor where he was found have to difficulty finding words when speaking. He commonly used vague words in place of the words he was trying to think of. Which type of aphasia does this patient most likely have?
    A) Wernicke's aphasia
    B) Broca's aphasia
    C) Global aphasia
    D) Conduction aphasia
    E) Anomic aphasia

19. The transcortical aphasias result from lesions within:
    A) Broca's area
    B) Wernicke's area
    C) Border zone
    D) Cerebellum

20. The language disorder that results from damage to the arcuate fasciculus, and results in good comprehension, good articulation but poor repetitions, word-finding difficulties, and oral reading that is paraphasic is called:
    A) Broca's aphasia
    B) Wernicke's aphasia
    C) Conduction aphasia
    D) Global aphasia

21. In a normal, healthy individual, esophageal motility takes how long to transport a bolus from the esophagus to the stomach?
    A) 1 second
    B) 3 to 5 seconds
    C) 8 to 20 seconds
    D) More than 60 seconds

22. Common anatomical sites that are observed in a modified barium swallow (MBS) study include all of the following **except**:
    A) Nasal sinuses
    B) Pyriform sinuses
    C) Valleculae
    D) Nasopharyngeal port

23. What is the most common cause of swallowing disorders?
    A) Mechanical
    B) Functional
    C) Behavioral/cognitive
    D) Neurological

24. The Mendelsohn maneuver involves:
    A) Performing a Valsalva maneuver and subsequent throat clearing in between swallows
    B) Tucking the chin to increase pharyngeal pressure before swallowing
    C) Holding a swallow midway for 3 to 5 seconds before completing the swallow
    D) Rotating the head to the weaker side before swallowing

25. Which muscle is an inferior pharyngeal constrictor?
    A) Cricopharyngeus muscle
    B) Cricothyroid muscle
    C) Pterygoid muscle
    D) Arytenoid muscle

26. The greatest amount of improvement in patients with aphasia occurs within what time frame?
    A) 3 weeks
    B) 3 months
    C) 6 months
    D) 1 year

27. A 75-year-old female with a history of hypertension, hyperlipidemia, and diabetes presents to the emergency department with new onset aphasia. On exam, she is able to complete fluent sentences but does not seem to comprehend when asked specific questions. Which type of aphasia does this patient most likely have?
    A) Wernicke's aphasia
    B) Broca's aphasia
    C) Global aphasia
    D) Conduction aphasia
    E) Anomic aphasia

28. Hypokinetic dysarthria is a result of:
    A) Parkinson's disease
    B) Alcohol toxicity

C) Depletion of dopamine
D) Choices (A) and (C)

29. The type of language disorder that results from a lesion in the frontal lobe and is characterized by relatively good comprehension but decreased verbal output, effortful speaking, dysprosody, difficulty in performing verbal repetitions, poor oral reading and writing, and right hemiparesis is called:
    A) Broca's aphasia
    B) Wernicke's aphasia
    C) Conduction aphasia
    D) Global aphasia

30. Where can residue pool in the pharynx?
    A) In the buccal cavity
    B) In the vallecular space
    C) In the pyriform sinuses
    D) Choices (A) and (B), but not (C)
    E) Choices (B) and (C), but not (A)

31. What problem(s) may result from a prolonged oral phase of swallowing?
    A) Esophageal dysmotility
    B) Nasal regurgitation
    C) Gastroesophageal reflux
    D) Fatigue/disinterest/improper nutrition

32. Dysphagia is often seen in patients who have experienced a stroke. Consequently, it may be associated with:
    A) Dementia
    B) Dysarthria
    C) Apraxia
    D) All of the above

33. The supraglottic swallow occurs in the following sequential order:
    A) Deep breath held in inspiration, swallow, throat clearing, swallow, breath
    B) Breath, deep breath held in inspiration, Valsalva, swallow, throat clearing, swallow
    C) Breath, deep breath held in inspiration, Valsalva, throat clearing, swallow, swallow
    D) Swallow, throat clearing, breath, deep breath held in inspiration, swallow

34. The time it takes for propulsion of food through the pharynx is:
    A) 0.3 seconds
    B) 0.6 seconds
    C) 0.9 seconds
    D) 1.2 seconds

35. Which type of aphasia may be improved with melodic intonation therapy?
    A) Conduction aphasia
    B) Transcortical sensory aphasia
    C) Wernicke's aphasia
    D) Broca's aphasia

36. A 65-year-old male presents to the rehab clinic 2 weeks after an acute cerebrovascular accident (CVA). His wife says that the patient has had a lot of difficulty speaking since the stroke. On exam, the patient has poor comprehension, as well as poor repetition and fluency. His wife also mentions that he tries to communicate using his hands and facial expressions. Which type of aphasia does this patient most likely have?
    A) Wernicke's aphasia
    B) Broca's aphasia
    C) Global aphasia
    D) Conduction aphasia
    E) Anomic aphasia

37. A patient with a brain stem lesion is likely to experience all of the following **except**:
    A) Poor anterior-posterior transport of a food/liquid bolus
    B) Decreased masseter tension
    C) Wet hoarseness
    D) Rigidity

38. The main branch of the arterial system that feeds the anterior portion of the brain comes from:
    A) Vertebral artery
    B) Basilar artery
    C) Internal carotid artery
    D) Posterior carotid artery

39. Where is the pharyngeal stage of swallowing triggered?
    A) In the oral cavity
    B) Anterior to the epiglottis
    C) At the anterior faucial pillars
    D) In the esophagus

40. A modified barium swallow (MBS) study:
    A) Is conducted in two views
    B) Is only used with adult patients
    C) Utilizes magnetic fields
    D) Requires nasoendoscopy to perform

41. During a modified barium swallow procedure, penetration of the laryngeal vestibule would be considered an example of:
    A) Oral stage disorder
    B) Pharyngeal stage disorder
    C) Esophageal stage disorder
    D) None of the above

42. The chin-tuck maneuver offers all of the following benefits for patients with pharyngeal-phase dysphagia **except**:
    A) Widening the vallecula
    B) Reducing the airway opening
    C) Reducing the space between tongue base and posterior pharyngeal wall
    D) Tucking food underneath the tongue base

**43.** Aspiration is most likely to occur during which phase of swallowing:
   A) Oral
   B) Pharyngeal
   C) Proximal esophageal
   D) Distal esophageal

**44.** The compensatory response of chin tuck involves tilting the head to the paretic side.
   A) True
   B) False

**45.** An 81-year-old male presents to the emergency room with slurred speech and right-sided weakness. He eventually undergoes an MRI of the brain, which reveals abnormal signals in a left middle cerebral artery (MCA) distribution. On evaluation of his speech, it is found that the patient has intact comprehension. However, his repetition, naming, and fluency abilities are all impaired. Which type of aphasia does this patient most likely have?
   A) Wernicke's aphasia
   B) Broca's aphasia
   C) Global aphasia
   D) Conduction aphasia
   E) Anomic aphasia

**46.** A patient presents with inappropriate commenting, left field neglect, and reduced affect. This patient has recently suffered from a:
   A) Right hemispheric stroke
   B) Brain stem infarct
   C) Left hemispheric stroke
   D) Trauma to the temporal lobe

**47.** In cerebral palsy, the syndrome that impairs one leg and one arm on the same side of the body is:
   A) Spastic hemiplegia
   B) Spastic diplegia
   C) Spastic triplegia
   D) Spastic quadriplegia

**48.** The three phases of swallowing are:
   A) Oral, pharyngeal, esophageal
   B) Tracheal, nasal, pharyngeal
   C) Esophageal, tracheal, epiglottic
   D) Oral, tracheal, pulmonary

**49.** Which of the following is **not** useful in evaluating a patient with a swallowing disorder?
   A) Electroencephalogram (EEG)
   B) Stethoscope
   C) Fluoroscopy
   D) Calorie count

**50.** Oral dysphagia signs and symptoms do **not** include:
   A) Orofacial asymmetry
   B) Difficulty holding food/liquid in mouth
   C) Nasal regurgitation
   D) Anterior-posterior (AP) transport to faucial pillars

51. You are consulted for a 65-year-old woman 6 weeks after a new-onset stroke. She is still having difficulty swallowing and requires evaluation for a feeding tube. Her infarct most likely arises from the:
    A) Brain stem
    B) Pons
    C) Anterior cerebral artery
    D) Middle cerebral artery

52. Anomic aphasia is likely to occur from a lesion within any of the following areas of the brain **except**:
    A) Angular gyrus
    B) Second temporal gyrus
    C) Juncture of the temporal lobes
    D) Frontoparietal junction

53. Which of the following choices depicts the pharyngeal phase of swallowing in sequential order?
    A) Tongue elevation, soft palate elevation, laryngeal elevation, pharyngeal constriction, and cricopharyngeal relaxation
    B) Tongue elevation, soft palate elevation, pharyngeal constriction and cricopharyngeal relaxation, laryngeal elevation
    C) Tongue elevation, laryngeal elevation, soft palate elevation, pharyngeal constriction, and cricopharyngeal relaxation
    D) Tongue elevation, pharyngeal constriction and cricopharyngeal relaxation, soft palate elevation, laryngeal elevation

54. The type of speech pathology due to a motor disorder is called:
    A) Aphasia
    B) Dysphagia
    C) Dysarthria
    D) Dysphonia

55. Voluntary movement, intellect, and speech are located in the:
    A) Parietal lobe
    B) Frontal lobe
    C) Temporal lobe
    D) Occipital lobe

56. A nonprogressive disorder of motion and posture due to brain injury or insult that occurs during early brain growth is:
    A) Dystonia
    B) Cerebral palsy (CP)
    C) Ataxia
    D) Dyskinetic

57. A patient was brought to the emergency department after a sudden onset of difficulty speaking. A neurological exam indicated that the patient was experiencing a subcortical aphasia. This would indicate that the patient possibly experienced a lesion in the:
    A) Thalamus
    B) Precentral gyrus
    C) Postcentral gyrus
    D) Occipital lobe

58. Dysphagia treatment is **not** intended to:
    A) Prevent obesity
    B) Prevent aspiration
    C) Improve nutrition
    D) Improve hydration

59. Anterior-posterior bolus propulsion:
    A) Is based on adequate oral-pharyngeal muscle strength and intraoral pressure
    B) Relies on cranial nerve VII
    C) Can be seen on fiberoptic endoscopic evaluation of swallow (FEES) exam
    D) All of the above

60. The most accurate way to visualize structural changes in the pharynx brought on by reflux would be:
    A) Modified barium swallow
    B) Esophagram
    C) Fiberoptic endoscopic evaluation of swallow (FEES)
    D) Manometry

61. The term *paraphasia* refers to:
    A) Paraplegia of the facial muscles
    B) Partial dysphagia not meeting criteria for any of the main categories of aphasias
    C) Jargon or nonsense vocalizations, or nonverbal or combinations of syllables
    D) Pseudodysphagia

62. What is the most common direct cause of dysphagia?
    A) Delayed pharyngeal swallow
    B) Gastroesophageal reflux disease (GERD)
    C) Unilateral weakness in one or more muscles of mastication
    D) Facial droop with incomplete lip closure

63. The distinguishing feature of the super supraglottic swallow when compared with the supraglottic swallow is:
    A) The patient performs a Valsalva maneuver concomitantly
    B) The patient provides an extra cough at the beginning of the maneuver
    C) The patient tilts the head posteriorly allowing superior displacement of the epiglottis
    D) The patient tilts the head anteriorly allowing the bolus to pass superior to the epiglottis

64. Aphasia traditionally has been attributed to cortical lesions of the:
    A) Parietal lobe
    B) Occipital lobe
    C) Left hemisphere
    D) Cerebellum

65. The response elicited in a neurologically impaired patient when the sole of the foot is firmly scratched and the toes fan out is called:
    A) Babinski reflex
    B) Rooting reflex
    C) Moro reflex
    D) Cough reflex

66. The valve that divides the airway into upper and lower regions is the:
    A) Esophagus
    B) Trachea
    C) Larynx
    D) Epiglottis

67. When the head and the tail of the bolus do not pass through the pharyngeal segment cohesively, this is:
    A) Cervical auscultation
    B) Piecemeal swallow
    C) Esophageal dysmotility
    D) A problem with mastication

68. What is the primary reason a person would require a jejunostomy?
    A) Surgeon's choice
    B) Religious reasons
    C) Uncontrolled reflux
    D) Tracheal penetration

69. In conducting an oral facial exam on a cleft palate infant, which would be of **least** concern regarding his or her feeding ability?
    A) Respiratory function
    B) Rooting reflex
    C) Bite reflex
    D) Hearing ability

70. Which of the following represents a nonfluent type of aphasia?
    A) Wernicke's aphasia
    B) Broca's aphasia
    C) Anomic aphasia
    D) Conduction aphasia

71. Which of the following is **not** a predictor of aspiration on bedside swallowing exam?
    A) Decreased pharyngeal peristalsis
    B) Dysphonia
    C) Dysarthria
    D) Cough or voice change after swallow

72. The benefits of the videofluoroscopic evaluation include:
    A) Diagnostic indications
    B) Therapeutic indications
    C) Choices (A) and (B)
    D) None of the above

73. In some cases, aphasia may:
    A) Progress owing to recurrent neurogenic pathology
    B) Be a static condition
    C) Be further influenced by coexisting medical problems
    D) Be all of the above

74. The specific aphasic symptom of lexical (word) retrieval deficit seen in patients is known as:
    A) Jargon
    B) Dyslexia
    C) Amnesia
    D) Anomia

75. Aphasia is a disorder of:
    A) Speech
    B) Language
    C) Both speech and language
    D) Swallowing

76. The procedure whereby the stomach is pulled up around the lower esophageal sphincter to control acid reflux is called:
    A) Esophageal dilation
    B) Gastrostomy
    C) Jejunostomy
    D) Fundoplication

77. A disordered narrowing of the esophagus is known as:
    A) Diverticulum
    B) Fistula
    C) Achalasia
    D) Sphincter

78. What is the **least** relevant factor when evaluating a patient suspected of having dysphagia?
    A) Cognitive disorder
    B) Cranial nerve VII deficit
    C) Cranial nerve I deficit
    D) Dysarthria

79. Which part of the brain is responsible for the interpretation of sensory information and proprioception?
    A) Frontal lobe
    B) Parietal lobe
    C) Temporal lobe
    D) Occipital lobe

80. What nerve innervates the muscles of mastication?
    A) Facial
    B) Laryngeal
    C) Vagus
    D) Trigeminal

81. The major voluntary pathway for speech, as well as all voluntary movement, is:
    A) Corticocerebellar tract
    B) Autonomic nervous system
    C) Pyramidal system
    D) Peripheral nervous system

82. The upper motor neuron consists of:
    A) Corticopontine, corticobulbar, and corticospinal fibers
    B) Cranial and spinal nerves
    C) Both of the above

83. Aphasia may be seen in:
    A) Adults
    B) Children
    C) Persons across the lifespan

84. With right-sided weakness that accompanies a left hemispheric stroke, what maneuver can be employed to prevent pooling of food or liquid in the right pyriform sinus?
    A) Chin tuck
    B) Mendelsohn maneuver
    C) Head turn to the right
    D) Head turn to the left

85. What can a person with apraxia for swallowing do to help improve the process of eating?
    A) Be fed small boluses by the speech-language pathologist or direct care provider
    B) Restrict the amount of salt used
    C) Use a swallowing maneuver called *effortful swallow*
    D) Feed themselves without listening to a lot of verbal directions

86. Esophageal dysphagia signs and symptoms do **not** include:
    A) Feeling of globus
    B) Heartburn
    C) Quick feeling of fullness
    D) Wet vocal quality

87. Oral-phase dysphagia may be a result of which of the following?
    A) Facial weakness
    B) Poor lingual control
    C) Choices (A) and (B)
    D) None of the above

88. Which nerve is responsible for salivation?
    A) Maxillary nerve
    B) Mandibular nerve
    C) Facial nerve
    D) Lingual nerve

# *Speech*

## ANSWERS

1. **B)** These symptoms describe the condition called *transcortical sensory aphasia*, a disorder that results from a lesion within the posterior aspect of the speech zone in the temporal lobe. Because such patients display disordered verbal abilities, marked by echolalia and paraphasias, it is considered a fluent type of aphasia.

2. **C)** Clonus occurs in cases of upper motor neuron (UMN) disease where muscles become spastic owing to increased tone. Athetosis is a slow writhing type of motion associated with damage to the basal ganglia. Fasciculations are small local, involuntary muscle contractions that may be visible under the skin. A tremor is an involuntary, somewhat rhythmic, muscle contraction involving to-and-fro movements of one or more body parts. It is differentiated from clonus by the fact that a tremor may occur without being elicited by holding a muscle or tendon in extension.

3. **D)** Swallowing disorders affect a wide range of people in different situations. It can occur throughout the lifespan, from infancy to advanced age.

4. **D)** Apraxia is a motor planning problem that results from a left anterior stroke in the frontal lobe. The result, depending on severity, is difficulty in planning the motor sequences needed for verbal speech (verbal apraxia), oral motor movements (oral apraxia, which could include apraxia for swallowing), as well as voluntary movements of the extremities (limb apraxia).

5. **D)** This phenomenon can occur when esophageal motility is affected. It may be due to poor sphincter control at the distal end of the esophagus, resulting in back flow, or due to a narrowing of the esophageal lumen. It is different from reflux in that the material that flows back has not initially entered the stomach and thus has not been mixed with stomach acids.

6. **D)** Thinned liquids would further decrease the time taken for the substance to pass through the pharyngeal musculature before the swallow reflex goes into effect.

7. **D)** FLASH-MRI is best for speech, tongue movements, and swallowing motion with multiple images able to be captured quickly at low angles. Although it is helpful in delineation of soft tissues, ultrasound can only capture the region of the tongue posterior to the hyoid level. Scintigraphy is not as useful in pharyngeal swallowing disorders as MRI. It may be useful in quantitative and qualitative evaluation of esophageal motility disorders and gastroesophageal reflux disease (GERD). However, these conditions are often best evaluated with manometry.

8. **C)** The nonfluent aphasias are Broca's, global, transcortical motor, and mixed transcortical. In transcortical motor, repetition can be intact. In mixed transcortical, there may be some comprehension, but repetition may be impaired (making it a nonfluent aphasia). The fluent aphasias are Wernicke's, conduction, anomia, and transcortical sensory. In transcortical sensory, there is no comprehension ability. Unlike Wernicke's aphasia, however, repetition is intact, making it a fluent aphasia.

9. **D)** Explanation: In conduction aphasia, comprehension and fluency are intact, but repetition and naming are impaired. This type of aphasia is commonly caused by damage to the arcuate fasciculus, which connects the Broca's and Wernicke's areas. As such, one would expect to see components from both Wernicke's and Broca's aphasia. The most common cause of this type of aphasia is a CVA, but can also be found in patients with traumatic brain injuries or brain tumors.

10. **C)** These symptoms describe the condition called *transcortical motor aphasia*, a disorder that results from a lesion within the anterior aspect of the speech zone in the frontal lobe. Because of the dysprosody and effortful speech that the patient exhibits, it is considered a nonfluent type of aphasia.

11. **B)** Persons with Huntington's disease often display psychiatric conditions as the first manifestation of their illness. Sometimes psychosis develops and depression is common. Movements may appear fidgety, but ultimately a choreoathetoid movement disorder develops. Speech rate and loudness become variable, and articulation becomes increasingly imprecise (hyperkinetic dysarthria).

12. **D)** In addition to these physical movements, the velopharyngeal port closes to prevent nasal regurgitation of food and the upper esophageal sphincter relaxes to allow movement of the bolus into the esophagus. All these things occur in the space of a single second, upon the triggering of the pharyngeal swallow stage with the passage of the bolus by the faucial pillars.

13. **C)** Typically, when a healthy individual inadvertently passes material into the trachea, a cough reflex is triggered. However, in some people who lack sensory awareness, the passage of food or liquid past the glottis into the trachea does not trigger a cough, which is the body's protective mechanism to rid itself of possible aspirant. As a result, a silent aspiration can occur.

14. **D)** The subcortical region of the brain (known as the *basal ganglia*) is also known as the *indirect activation pathway*, meaning that it is responsible for the proximal muscles of the body that control such things as tone and posture. Persons with basal ganglia problems may experience both postural instabilities (standing or sitting upright) as well as muscle tone issues (including hypertonicity) that can lead to muscle rigidity. Tongue rigidity can affect how well a person moves the bolus in an anterior-posterior direction.

15. **B)** There are three phases of swallowing: the oral phase, the pharyngeal phase, and the esophageal phase. Pharyngeal-phase dysphagia is the most common. It is usually the shortest phase with the least amount of time for compensation or correction, yet it requires the most precise coordination from multiple muscle groups. It is most often appreciated on physical exam by a wet, gurgly voice with coughing. Answer choice (C) is not considered a separate phase of swallowing.

16. **A)** Agents that are water soluble often are highly osmolar. This property leaves them highly susceptible for causing pulmonary edema if accidentally aspirated into the lungs.

17. **B)** Global aphasia describes the most severe form of language deficits in which both written and spoken language are impaired. It often involves both Broca's and Wernicke's areas and spans over both anterior and posterior regions of the brain. The MCA is the only vessel of the four answer choices that affects both anterior and posterior regions of the cerebrum, and is often associated with global aphasia.

18. **E)** Anomic aphasia is characterized by an individual's inability to find the particular words that they would like to say. Patients will commonly say vague words in place of the words they are

trying to think of. They usually have the most trouble with nouns and verbs. Anomia is viewed as one of the more mild types of aphasia as comprehension, fluency, repetition and reading ability are all preserved. Patients usually have the same difficulty findings words while writing. Most types of aphasia have some component of anomia.

19. **C)** The border zone refers to a region of the cortex that takes in Broca's area in the frontal lobe and Wernicke's area in the temporal lobe, as well as the arcuate fasciculus (a connecting bundle of association fibers that joins the two). Damage within that zone could result in either transcortical motor aphasia (more anterior lesion) or transcortical sensory aphasia (more posterior lesion).

20. **C)** The arcuate fasciculus is a neural association pathway that connects Broca's area in the frontal lobe to Wernicke's area in the temporal lobe. As such the patient with this condition can generally understand routine conversational interactions and demonstrate good comprehension, but has word-finding problems marked by pausing and hesitations. In addition, this patient may exhibit poor spelling as well as poor writing skills.

21. **C)** The average time it takes for a healthy person to clear the food through the esophagus is between 8 and 20 seconds.

22. **A)** The valleculae are visualized in the lateral aspect during an MBS study, whereas the pyriform sinuses are visualized in the anteroposterior view. The nasopharyngeal port can be similarly viewed when the patient is positioned in the lateral aspect. The MBS procedure is not designed, nor is it sufficiently sensitive, to view the nasal sinuses.

23. **D)** Swallowing is the physical ability we possess to sense the texture, taste, and temperature of foods and liquids that are introduced into our mouths so that we can then perform the proper motoric movements necessary to chew and/or otherwise prepare the bolus before swallowing it. It includes both motor and sensory functions, both of which are controlled by the upper and lower motor neurons of the neurological system.

24. **C)** The Mendelsohn maneuver involves holding a swallow midway for 3 to 5 seconds before completing the swallow. This allows more complete cricopharyngeal relaxation, improving pharyngeal clearance in patients with incomplete relaxation or premature closing of the cricopharyngeus. Choice (A), performing Valsalva maneuver and subsequent throat clearing in between swallows, is part of the super supraglottic swallow technique. Choices (A) and (B) are useful for patients with pharyngeal-phase dysphagia owing to reduced laryngeal closure. In choice (D), rotating the head to the weaker side before swallowing also aids patients with pharyngeal-phase dysphagia, but it is most helpful when the problem is specifically due to delayed swallow reflex, not incomplete cricopharyngeal relaxation.

25. **A)** The cricopharyngeus muscle is an inferior pharyngeal constrictor. It is unique in that it constricts as the other muscles of the inferior pharynx relax. It is the only muscle serving as a closed mechanism to prevent esophageal reflux into the pharynx.

26. **B)** The greatest level of improvement in patients with aphasia occurs in the first 2 to 3 months after the onset. By 6 months, there is a significant drop in the rate of recovery. The majority of cases of patients with aphasia do not recover spontaneously after 1 year.

27. **A)** Wernicke's aphasia is a type of fluent aphasia where fluency is intact but comprehension is impaired. Wernicke's area is usually located in the posterior superior temporal gyrus. Similar to Broca's area, it is also supplied by the middle cerebral artery (MCA).

28. **D)** Hypokinetic dysarthria is the motor speech problem typically seen in patients who suffer from Parkinson's disease. This results directly from a depletion of dopamine in the substantia nigra of the basal ganglia. The disease is characterized by bradykinesia or akinesia, rigidity, tremors, and a loss of postural reflexes. Patients characteristically have a "masked" and inexpressive face. Their speech is hypokinetic (less articulatory movement), monotone, and monoloud.

29. **A)** Typically the result of damage to the frontal lobe of the left hemisphere, this nonfluent type of aphasia is marked by all the symptoms noted, as well as (possibly) an accompanying motor speech problem, such as apraxia or dysarthria. Both Wernicke's and conduction aphasia are considered fluent types of aphasia, as the site of lesion is more posterior in the brain and so articulation is generally intact. Global aphasia often results from more diffuse types of lesions and usually affects both comprehension and production.

30. **E)** Both the valleculae and the pyriform sinuses are regions within the pharynx where residue can accumulate if the patient is not able to pass the bolus cohesively. Although food may also pool in the buccal cavities or cheeks, this is considered part of the oral cavity, not the pharynx.

31. **D)** Both esophageal dysmotility and gastroesophageal reflux occur during the final stage of swallowing, not the first (oral) stage. In addition, nasal regurgitation would occur if the velopharyngeal port does not properly close off the nasopharynx during the second (pharyngeal) stage of swallowing. Food remaining too long in the oral cavity may lead to fatigue, as well as disinterest on the part of the patient to continue with his or her meal. Thus, improper nutrition may result.

32. **D)** Both dysarthria and apraxia (motor speech disorders) may occur in cases of stroke. Furthermore, a person who has had multiple strokes may suffer from dementia. Swallowing problems are quite prevalent in the neurologically impaired patient.

33. **A)** The supraglottic swallow is composed of five main sequential steps: the patient holds a deep breath, swallows, clears the throat, then swallows again, before resuming breathing. This allows the minimal amount of time possible for airway opening to reduce the risk of aspiration. Choices (B) and (C) include Valsalva, which is characteristic of a super supraglottic swallow.

34. **B)** Propulsion of a bolus of food through the pharynx during the pharyngeal phase of swallowing takes 0.6 seconds. If this function is slowed or delayed, there is increased exposure of the bolus to the larynx and therefore increased chance of aspiration through the laryngeal opening.

35. **D)** Melodic intonation therapy recruits the right hemisphere for communication by incorporating melodies or rhythms with simple statements. It is helpful in patients with nonfluent aphasia. Broca's aphasia is the only answer choice that describes a nonfluent aphasia.

36. **C)** Global aphasia is a severe type of aphasia affecting both fluency and comprehension. It usually results from damage to multiple speech areas of the brain, including Wernicke's area and Broca's area. Patients commonly have difficulty reading and writing but may be able to communicate through hand gestures and facial expressions.

37. **D)** Brain stem lesions will affect the function of cranial nerves, which, in turn, control such things as chewing, bolus movement, and swallowing. Muscle rigidity, on the other hand, is typically associated with either an upper motor neuron lesion in the cortex or damage to the basal ganglia, a subcortical structure.

38. **C)** The two internal carotid arteries each branch off into the anterior and middle cerebral arteries. The two vertebral arteries join together in the ventral brain stem to form the basilar artery, and then split again to form the posterior vertebral arteries.

39. **C)** As the food bolus leaves the oral cavity and moves backward, it must pass the faucial pillars (where tonsils are located). This region contains sensory receptors that detect the presence of the bolus, which sets into motion a chain of events that result in the bolus moving through the pharynx and entering the esophagus.

40. **A)** A patient is viewed in both the lateral and anteroposterior fields to get a good sense of how well they are able to swallow. The two fields allow for better visualization of anatomical structures that provide the clinician with useful information regarding the tolerance the patient exhibits for the different food and liquid consistencies provided.

41. **B)** Pooling or penetration of the bolus above the glottis is considered a pharyngeal stage problem of swallowing. If left unchecked, penetration may lead to aspiration, which is migration of the bolus past the glottis and into the trachea itself.

42. **D)** The chin-tuck maneuver provides several mechanical advantages for the patient with pharyngeal-phase dysphagia. It widens the vallecula, allowing the bolus to rest there while the reflex is triggered. It reduces the airway opening. Finally, it reduces the space between tongue base and posterior pharyngeal wall, therefore increasing pharyngeal pressure to more effectively propel the bolus through the pharynx.

43. **B)** During the pharyngeal phase of swallowing, breathing is interrupted and the laryngeal opening is exposed. The laryngeal opening is protected by the folding of the epiglottis, the closure of the vocal cords, and elevation and anterior displacement of the larynx. Dysfunction at any of these locations results in risk of aspiration.

44. **B)** Rotating the head to the paretic side closes the ipsilateral pharynx, forces the bolus into the contralateral pharynx, and decreases cricopharyngeal pressures. Head tilt, on the other hand, involves side bending to guide the bolus into the ipsilateral pharynx with gravity. The question describes the compensatory response of head tilt. Chin tuck involves forward flexion of the neck, widening the vallecula, and reducing the chance of aspiration.

45. **B)** Broca's aphasia is a type of expressive, or nonfluent, aphasia and is most commonly caused by a cerebrovascular accident (CVA). The Broca's area in the brain is usually located in the left lateral frontal lobe, which is supplied mainly by the MCA. Patients will have difficulty constructing complete sentences, and commonly become frustrated as comprehension remains intact but they have difficulty speaking coherently. Treatment includes intensive speech therapy starting as soon as possible. Most recovery occurs within 4 weeks of the CVA.

46. **A)** Whereas the left hemisphere is considered the language hemisphere for the majority of all individuals, the right hemisphere is considered the center for visuospatial orientation and constructional skills. Right hemisphere brain damage (RHBD) results in a variety of symptoms, as noted, although on the surface an overt language problem that compromises the ability of the patient to speak in a grammatically correct manner is not one of them. Rather, they may exhibit a lack of awareness concerning their subtle problems in social interactions, have difficulty navigating their way around a room, and do poorly on drawing tasks.

47. **A)** Hemiplegia refers to one symmetrical half of the body, either the left or the right side. Diplegia affects all four extremities, but the legs are more affected than the arms or hands. Triplegia involves three extremities, usually both legs and one arm. Quadriplegia affects the entire body, including the trunk and all four extremities.

48. **A)** When we eat, food is formed into a bolus, which must then pass through the oral, pharyngeal, and esophageal cavities before depositing into the stomach.

49. **A)** An EEG measures brain activity, but not what happens during the course of normal or disordered swallowing. A stethoscope can be used to perform cervical auscultation at the throat while a person is swallowing to hear the quality of the swallowing event. A fluoroscope can be used during a modified barium swallow procedure. A speech-language pathologist may recommend a calorie count over 3 days to determine how much food a patient consumes by mouth.

50. **C)** Orofacial asymmetry may result from left or right hemiparesis secondary to a stroke, which is an indication that the mouth may be incapable of holding food or liquid intraorally; both are oral stage signs of dysphagia. AP transport is the movement of the food or liquid back to the threshold of the throat at the faucial pillar region, another sign of oral stage dysphagia. Nasal regurgitation results from poor velopharyngeal closure that allows the bolus, after coughing, to shoot upward and enter the nasal cavity posteriorly—a sign of pharyngeal stage dysphagia.

51. **A)** Patients with dysphagia from a unilateral stroke usually improve rapidly within the first few weeks after the onset of symptoms. Only ~2% of patients still have difficulty at 1 month post-stroke. However, patients with brain stem strokes may progress more slowly and require tube feeding. A patient with continued difficulty feeding or swallowing more than 4 weeks after a stroke is likely to have undergone damage to the brain stem.

52. **D)** This variety of fluent aphasia may be caused by lesions in one or more different regions of the *temporaparietal junction?* brain, including the angular gyrus, the second temporal gyrus, or at the juncture of the temporal lobes. With this type of language disorder, a patient is typically unable to verbalize the names of objects. However, the condition does allow most other language functions aside from naming to remain intact, such as auditory comprehension. Therefore, the frontoparietal junction, which is involved in auditory comprehension, would not likely be affected.

53. **A)** Soft palate elevations, also seen in the oral phase of swallowing and velopharyngeal port closure, serve to close off the nasal cavity and prevent regurgitation into the nasopharynx. Laryngeal elevation with folding of epiglottis and vocal cord adduction works to prevent aspiration. Coordinated pharyngeal constriction and cricopharyngeal in the upper esophageal sphincter relaxation facilitate bolus transport into the esophagus.

54. **C)** Dysarthria is a speech disorder owing to the motor efferent pathway of speech production. Aphasia, on the other hand, is a speech disorder owing to the cognitive pathway of speech production that involves processing of language. Dysphagia refers to a swallowing disorder, and dysphonia represents inability to produce sounds with tone regardless of whether those sounds are words with meaning. Often a patient with dysphonia will present with a hoarse voice.

55. **B)** It has long been known that different regions of the brain are responsible for different functions. The frontal lobe is known as the motor cortex. As such, it is responsible for voluntary movements, as well as intellect and speech-language. The parietal lobe is the sensory cortex, the temporal lobe is the auditory cortex, and the occipital lobe is the visual cortex.

56. **B)** Cerebral palsy may result from lack of oxygen to the brain and can manifest as spastic CP if the cortical region of the brain is affected, athetoid CP if the basal ganglia is affected, or ataxic CP if the cerebellum is affected.

57. **A)** The thalamus is a subcortical structure, located in the diencephalon at the top of the brain stem. Both precentral and postcentral gyri are located adjacent to the central sulcus on the surface of the cortex, whereas the occipital lobe is located in the posterior aspect of the cortex.

58. **A)** Helping a person improve their swallowing ability is helping to ensure good health. In no way is it intended to keep a person from becoming overweight. Dysphagia treatment helps a person to learn how to swallow safely and to prevent aspiration events, while ensuring good nutrition and hydration.

59. **A)** To swallow, a person must move the bolus from a forward to backward position. The VII (facial) cranial nerve, while it has both a sensory and motor component, is not responsible for bolus movement. The oral cavity cannot be viewed on a FEES examination, as only the pharyngeal stage of swallowing is visualized (based on the positioning of the probe).

60. **C)** The FEES test allows the examiner to view the larynx from a position above the glottis. The test can assess for spillage into the glottal opening, pooling in the vallecular space or pyriforms, or reflux back up from the esophagus. A modified barium swallow and an esophagram are procedures done in an x-ray suite and allow the examiner a radiologic view of barium traces. Manometry is a procedure whereby any narrowing of the esophageal lumen can be made wider through tube and balloon manipulation.

61. **C)** The definition of paraphasia is a group of jargon or nonsense vocalizations, or nonverbal or combinations of syllables. This pattern of speech often presents in patients with Wernicke's aphasia.

62. **A)** The most common cause of dysphagia occurs during the pharyngeal phase of swallowing. Choices (C) and (D) occur during the oral phase of swallowing, and choice (B) occurs at the esophageal level.

63. **A)** The super supraglottic swallow is designed to close the entrance to the airway voluntarily by tilting the arytenoid cartilage anteriorly to the base of the epiglottis before and during the swallow. Bearing down helps to tilt the arytenoid anteriorly and close the entrance to the airway earlier in the swallowing sequence. This strategy is used in patients with reduced closure of the airway entrance, such as those who have undergone a supraglottic laryngectomy. The supraglottic swallow, on the other hand, uses holding of the breath without adding Valsalva. This technique may be used in patients whose vocal folds may or may not achieve full closure.

64. **C)** The left hemisphere is traditionally viewed as the language center of the brain. When lesions occur in the left hemisphere, the result could be different types of aphasia spanning a continuum from nonfluent to fluent, based on site of lesion. The frontal lobe itself is associated with voluntary movements in the body, which includes speech production. If a lesion were to occur there, a particular type of aphasia may result from among the nonfluent varieties. But in general, any aphasia that occurs in a patient population would be the direct result of cortical damage to the left hemisphere.

65. **A)** The Babinski reflex is typically seen in infants. This reflex diminishes over time through cortical control arising from progressive myelinization of the corticospinal tract. This reemergent reflex is associated with upper motor neuron (UMN) lesions.

66. **C)** The larynx divides the airway into upper and lower regions. Any condition that affects the functionality of the larynx may result in either swallowing problems, voice problems, or both. The trachea is the airway that actually extends from the larynx inferiorly to the lungs. The esophagus is the tube that carries nutrition to the stomach. The epiglottis, which is part of the larynx, serves a protective function by folding over the vocal fold area during swallowing to protect the airway from infiltration.

67. **B)** Piecemeal refers to the noncohesive manner in which people sometimes swallow food and liquid. It may take them several attempts, gulp after gulp after gulp, before what they have put into their mouths has been completely cleared.

68. **C)** A J-tube, or jejunostomy, is required when a person has uncontrolled reflux and poor absorption of stomach contents. The J-tube bypasses the stomach lining and introduces tube feedings directly into the jejunum to aid in nutritional absorption.

69. **D)** A hearing impairment would not affect the feeding ability of a child (with or without cleft palate). On the other hand, it would be essential to assess its rooting and bite reflexes, as these contribute greatly to how a child takes nourishment orally. Furthermore, it would be very important to track that child's respiratory function, if simply to determine that the child is not aspirating on foods and liquids while feeding.

70. **B)** Nonfluent aphasia differs from fluent in that the patient is unable to connect words and sentences in a smooth, fluid manner. Broca's aphasia is an injury to the third frontal convolution of the left, or language dominant, hemisphere (Broca's area). The speech of these patients is characteristically disconnected and "broken" with many occurrences of the patient not being able to remember the words he or she is trying to say. Another nonfluent aphasia is global aphasia, in which the patient is marked by deficits in both comprehension and production of language and usually is affected by lesions involving both Broca's and Wernicke's areas. The other answer choices all represent fluent aphasias. Wernicke's aphasia produces deficits in auditory comprehension, with produced words mixed with jargon or nonsense syllabic combinations called *paraphasias*. Anomic aphasia presents with a patient unable to produce the names of objects, but has intact auditory comprehension.

71. **A)** Decreased pharyngeal peristalsis can be reliably diagnosed on videofluoroscopic swallowing study (VFSS). All of the other answer choices can be appreciated on physical exam. In contrast to the other answer choices, decreased pharyngeal peristalsis can actually protect against aspiration by giving the airway more time to close. Voice changes (either wet or gurgling) can increase the suspicion for aspiration.

72. **C)** The videofluoroscopic evaluation is a radiographic tool used to diagnose causes of swallowing disorders. Food particles mixed with barium are swallowed as x-ray imaging of the process is obtained. Because the images are moving (and therefore able to evaluate function), the evaluation can be therapeutic as well. A speech pathologist can work with the physiatrist to try different compensatory maneuvers by the patient and see immediate results of the efforts recorded by the radiologist. Alternative sizes and textures of foods can be trialed during the procedure. In this way, the videofluoroscopic evaluation can be both diagnostic and therapeutic.

73. **D)** Aphasia is the language disorder that results from damage in the left hemisphere of the brain. The condition can remain unchanged, worsen in the face of additional neurogenic or medical conditions, or improve with medical and therapeutic intervention.

74. **D)** Anomia comes from Latin, which means "no name." Jargon is a different speech characteristic that is marked by excessive, nonsensical verbiage. Dyslexia is a reading disorder. Amnesia is a generalized loss of memory for people, places, and things.

75. **B)** Following a stroke or brain injury, a person may undergo dramatic changes in how they are able to communicate. Aphasia is the language-based disorder that may occur as a result of such neurological events. Speech disorders, on the other hand, are considered different types of ailments, where either the planning centers for formulating the correct sequence of movements to

form speech sounds (phonemes) are hampered (known as the *motor speech disorder of apraxia*), or the different subsystems that combine to create verbal speech (the respiratory, phonatory, resonatory, and articulatory systems) are unable to complete the tasks that are programmed, resulting in the motor-speech disorder of dysarthria. Dysphagia is a swallowing disorder.

76. **D)** Dilation is performed to help increase the lumen of the esophageal tube, whereas gastrostomy and jejunostomy procedures are performed to help provide nutrition to a patient nonorally. Fundoplication is a surgical procedure employed to help control severe reflux.

77. **C)** A diverticulum does not describe narrowing—it is an outpocketing of the esophagus where small bolus particles may accumulate. A fistula is an opening between two structures (the esophagus and the trachea). A sphincter is a ring of muscles that opens and/or closes the top and bottom ends of the esophagus.

78. **C)** The first cranial nerve is the olfactory nerve, a sensory nerve responsible for our sense of smell. Although it may be a benefit to smell our food before or while eating it, it does not contribute to a swallowing problem. Cognitive problems, problems with cranial nerve VII (facial nerve), and dysarthria (a motor-speech problem that results from neurological problems) all may contribute to a swallowing problem.

79. **B)** The cerebrum can be spatially organized into lobes on the basis of the function each provides. The frontal lobe is responsible for voluntary motor function. The parietal lobe allows interpretation of sensory information and proprioception. The temporal lobe provides long-term memory storage, and the occipital lobe interprets visual information.

80. **D)** The mandibular division of the trigeminal nerve controls the muscles of mastication, which is involved in the oral phase of swallowing. These muscles include the temporalis, masseter, and medial and lateral pterygoids. The mandibular division also sends fibers to the tensor veli palatini muscle, which tenses the palate.

81. **C)** The pyramidal system includes the corticopontine, corticobulbar, and corticospinal pathways. This pathway provides the network of neural connections necessary to ensure that communication between the speech planning centers in the frontal lobe is relayed to the various subsystems of speech to create a verbal message. Those subsystems include the respiratory, phonatory, resonatory, and articulatory subsystems.

82. **A)** The upper motor neuron (UMN) is associated with the central nervous system that structurally includes the brain and spinal cord, or neuraxis. The pathways indicated help to create the neural connections between the cortex and pons, medulla oblongata, and spinal cord. The UMN is the first-order neuron, meaning that it functions to plan out and organize the instructions needed to carry out voluntary movements seen in speech, swallowing, or limb motion. The cranial and spinal nerves are part of the peripheral nervous system, which comprises the lower motor neuron (LMN). The LMN is considered the second-order neuron, which actually carries out the commands sent to it by the UMN.

83. **C)** Aphasia, the language deficit that results from cortical damage to the speech-language centers of the brain, may affect persons both young and old. Unfortunately, there is no protection against the devastation that is wrought by such a condition on the basis of one's age.

84. **C)** Advances in swallow therapy over the years have shown the benefit of having patients with right hemiparesis turn their heads to the weaker side (in this case, the right) to prevent food buildup that could cause penetration and/or aspiration if left unchecked.

85. **D)** Apraxia is a disorder in motor planning, not motor execution. This implies that a person can follow through on motor movements as long as the patient is not thinking about what they are doing. If the movement required for completion of the task (eg, chewing) becomes a conscious thought and no longer an automatic one, the patient may begin to stumble and/or grope about and be unable to complete the motoric sequence.

86. **D)** A wet vocal quality is indicative of bolus pooling in the vicinity of the glottis, or vocal fold region (a pharyngeal stage sign of dysphagia). Globus, or the sensation of food being stuck, is usually reported by patients to occur in an area that is actually not the true location of the material. Heartburn, or reflux, is the feeling that patients report when stomach contents spill back into the esophagus and cause a burning sensation. The feeling of fullness that some patients report long before the meal is over is due to a narrowing of the esophageal lumen that causes food and liquid to build up in the esophageal column.

87. **C)** Oral-phase dysphagia can arise from facial weakness, poor lingual control, or both. Several compensation mechanisms can be taught in therapy for this condition. For facial weakness, food texture can be modified and food can be placed at the back of the mouth or on the stronger side of the face. The head can also be tilted toward the stronger side. Sucking/blowing exercises may be helpful. Electromyogram (EMG) biofeedback performed by the physician may be helpful as well. For poor lingual control, tongue active range of motion and strengthening can be prescribed. Precise articulation should be encouraged in conjunction with this technique.

88. **C)** The facial nerve, cranial nerve (CN) VII, is responsible for activation of the salivary glands. The branches of CN VII that innervate the salivary glands are general visceral efferent nerves that carry parasympathetic fibers to the submandibular and sublingual glands. The maxillary and mandibular nerves are branches of CN V, the trigeminal nerve. The lingual nerve is a branch of the mandibular nerve, providing sensation to the tongue. During the oral phase of swallowing, insufficient or overproduction of saliva can cause problems with the swallowing sequence.

# Neuromuscular Disorders

1. Which of the following pharmacologic agents is a first-line treatment for spasticity in patients with amyotrophic lateral sclerosis (ALS)?
   A) Tizanidine
   B) Dantrolene
   C) Benzodiazepine
   D) Baclofen

2. A 4-year-old boy is brought into your office because his mother has noticed that he has difficulty getting up from a seated position on the floor while playing with his toys. On physical exam, there is increased gastrocnemius calf circumference bilaterally. You think the child may have dystrophic myopathy. The maneuver the child performs to assist him in standing is caused by:
   A) Proximal leg weakness
   B) Distal leg weakness
   C) Proximal arm weakness
   D) Distal arm weakness

3. In central core disease, all of the following may be present **except**:
   A) Floppy infant
   B) Congenital hip dislocation
   C) Mitochondria present on muscle biopsy
   D) Association with malignant hyperthermia

4. A common side effect of anti-Parkinson's drugs (eg, Sinemet, Requip) is:
   A) Facial flushing
   B) Erectile dysfunction
   C) Tachycardia
   D) Postural hypotension

5. Of the following choices, which is **not** a major problem affecting activities of daily living (ADLs) reported by multiple sclerosis (MS) patients?
   A) Sensory disturbance
   B) Fatigue
   C) Balance difficulties
   D) Weakness

6. Which of the following statements regarding constraint-induced movement therapy (CIMT) is true?
   A) It requires constraint of the affected extremity
   B) It is based on principles of repeated practice and intense activity
   C) It utilizes a passive nonintensive approach
   D) It aims to increase the use of the unaffected extremity

ANSWERS TO THIS SECTION CAN BE FOUND ON PAGE 139

7. Which of the following is **not** used in the treatment of multiple sclerosis (MS)?
   A) Corticosteroids
   B) Interferon beta
   C) Glatiramer acetate
   D) Rituximab

8. Which of the following statements regarding Duchenne muscular dystrophy is true?
   A) Usually diagnosed by age 5 years
   B) X-linked recessive condition
   C) Patients generally lose the ability to ambulate at 8 to 12 years of age
   D) All of the above

9. In myasthenia gravis (MG), early monitoring of which of the following can help prognosticate?
   A) Exertion-related fatigue
   B) Spirometry
   C) Response to edrophonium
   D) Onset of diplopia

10. Amyotrophic lateral sclerosis (ALS) is a lesion of:
    A) Upper motor neurons
    B) Lower motor neurons
    C) Upper and lower motor neuron
    D) The neuromuscular junction

11. Duchenne muscular dystrophy (DMD) is a disorder of:
    A) Dystrophin
    B) Axon
    C) Myelin
    D) Schwann cells

12. Parkinson's disease is characterized by which of the following tremors?
    A) Intention tremor
    B) Resting tremor
    C) Essential tremor
    D) Myoclonus

13. A 12-year-old male presents to your office with difficulty walking. The patient's mother says that over the last few months, he has had three falls owing to losing his balance while walking. His past medical history is positive for diabetes mellitus and scoliosis. On physical exam, you notice weakness in both the upper and lower extremities, as well as absent deep tendon reflexes. Which of the following diseases is the most likely diagnosis?
    A) Amyotrophic lateral sclerosis (ALS)
    B) Friedreich's ataxia
    C) Ataxia telangiectasia
    D) Fazio-Londe disease

14. Which of the following motor neuron diseases has the best prognosis?
    A) Kugelberg-Welander disease
    B) Chronic Werdnig-Hoffmann disease

C) Werdnig-Hoffmann disease

D) Both (B) and (C), as their clinical course is similar

15. Symptoms of botulism present how soon after spore ingestion?

A) 1 hour

B) 2 to 4 hours

C) 1 day

D) 1 month

16. All of the following are clinical features of facioscapulohumeral dystrophy (FSHD) **except**:

A) Inability to extend the wrist

B) Inability to whistle

C) Deltoid muscle weakness

D) Protruding shoulder blades

17. Parkinson's disease can be effectively medically treated with all of the following **except**:

A) L-Dopa

B) Dopamine receptor agonist

C) Dopamine receptor antagonist

D) Anticholinergic agents

18. The following are all common symptoms in patients with multiple sclerosis (MS), **except**:

A) Bowel/bladder dysfunction

B) Decreased IQ

C) Pain

D) Fatigue

19. Neuroplasticity is a concept that refers to all of the following **except**:

A) The potential ability of the central nervous system (CNS) to modify its structural and functional organization

B) Partial recovery is possible long after sustaining a brain injury

C) The brain remains capable of changing in response to experience and injury

D) Insult or injury to the CNS is permanent and functional ability cannot be altered with any type of intervention

20. Although a multitude of tests can be done to help diagnose multiple sclerosis (MS), which of the following is **not** suggestive of this diagnosis?

A) Multifocal bright T2-weighted periventricular images

B) Increased latency seen in somatosensory evoked potentials (SSEP)

C) Increased cerebrospinal fluid (CSF) protein with oligoclonal bands

D) Decreased amplitudes of sensory nerve action potentials (SNAPs) and compound motor action potentials (CMAPs) in nerve conduction studies (NCSs)

21. Which option describes the pulmonary dysfunction seen in patients with Duchenne muscular dystrophy (DMD)?

A) Decreased lung compliance and increased atelectasis secondary to loss of surfactant

B) Restrictive lung disease due to weakness of the diaphragm, chest, and abdominal walls

C) Hyperventilation with signs of respiratory alkalosis due to hyperreactive diaphragm

D) Impaired innervation of the phrenic nerve

22. Which condition is characterized by onset before age 20 years, gait ataxia, and progressive paralysis?
    A) Guillain-Barré syndrome (GBS)
    B) Spinal muscular atrophy (SMA)
    C) Friedreich's ataxia
    D) Becker's muscular dystrophy (BMD)

23. Becker's muscular dystrophy may present with:
    A) Weakness in the first few days of life
    B) Calf pseudohypertrophy
    C) Rapid progression to death by age 4 years
    D) Costochondritis

24. What is the leading cause of mortality in children with neuromuscular diseases?
    A) Neurologic complications
    B) Renal complications
    C) Pulmonary complications
    D) Cardiac complications

25. Which of the following disorders is exacerbated with rest?
    A) Lambert-Eaton myasthenic syndrome (LEMS)
    B) Botulism
    C) Myasthenia gravis (MG)
    D) Amyotrophic lateral sclerosis

26. A 25-year-old female presents to your office with complaints of double vision, particularly after watching television for a prolonged period of time or at the end of a long day. She also complains of difficulty chewing food, even describing eating as "tiring." Which drug can be given to help establish the most likely diagnosis?
    A) Neostigmine
    B) Prednisone
    C) Pyridostigmine
    D) Edrophonium

27. A patient with spinal muscular atrophy (SMA) type II (chronic Werdnig-Hoffmann) can usually achieve which of the following childhood milestones?
    A) Assisted sitting
    B) Independent sitting
    C) Independent standing
    D) Independent ambulation

28. A 49-year-old female presents to your clinic with complaints of fluctuating double vision and droopy eyelids. The patient is sent for a test where edrophonium chloride is injected, and there is brief improvement in her symptoms. Which of the following treatments is most appropriate?
    A) Trivalent antitoxin
    B) Guanidine
    C) Treat the malignancy
    D) Mestinon (pyridostigmine)

29. A teenager presents with an elbow flexion contracture and mild weakness that has affected his ability to walk. On physical exam, you also notice a neck extension contracture. Which of the following is he most likely to have?
    A) Becker's muscular dystrophy (BMD)
    B) Emery-Dreifuss muscular dystrophy (EMD)
    C) Facioscapulohumeral dystrophy (FSHD)
    D) Limb-girdle muscular dystrophy (LGMD)

30. A patient with advanced Parkinson's disease comes to your clinic hoping to decrease his symptoms. He has tried antiparkinsonian drugs, but still has resting tremor, rigidity, and bradykinesia that interfere with his quality of life. What can you recommend that may help reduce his symptoms?
    A) Subthalamic deep-brain stimulation
    B) Thalamotomy
    C) Pallidotomy
    D) There is nothing more you can offer

31. The following are all considered good prognostic factors in multiple sclerosis (MS) **except**:
    A) Age of onset ~~greater~~ *less than* than 35 years
    B) Optic neuritis at onset
    C) Monosynaptic symptoms
    D) Ataxia and tremor

32. Medial medullary syndrome characteristically presents with the following signs and symptoms **except**:
    A) Ipsilateral tongue deviation
    B) Contralateral hemiparesis
    C) Contralateral proprioception and position sense loss
    D) Contralateral decreased pain and temperature

33. Lhermitte's sign is produced by:
    A) Passive neck flexion causing electrical shock–like sensation radiating to the spine, shoulders, and other areas
    B) Axial load placed by pressing downward force on top of the patient's head causing reproducible numbness to one or both limbs
    C) Rotating head to side with neck extended with ipsilateral shoulder abducted at 45° and elbow extended with patient inhaling and holding inspiration
    D) None of the above

34. Which of the following is **not** true regarding spina bifida?
    A) Complicated by hydrocephalus in 90% of cases
    B) Of those with Arnold-Chiari malformation, more than 80% of children will require ventriculoperitoneal shunting
    C) Threefold increase in the incidence of patients with lower IQ than the normal population
    D) Most common cause of death is cardiovascular complications

35. Cerebral palsy (CP) is associated with nonprogressive lesions in the immature brain. One of the more common pathognomonic lesions seen in CP is:
    A) Hydrocephalus
    B) Periventricular leukomalacia (PVL)
    C) Arnold-Chiari malformation
    D) Central pontine myelinolysis

36. Edrophonium (or Tensilon) test is used to help diagnose:
    A) Myasthenia gravis
    B) Botulism
    C) Lambert-Eaton myasthenic syndrome
    D) Amyotrophic lateral sclerosis

37. Which of the following is **not** a symptom of Friedreich's ataxia?
    A) Absent deep tendon reflexes (DTRs)
    B) Scoliosis
    C) Seizures
    D) Nystagmus

38. Guillain-Barré syndrome (GBS) may be treated with all of the following **except**:
    A) Rehabilitation
    B) Plasmapheresis
    C) Steroids
    D) IV immunoglobulins (IVIgs)

39. A 16-year-old boy presents to your office with complaints of progressive numbness in both feet. He also says that he has been tripping over himself a lot lately, which is unusual as he is very active. On physical exam you notice that he has high arches in both feet, decreased strength in ankle dorsiflexion, and has decreased sensation to light touch in both feet. When asked to walk across the room, you notice that he has a steppage gait pattern. Which of the following is the most likely diagnosis?
    A) Becker's muscular dystrophy
    B) Charcot-Marie-Tooth disease
    C) Werdnig-Hoffmann disease
    D) Amyotrophic lateral sclerosis

40. A 16-year-old male presents to your office with concerns that recently he uses his hands and arms to "walk" up his own body from a squatting position. He states that he was otherwise independent with standing and walking and has been doing well as a student and plans on attending college. Which lower motor neuron disease does he most likely have?
    A) Spinal muscular atrophy (SMA) type I
    B) SMA type II
    C) SMA type III
    D) Amyotrophic lateral sclerosis (ALS)

41. A 49-year-old woman presents to your clinic with complaints of fluctuating double vision and droopy eyelids. The patient is sent for a test where edrophonium chloride is injected, and there is brief improvement in her symptoms. Which of the following does she most likely have?
    A) Myasthenia gravis (MG)
    B) Lambert-Eaton myasthenic syndrome (LEMS)
    C) Botulism
    D) Amyotrophic lateral sclerosis (ALS)

42. A 19-year-old female presents to your outpatient office with complaints of not being able to smile or close her eyes. She is not able to whistle and has some hearing difficulties. On physical exam, scapula winging is present. Which of the following is she most likely to have?
    A) Becker's muscular dystrophy (BMD)
    B) Duchenne muscular dystrophy (DMD)

C) Facioscapulohumeral dystrophy (FSHD)
D) Limb-girdle muscular dystrophy (LGMD)

43. The movement disorder that results from a decrease in dopamine input in the striatum and an increase in cholinergic input is:
    A) Multiple sclerosis
    B) Friedreich's ataxia
    C) Parkinson's disease (PD)
    D) Huntington's disease

44. Of the several patterns of multiple sclerosis, which is most common?
    A) Secondary progressive
    B) Progressive-relapsing
    C) Relapsing-remitting
    D) Primary progressive

45. A patient presents to the emergency department with loss of muscle strength in his right upper and lower extremities. He has loss of proprioception and position sense on his right side and has left-side tongue deviation. What does he most likely have?
    A) Lateral medullary syndrome
    B) Medial medullary syndrome
    C) Benedikt's syndrome
    D) Weber's syndrome

46. All of the following symptoms are seen in multiple sclerosis (MS) **except**:
    A) Impairment of deep sensation, proprioception
    B) Scanning speech
    C) Impaired convergence
    D) Bowel and bladder incontinence

47. Arnold-Chiari malformation type II (the downward displacement of the medulla and brain stem through the foramen magnum causing kinking of the brain stem) is associated with which condition?
    A) Spina bifida occulta
    B) Meningocele
    C) Myelomeningocele
    D) Alzheimer's disease

48. Which of the following complications listed below is the most common risk factor for cerebral palsy (CP)?
    A) Toxoplasmosis, other (syphilis, varicella-zoster, parvovirus B19), rubella, cytomegalovirus and herpes (TORCH) congenital infections
    B) History of maternal seizures
    C) Maternal bleeding
    D) Premature birth

49. What is a requirement for the diagnosis of botulism?
    A) Muscle biopsy
    B) Botulinum toxin found in stool or blood
    C) Chest x-ray
    D) MRI

50. A baby with spinal muscular atrophy (SMA) type I (Werdnig-Hoffmann disease) may present with:
    A) Weak cry, dysphagia, weak suck
    B) Normal developmental milestones until age 3 years

    C)  Mild weakness of proximal muscles at birth
    D)  Decreased sensation

51.  Which of the following can trigger Guillain-Barré syndrome (GBS)?
    A)  Bacterial pneumonia
    B)  Gastrointestinal viral infection
    C)  Blood transfusions
    D)  Syphilis

52.  A 5-year-old boy presents to his pediatrician with difficulty standing up from the floor. The patient's mother notes that the child uses his hands to "walk up" the floor to stand up. She has also noticed that his calves have grown in size over the past few months. What test can be used to make a definitive diagnosis?
    A)  Electrodiagnostic testing (nerve conduction studies [NCS]/electromyography [EMG])
    B)  Muscle biopsy
    C)  Creatine phosphokinase (CPK) level
    D)  MRI

53.  Which of the following motor neuron diseases typically causes lower motor neuron signs and has the earliest disease onset?
    A)  Kugelberg-Welander disease
    B)  Primary lateral sclerosis (PLS)
    C)  Amyotrophic lateral sclerosis (ALS)
    D)  Werdnig-Hoffmann disease

54.  A 45-year-old man presents to your office with complaints of fatigue and weakness that are exacerbated with rest and often improved with exercise. He denies vision disturbances bilaterally. On physical exam, there is notable weakness in bilateral quadriceps. Which neuromuscular junction disorder may he have, and which location is affected?
    A)  Myasthenia gravis (MG); postsynaptic
    B)  Lambert-Eaton myasthenic syndrome (LEMS); presynaptic
    C)  MG; presynaptic
    D)  LEMS; postsynaptic

55.  An 18-year-old boy with an X-linked genetic disease has a mild functional disability, proximal muscles weakness, prominent calves, lordosis, and a waddling gait. He is not a wheelchair user. Which of the following conditions is he most likely to have?
    A)  Becker's muscular dystrophy (BMD)
    B)  Duchenne muscular dystrophy (DMD)
    C)  Facioscapulohumeral dystrophy (FSHD)
    D)  Limb-girdle muscular dystrophy (LGMD)

56.  Which of the following is **not** a sign/symptom of Parkinson's disease?
    A)  Impaired vibration or position sense
    B)  Resting tremor
    C)  Slowing of movements
    D)  Tremor superimposed on muscular rigidity

57.  Which of the following is **false** regarding multiple sclerosis?
    A)  Affects males more frequently than females
    B)  Affects Whites more frequently than African Americans

C) Increased incidence in higher socioeconomic class

D) There is no change in long-term relapses in pregnancy

58. In lateral medullary (Wallenberg's) syndrome, all of the following can be seen **except**:
    A) Decrease in pain and temperature sensation on the ipsilateral side of the face
    B) Decreased pain and temperature on the contralateral body
    C) Decreased muscle strength on the contralateral side
    D) Ptosis, anhidrosis, and miosis on the ipsilateral side

59. Which of the following features is considered a good prognosis indicator in patients with multiple sclerosis?
    A) Age at onset greater than 35 years
    B) Rapidly progressive onset
    C) Sensory findings/optic neuritis at onset
    D) Male sex

60. A 12-year-old boy comes into your office complaining of progressive hearing deficits. He is having difficulty whistling a tune he is listening to on headphones on his good ear. On examination, he is noted to have some hyperlordosis of his spine. Which condition do you suspect the boy may have?
    A) Duchenne muscular dystrophy (DMD)
    B) Emery-Dreifuss muscular dystrophy (EMD)
    C) Facioscapulohumeral dystrophy (FSHD)
    D) Limb-girdle syndromes

61. In the Miller Fisher variant (MFV) of Guillain-Barré syndrome (GBS), what are the classical findings?
    A) Ophthalmoplegia, ataxia, and areflexia
    B) Dysrhythmias, impaired diaphoresis, photophobia
    C) Dysphagia, nausea, diarrhea
    D) Dysrhythmias, hyperreflexia, and nausea

62. Which of the following is associated with small-cell (oat-cell) carcinoma of the lung?
    A) Lambert-Eaton myasthenic syndrome
    B) Botulism
    C) Myasthenia gravis
    D) Amyotrophic lateral sclerosis

63. Patients with facioscapulohumeral dystrophy (FSHD) may exhibit which of the following signs on physical examination?
    A) Hand weakness
    B) Scapular winging
    C) Spasticity
    D) Decreased sensation in the face

64. Pompe's disease presents with all of the following **except**:
    A) Dermatomyositis
    B) Respiratory insufficiency
    C) Hypotonia
    D) Cardiomegaly

65. The only medication that has been proven to slow disease progression and delay the onset of ventilator dependency in patients with amyotrophic lateral sclerosis (ALS) is:
    A) Pyridostigmine
    B) Baclofen
    C) Riluzole
    D) Modafinil

66. Which of the following pharmacologic agents has been approved for patients with amyotrophic lateral sclerosis (ALS) to slow the progression and improve survival?
    A) Levodopa
    B) Riluzole
    C) Baclofen
    D) Rebif

67. What is the etiology of Lambert-Eaton myasthenic syndrome (LEMS)?
    A) Disorder of neuromuscular transmission caused by *Clostridium botulinum* toxins blocking exocytosis of acetylcholine from the nerve terminal
    B) Disorder of neuromuscular transmission caused by *C. botulinum* toxins blocking endocytosis of acetylcholine from the nerve terminal
    C) Disorder resulting in a decreased quantal response because of an autoimmune response against acetylcholine receptors on the postsynaptic membrane
    D) Disorder of neuromuscular transmission due to an autoimmune response against the active sites on the presynaptic membrane

68. A patient with Duchenne muscular dystrophy (DMD) is most at risk to have which of the following as the disease progresses?
    A) Sudden cardiac death
    B) No contractures because of flaccid limbs
    C) Fecal incontinence
    D) Progressive mental deterioration

69. Which of the following is an ergot derivative and stimulates D2 receptors in the treatment of Parkinson's disease?
    A) Pergolide
    B) Bromocriptine
    C) Ropinirole
    D) Pramipexole

70. The etiology of which disease is thought to be an autoimmune response causing demyelination, axonal damage, and brain atrophy?
    A) Parkinson's disease
    B) Huntington's disease
    C) Multiple sclerosis (MS)
    D) Guillain-Barré syndrome

71. A patient presents to the emergency department with ptosis, anhidrosis, and miosis on the left side of his face. He has difficulty walking and recently fell to his left side. On physical exam, there is decrease in pain and temperature sensation on the left side of his face and on the right side of his body. There is no muscle weakness. He most likely has:
    A) Lateral medullary syndrome
    B) Medial medullary syndrome

C) Benedikt's syndrome

D) Weber's syndrome

72. Huntington's disease is characterized by all the features listed below **except**:

A) Evidence of chorea and dementia/personality disorders

B) Trinucleotide repeat sequence of cytosine, adenine, and guanine (CAG) in the DNA

C) Markedly decreased amount of gamma-aminobutyric acid (GABA) in the basal ganglia

D) Microscopically noted to have intracytoplasmic eosinophilic inclusions called Lewy bodies in damaged cells

73. Which of the following medications used for spasticity has the least amount of sedation and cognitive impairment?

A) Diazepam

B) Dantrolene sodium

C) Baclofen

D) Clonidine

74. Botulism in an infant is associated with ingestion of:

A) Mayonnaise

B) Pasta

C) Honey

D) Strawberries

75. Children with which disorder are at an increased risk for developing hip dislocations, scoliosis, and hydrocephalus?

A) Child abuse

B) Down syndrome

C) Werdnig-Hoffmann disease

D) Congenital muscular dystrophy (CMD)

76. What is the most common type of cerebral palsy (CP)?

A) Mixed type

B) Dyskinetic

C) Flaccid

D) Spastic

77. Which of the following is considered an inflammatory myopathy?

A) Cerebral palsy (CP)

B) Inclusion body myositis (IBM)

C) Meralgia paresthetica

D) Charcot-Marie-Tooth disease

78. What is the prognosis for patients with amyotrophic lateral sclerosis?

A) 50% die within 3 years

B) 100% die within 3 years

C) 50% live up to 7 years

D) 50% live up to 10 years

79. Of the following, which is a disorder of neuromuscular transmission due to an autoimmune response against acetylcholine receptors on the postsynaptic membrane?

A) Myasthenia gravis

B) Lambert-Eaton myasthenic syndrome (LEMS)

C) Botulism

D) Amyotrophic lateral sclerosis (ALS)

80. Cognition may be impaired in which of the following myopathies?

A) Becker's muscular dystrophy (BMD)

B) Duchenne muscular dystrophy (DMD)

C) Facioscapulohumeral dystrophy (FSHD)

D) Limb-girdle muscular dystrophy (LGMD)

81. Which of the following inflammatory myopathies is **not** treated primarily with corticosteroids or other immunosuppressive medications?

A) Childhood dermatomyositis

B) Adult dermatomyositis

C) Polymyositis

D) Inclusion body myositis (IBM)

82. Which of the following is true of multiple sclerosis (MS) in women and pregnancy?

A) Interferon beta is a safe treatment option during pregnancy

B) Glatiramer acetate is a safe treatment option during pregnancy

C) Breastfeeding increases relapse rate in the first 6 months postpartum

D) Restarting disease-modifying agents during breastfeeding is recommended

83. Which first-line treatment choice can reduce relapse in multiple sclerosis (MS) patients?

A) Corticosteroids

B) Immunomodulator agents

C) Intravenous immunoglobulin

D) Immunosuppressive agents

84. Side effects from all of the following medications should be considered in the differential diagnosis of Parkinson's disease **except**:

A) Metoclopramide (Reglan)

B) Lithium

C) Haloperidol

D) Amantadine

85. Which of the Parkinson's plus syndromes is characterized by onset at 40 to 60 years of age, involving weakness in lower extremities (LE) with possible intention tremor of LE, and ataxia plus dysarthria?

A) Multiple system atrophy (Shy-Drager syndrome)

B) Supranuclear palsy

C) Olivopontocerebellar atrophy

D) Striatonigral degeneration

86. Which of the following is considered to be a lacunar syndrome?

A) Pure motor hemiplegia

B) Pure sensory stroke

C) Clumsy hand syndrome

D) All of the above

87. Botulism is caused by:

A) *Clostridium botulinum* toxin

B) *C. botulinum* colonies

    C) *Staphylococcus aureus*
    D) *Campylobacter jejuni*

88. Fatigue in a patient with multiple sclerosis (MS) will increase with:
    A) Heating
    B) Cooling
    C) Wetness
    D) Dryness

89. Which of the following disorders is the leading cause of childhood disability?
    A) Muscular dystrophy
    B) Cerebral palsy (CP)
    C) Osgood-Schlatter disease
    D) Charcot-Marie-Tooth disease

90. Patients with this particular syndrome report a strong, sometimes irresistible urge to move their legs:
    A) Restless leg syndrome (RLS)
    B) Cerebral palsy (CP)
    C) Amyotrophic lateral sclerosis (ALS)
    D) Spinal muscular atrophy (SMA)

91. Which of the following is considered a poor prognostic factor in patients with amyotrophic lateral sclerosis (ALS)?
    A) Predominance of upper motor neuron (UMN) findings at diagnosis
    B) Long period from symptom onset to diagnosis
    C) Younger age of onset
    D) Pulmonary dysfunction early in the clinical course

92. Which virus has been implicated in the development of poliomyelitis?
    A) Herpes virus
    B) Papillomavirus
    C) Picornavirus
    D) Poxvirus

93. Which of the following myopathies is **not** associated with cardiac abnormalities?
    A) Becker's muscular dystrophy (BMD)
    B) Duchenne muscular dystrophy (DMD)
    C) Facioscapulohumeral dystrophy (FSHD)
    D) Limb-girdle muscular dystrophy (LGMD)

94. A patient presents to your office with malaise, fever, weight loss, and proximal muscle weakness and tenderness. On physical examination, he is noted to have a heliotrope rash with periorbital edema. Which of the following does he most likely have?
    A) Primary idiopathic polymyositis
    B) Primary idiopathic dermatomyositis
    C) Rheumatoid arthritis
    D) Childhood dermatomyositis or polymyositis

95. Which of the following is **false** regarding multiple sclerosis (MS) in women and pregnancy?
    A) Relapses decrease during pregnancy
    B) Higher relapse rate in the first 3 months postpartum
    C) Women should not worry about pregnancy worsening their disease process
    D) Increased incidence of MS by over 50% among their offspring

96. Corticosteroid use in multiple sclerosis (MS) is considered:
    A) Effective in long-term use
    B) Most responsive in cerebellar and sensory symptoms
    C) To speed recovery
    D) To prevent further attacks

97. Neuroplasticity is **not** positively influenced by:
    A) Environment and stimulation
    B) Repetition of tasks
    C) Motivation
    D) Compensation strategies

98. Which of the following is **not** a characteristic of ~~myasthenic syndrome of~~ Lambert-Eaton syndrome (LES)?
    A) Paraneoplastic syndrome associated with small-cell lung cancer
    B) Involves antibodies to presynaptic Ca+ ion channels
    C) Proximal muscle weakness that improves with further exertion
    D) Extraocular weakness

99. A patient seen in the stroke recreational unit is told to draw a clock. After examining his illustration, you note that all the numbers of the clock are written and squeezed to the right side. Where do you suspect is his lesion?
    A) Left middle cerebral artery (MCA)
    B) Right MCA
    C) Left anterior cerebral artery (ACA)
    D) Right ACA

100. In myasthenia gravis, there is an autoimmune response against:
    A) Calcium channels
    B) Acetylcholine receptors
    C) Sodium channels
    D) Sodium potassium pump

101. Lhermitte's sign is classically seen, but is not pathognomonic, for this disease:
    A) Multiple sclerosis (MS)
    B) Amyotrophic lateral sclerosis (ALS)
    C) Duchenne muscular dystrophy
    D) Poliomyelitis

102. Which of the following is the overall leading cause of cerebral palsy (CP)?
    A) Prematurity
    B) Iodine deficiency
    C) Child abuse
    D) Tetralogy of Fallot

103. A 60-year-old man without any significant past medical history presents to your outpatient office with asymmetric atrophy, weakness, and fasciculations. He also complains of some difficulty swallowing his meals and complains of a strained and strangled quality in his speech. He describes normal bowel and bladder function. Which of the following is most likely his diagnosis?
    A) Amyotrophic lateral sclerosis (ALS)
    B) Spinal muscle atrophy III

C) Primary lateral sclerosis (PLS)

D) Poliomyelitis

104. Which of the following is **not** included in the Halstead and Rossi (1987) criteria in defining Post-polio syndrome?
   A) History of previous diagnosis of polio
   B) Stability for approximately 5 years
   C) Recovery of function
   D) No other medical problem to explain new symptoms of weakness/atrophy

105. Becker's muscular dystrophy is characterized by:
   A) Autosomal dominant condition
   B) Autosomal recessive condition
   C) X-linked, absent dystrophin
   D) X-linked, reduced dystrophin

106. The age of onset for idiopathic inflammatory myopathies is:
   A) Bimodal
   B) Early
   C) Late
   D) Not specific and can occur at any time

107. A 32-year-old man presents to your office with hyperkinetic, involuntary, jerky movements. His sister states that she fears he also has dementia and that he is acting like her deceased father, uncle, and grandfather. They all passed away after having similar symptoms. This patient most likely has:
   A) Parkinson's disease
   B) Multiple sclerosis
   C) Huntington's disease
   D) Friedreich's ataxia

108. The pathognomonic test for multiple sclerosis (MS) includes:
   A) Increased cerebrospinal fluid (CSF) protein, oligoclonal IgG bands
   B) Multifocal "bright" areas of hyperintensity on T2-weighted images
   C) Both of the above
   D) None of the above

109. Benefits of partial body weight–supported gait training include:
   A) Addressing ambulation issues for patients who have sufficient strength and balance
   B) Enhancing development of compensatory gait strategies
   C) Providing earlier weight bearing to increase strength and increase spasticity
   D) Allowing for the simulation of task-specific walking movements

110. What are the typical features of amyotrophic lateral sclerosis (ALS) associated with lower motor neuron disease?
   A) Babinski sign
   B) Increased tone
   C) Spasticity
   D) Fasciculations

111. A patient is noted to have ptosis of his right eyelid. When the eyes are opened, his pupil is noted to be dilated and faced downward and out. He is also noted to have weakness of his left side with signs of ataxia. He is likely to have?
    A) Weber's syndrome
    B) Millard-Gubler syndrome
    C) Wallenberg's syndrome
    D) Medial medullary syndrome

112. Which of the following is a postsynaptic neuromuscular junction disorder?
    A) Myasthenia gravis
    B) Botulism type A
    C) Lambert-Eaton myasthenic syndrome
    D) Botulism type E

113. In a patient with multiple sclerosis (MS), pregnancy usually results in:
    A) Death
    B) Symptom relapse
    C) Complete recovery
    D) Decreased relapses

114. Which of the following disorders gives a patient an "inverted champagne bottle" or "stork leg" appearance?
    A) Duchenne muscular dystrophy (DMD)
    B) Charcot-Marie-Tooth (CMT) disease
    C) Myasthenia gravis
    D) Spinal muscular atrophy

115. Which of the following motor neuron diseases typically causes **both** upper and lower motor neuron signs?
    A) Spinal muscle atrophy II
    B) Primary lateral sclerosis (PLS)
    C) Amyotrophic lateral sclerosis (ALS)
    D) Poliomyelitis

116. Which of the following is the most common presenting form of motor neuron disease in adults?
    A) Amyotrophic lateral sclerosis (ALS)
    B) Poliomyelitis
    C) Spinal muscular atrophy (SMA)
    D) Primary lateral sclerosis (PLS)

117. Which myopathy is characterized by a steadily progressive, X-linked muscular dystrophy that is characterized by absent dystrophin or less than 3% that is normal?
    A) Becker's muscular dystrophy (BMD)
    B) Duchenne muscular dystrophy (DMD)
    C) Limb-girdle muscular dystrophy (LGMD)
    D) Facioscapulohumeral dystrophy (FSHD)

118. A judicious workup for carcinoma is recommended in adult patients with newly diagnosed:
    A) Inclusion body myositis
    B) Polymyositis

    C) Steroid myopathy
    D) Dermatomyositis

119. Of the following, which does **not** cause drug-induced parkinsonism?
    A) Metoclopramide
    B) Interferon beta-1a
    C) Amiodarone
    D) Haloperidol

120. Which of the following can be seen in patients with multiple sclerosis (MS)?
    A) Pill rolling tremor
    B) Lower motor neuron signs
    C) Adson's sign
    D) Weakness and/or Lhermitte's sign

121. Neural strategies of functional improvement after central nervous system injury include all of the following **except**:
    A) Restoration
    B) Redacting
    C) Recruitment
    D) Retraining

122. What is Uhthoff's phenomenon?
    A) Passive neck flexion causing shock-like symptoms radiating to the spine and shoulders
    B) Inability to adduct the left eye on right lateral gaze and inability to adduct the right eye on left lateral gaze with intact convergence
    C) Worsening of neurological symptoms including visual problems seen with increased body temperature
    D) Ptosis of both eyes

123. A patient seen in the traumatic brain injury (TBI) unit is noted to have a constricted pupil on the left side that is nonresponsive to light. Also, he is noted to not appreciate pinprick sensation on the left side of his face and right side of his body. What condition does this patient have?
    A) Benedikt's syndrome
    B) Lateral medullary syndrome
    C) Weber's syndrome
    D) Millard-Gubler syndrome

124. Which type of aphasia would you expect to see in a patient who is noted to have fluent speech, with signs of comprehension, but unable to repeat?
    A) Anomic aphasia
    B) Transcortical sensory aphasia
    C) Conduction aphasia
    D) Transcortical motor aphasia

125. Lower motor neuron (LMN) signs include all of the following **except**:
    A) Spasticity
    B) Atrophy
    C) Hyporeflexia
    D) Fasciculations

126. Which of the following is true about children with neuromuscular scoliosis?
    A) It is common in children with neuromuscular disorders who are able to walk
    B) In Duchenne muscular dystrophy, scoliosis is unusual until the child becomes a wheel-chair user
    C) In cerebral palsy, scoliosis is usually seen in patients who are able to stand and walk
    D) It usually presents before age 1 year

127. Locked-in syndrome (tetraparesis in a completely conscious patient with only the ability to move eyes vertically and blink) is suggestive of an occlusion in which artery(ies)?
    A) Bilateral vertebral artery
    B) Posterior inferior cerebellar artery
    C) Posterior cerebral artery
    D) Basilar artery

# Neuromuscular Disorders

## ANSWERS

1. **D)** Baclofen is a gamma-amino butyric acid (GABA) analogue used to facilitate motor neuron inhibition at spinal levels and is the first-line treatment. Dosing can be started at 5 to 10 mg two to three times per day. It can be titrated up to 20 mg four times per day. Potential side effects include weakness, fatigue, and sedation. Patients must be informed that abrupt discontinuation of baclofen may cause withdrawal seizures. Tizanidine is an alpha-2 agonist. Benzodiazepine can be helpful, but can cause respiratory depression and somnolence. Dantrolene blocks calcium release in the sarcoplasmic reticulum and is ineffective at reducing muscle tone, but can cause generalized muscle weakness.

2. **A)** The maneuver noted here is Gower's sign, which is the inability to rise from a seated position on the floor. The patient has to use his hands and knees for assistance in a four-point stance. He will bridge the knees into extension and lean the upper extremity forward. This will substitute hip extension weakness (proximal leg weakness) and lean the upper extremities forward. The patient then moves the upper extremities up the thigh, and a full hip extension is achieved in an upright stance. The Gower's sign indicates proximal muscle weakness. Also, this patient has pseudohypertrophy, which is seen in patients with either Duchenne or Becker's muscular dystrophy. The enlargement in the calf is not due to increased muscle. It is a result of increased fat and connective tissue.

3. **C)** Central core disease is an autosomal dominant congenital myopathy. Onset is shortly after birth, and the infant is noted to be floppy and attains milestones slowly. Congenital hip dislocation is often noted, and as the child ages, he or she cannot run and jump like their peers. Weakness is more pronounced in the proximal muscles, and patients can show a Gower's sign. It is important to note that there is an association with malignant hyperthermia when receiving general anesthesia. This is because central core disease's gene locus is at 19q13.1, which is the same gene locus as the malignant hyperthermia gene. On light microscopy, the muscle cells have cores that lack mitochondria.

4. **D)** Postural hypotension is a common problem in many anti-Parkinson's drugs. Postural hypotension can be treated with salt tablets or mineralocorticoids (such as fludrocortisone or midodrine). Other side effects of these medications include confusion and hallucinations. L-dopa may cause nausea, abdominal cramping, and diarrhea.

5. **A)** Fatigue is more problematic in patients in the afternoon and can be experienced in 77% of patients with MS. Energy conservation techniques can be used to treat fatigue, and medications such as methylphenidate and amantadine can also be used. Balance difficulties and weakness can contribute to falls in this patient population.

6. **B)** CIMT is an intervention directed at improving the function of the affected upper extremity after a brain injury. It involves intensive motor training of up to 6 hours daily and motor restriction (constraint) of the unaffected extremity. CIMT is based on research findings that the affected limb is negatively impacted by learned nonuse because of increased dependence on the intact limb.

7. **D)** All of the answer choices are used in the treatment of MS except for choice (D), which is used in Devic's disease or neuromyelitis optica. Corticosteroids are often used in acute attacks and are used in high doses and tapered down. Interferon beta and glatiramer acetate are immunomodulating agents that help in decreasing the progression of the disease. Rituximab is a monoclonal antibody against B-cell CD20 antigen used in hematological diseases (lymphomas) and many autoimmune diseases, but not in MS.

8. **D)** All of the listed statements are true regarding Duchenne muscular dystrophy.

9. **B)** It is vital to do pulmonary function tests (PFTs) in patients diagnosed with MG. The forced vital capacity is probably the most important PFT, as it correlates to the function of the pulmonary muscles, including the diaphragm. Severe myasthenia may cause respiratory failure due to exhaustion of the respiratory muscles. Choice (C) is one of the tests done to diagnose MS. In the Tensilon test, edrophonium or neostigmine is administered (acetylcholinesterase inhibitors), which temporarily relieves symptoms of MG. Choices (A) and (D) are common symptoms of MG and provide little prognostic value.

10. **C)** In ALS, there is weakness and muscle atrophy caused by degeneration of upper and lower motor neurons.

11. **A)** Patients with DMD have an absence of dystrophin, which leads to progressive muscle weakness and fatigability. Most DMD patients become wheelchair users early in life. When dystrophin is partially functioning, the disorder is known as Becker's muscular dystrophy (BMD).

12. **B)** Parkinson's disease results from the death of dopamine-generating cells in the substantia nigra. The resting tremor, which occurs only at rest, is characteristic of Parkinson's. Intention tremor occurs during voluntary movement, and essential tremor occurs during sustained muscle contraction.

13. **B)** Friedreich's ataxia is an autosomal recessive disease that affects mitochondrial function, which leads to cerebellum and spinal cord degeneration. Patients exhibit abnormal gait, which leads to frequent falls. Patients also usually develop early insulin resistance, cardiomyopathies, dysarthria, scoliosis, and pes cavus. They will have bilateral muscle weakness affecting upper and lower extremities, as well as have impaired proprioception/vibratory senses. Treatment involves physical/occupational therapy and surgery if needed. ALS is a progressive motor neuron disease affecting voluntary muscles. Patients will exhibit both upper and lower motor neuron signs on physical exam. ALS usually presents later in life with progressive muscle weakness.
Ataxia telangiectasia is an autosomal recessive disease affecting the cerebellum, which also causes difficulty with ambulation and movement. Symptoms usually develop around the age of 2 years. Patients will commonly have difficulty walking and frequent infections, and exhibit telangiectasias (dilations of small blood vessels, usually in the eye or around the face).
Fazio-Londe disease is an autosomal recessive neuromuscular disorder, also presenting in childhood, which usually affects the cranial nerves. Patients will develop progressive weakness of the tongue and facial muscles that eventually lead to dysarthria and dysphagia. Difficulty ambulating is usually not one of the symptoms of the disease.

14. **A)** Spinal muscular atrophy (SMA) type I is also known as Werdnig-Hoffmann disease. Death usually occurs by 2 to 3 years of age. The progression is rapid and fatal. Patients with SMA type II, known as chronic Werdnig-Hoffmann, usually die by about 10 years of age. Again, the progression is fatal. Patients with SMA type III, known as Kugelberg-Welander disease, have a normal life expectancy with a slow progression.

15. **C)** Symptoms such as blurred vision and diplopia can occur, along with nausea and vomiting, between 12 and 36 hours after consuming raw meat, fish, canned vegetables, or honey, making answer choice (C) the best answer. Bulbar symptoms are noted first and include ptosis, dysphagia, or dysarthria. Gastrointestinal symptoms include nausea and vomiting, and then there may be widespread paralysis or flaccidity. If severe, there may be respiratory dysfunction. Lab work may reveal botulinum toxin in the stool or blood serum. Recovery occurs from collateral sprouting of nerves.

16. **C)** Although the term facioscapulohumeral dystrophy would imply that all the muscles of the shoulder and upper arm are atrophic, the deltoid is surprisingly well preserved in many cases. This can be overlooked because scapular fixation prevents the deltoid from exerting its maximal effect. It is best to have the patient lying down with the examiner's hand pressing down on the thorax backward to prevent the scapula from moving. When examined in this manner, the deltoid is normal in strength or only slightly weak. The inability to extend the wrist is a characteristic posture adopted by these patients. Answer choices (B) and (D) are cardinal clinical signs. Other clinical presentations may include lordosis and pelvic girdle weakness, deafness, and fundal changes. Some patients may benefit from surgery that fixes the scapula to facilitate abduction of the arms.

17. **C)** An example of a dopamine receptor antagonist is haloperidol. This medication is used in movement disorders such as Huntington's disease, but has extrapyramidal and anticholinergic side effects. These side effects can mimic parkinsonian-like symptoms, making answer choice (C) incorrect. All other answer choices can be effectively used in the treatment of Parkinson's disease. Other treatment options can also include amantadine and selective monoamine oxidase B (MAO-B) inhibitors.

18. **B)** The classic symptoms of MS include bowel/bladder dysfunction, fatigue (which is central in nature), and pain. Other symptoms that patients may report are balance problems, weakness/paralysis, numbness/tingling, spasticity, cognitive problems, depression, emotional lability, and tremor. MS produces a wide variety of problems depending on the location of the lesion in the central nervous system. However, IQ is not usually affected.

19. **D)** "Insult or injury to the CNS is permanent and functional ability cannot be altered with any type of intervention" is not part of the concept of neuroplasticity. Neuroplasticity refers to the dynamic nature of the brain and the CNS and its ability to change in response to experience and injury.

20. **D)** All of the answer choices are suggestive findings of MS except for choice (D). Often, clinical evidence alone is diagnostic of MS if there is an apparent history of repeated attacks and signs of more than two lesions. However, in other cases, MRI findings and spinal tap can help assist in the diagnosis. MRI has the greatest sensitivity, as lesions of white matter are seen in approximately 85% of the cases involving the optic nerves, spinal cord, and brain. Enhancement with gadolinium is a sensitive indicator of disease activity. CSF tap will show increased protein because of the lost myelin and increased amount of IgG. SSEPs are frequently delayed, because MS is a central process and generally involves the cord. As NCSs test peripheral nerves, they are generally not affected.

21. **B)** In DMD, restrictive pulmonary disease is manifested by exertion and fatigue. This causes hypoventilation with elevation of $CO_2$ levels, which can result in daytime somnolence and headache. Noninvasive devices are the preferred form of pulmonary management.

22. **C)** Friedreich's ataxia is a type of spinocerebellar degeneration disease. It has an autosomal recessive genetic predisposition. All the features listed are associated with cerebellar injury. GBS is generally preceded by a viral etiology and then develops a spontaneous ascending paralysis that usually resolves without any of the cerebellar symptoms. In SMA, there is generalized proximal muscle weakness and wasting of upper and lower extremities, with signs of upper and lower motor neurons (degeneration of spinal cord and anterior horn cells).

23. **B)** Becker's muscular dystrophy is an X-linked muscular dystrophy that has a slower progression and milder symptoms than Duchenne muscular dystrophy. Calf pseudohypertrophy can be seen in both Duchenne and Becker's muscular dystrophy and reflects destruction of the gastrocnemius muscle tissue by connective and fat tissue.

24. **C)** Pulmonary complications are the number one cause of mortality. This is due to respiratory muscle weakness and fatigue along with impaired central control of respiration.

25. **A)** The symptoms of LEMS are the result of an insufficient release of neurotransmitter by nerve cells. Continued use of the muscles may lead to a buildup of the neurotransmitter to normal levels, so symptoms of LEMS can often be lessened or alleviated. Symptoms of myasthenia gravis do not improve with continued muscle use.

26. **D)** This patient most likely has myasthenia gravis (MG). MG is a neuromuscular disorder affecting postsynaptic acetylcholine receptors. It can present with muscle weakness, especially with repetitive movements. Edrophonium is a rapidly acting reversible acetylcholinesterase inhibitor which, when given, will block acetylcholinesterase enzymes and allow acetylcholine to bind to its receptor. The Tensilon test is when edrophonium is given via IV. The patient's muscle strength is observed for improvement over the next few minutes. Patients with severe ptosis from MG may see their ptosis completely resolve for a short period of time. Neostigmine, pyridostigmine, and prednisone are all medications used in the treatment of MG. Neostigmine and pyridostigmine are both longer-acting acetylcholinesterase inhibitors, compared to edrophonium. Prednisone is an immunosuppressant that is used in some MG exacerbations.

27. **B)** SMA type II is also known as chronic Werdnig-Hoffmann. The disease onset is between 2 and 12 months of age, and death (often by respiratory failure) occurs by 10 years of age. These patients can usually achieve milestones including independent sitting. They may be able to stand or walk with an assistive device. Answer choice (D) is therefore incorrect and refers to someone with SMA type III. SMA type I patients never attain the ability to sit independently, and this severe disorder usually results in death by the age of 2 years.

28. **D)** Mestinon (pyridostigmine) reversibly binds to and inactivates acetylcholinesterase, which is a cholinesterase inhibitor. This patient has myasthenia gravis (MG). Mestinon 60 to 120 mg orally every 3 to 8 hours can be used to treat MG. Other treatment options for MG include thymectomy, corticosteroids, immunosuppressive agents, and plasmapheresis. Answer choice (C) is correct in Lambert-Eaton myasthenic syndrome (LEMS) patients with malignancy. Initial treatment should be aimed at the neoplasm because weakness frequently improves with effective cancer therapy. No further LEMS treatment may be necessary in some patients. Answer choice (A) is used for patients with botulism.

29. **B)** This is an X-linked and slowly progressive myopathy caused by an abnormality of the protein emerin with a gene locus identified at Xq28. Patients usually present in the teenage years, and early elbow flexion contractures are the hallmark of the disease. Ankle equinus, rigid spine, and neck extension contractures can also be seen and are often more limiting than the weakness. This

disease is also associated with cardiac arrhythmias and almost always present by the age of 40 years. Twenty-four–hour Holter monitoring is required, as arrhythmias may not be obvious clinically or on routine ECG. EMD is managed by promotion of ambulation, prevention of deformities or their progression, monitoring cardiac status, and assessment of respiratory function.

30. **A)** Subthalamic deep-brain stimulation has been effective in reducing symptoms and has been shown to reduce the need for antiparkinsonian medications by at least half. This is the most common surgical procedure used in patients with Parkinson's, although destructive surgery is another option. Thalamotomy is surgical destruction of cells in the thalamus and can alleviate tremor on the contralateral side. Pallidotomy is the permanent ablation of part of the globus pallidus. This can be used in alleviating dyskinesias, stiffness, and the inability to perform or restart certain tasks.

31. **D)** Ataxia and tremor have a poorer prognosis for MS patients. All other choices are good prognostic factors. Optic neuritis is inflammation of the optic nerve. It may cause sudden, reduced vision in the affected eye and is considered a good prognostic factor when presenting at onset in MS patients.

32. **D)** Medial medullary syndrome is caused by an infarction of the medial medulla secondary to occlusion of penetrating branches of vertebral arteries or anterior spinal artery. This syndrome is rare and happens far less than lateral medullary syndrome (1–2:10). Signs and symptoms can include ipsilateral hypoglossal palsy, contralateral hemiparesis, and contralateral lemniscal sensory loss.

33. **A)** Lhermitte's sign is commonly seen in multiple sclerosis (MS), but is not universally seen in all cases. This test assesses for increased sensitivity of the myelin to traction and is similar to an upper motor neuron sign. Choice (B) refers to Spurling's test, which is done to test for radiculopathies. Choice (C) is Adson's maneuver, which is done to assess for neurogenic thoracic outlet syndrome by causing scalene compression of the brachial plexus.

34. **D)** All of the statements are correct except for choice (D). The most common cause of death in spina bifida is central respiratory dysfunction.

35. **B)** PVL is highly predictive of cerebral palsy. It is seen in hemorrhagic infarction and is due to hemorrhagic lesions adjacent to the lateral ventricle. As this bleeding resolves, symmetric necrosis of the white matter bordering the external angle of the lateral ventricles can develop. Choice (C) is often seen in syringomyelia, and choice (D) is seen after rapid treatment of hyponatremia with hypertonic saline.

36. **A)** Edrophonium (or Tensilon) test will show improvement in myasthenia gravis. Edrophonium is a reversible acetylcholinesterase inhibitor.

37. **C)** Friedreich's ataxia is a type of spinocerebellar degeneration syndrome that usually starts with gait ataxia and progresses to the rest of the body from the lower extremities upward. Symptoms may include weakness and muscle atrophy, nystagmus, dysarthria, fatigue, scoliosis, absent DTRs, and gradual loss of proprioception and vibratory sense.

38. **C)** Steroids have not proven to be an effective treatment for GBS. IVIg is usually started first owing to the ease of administration and safety profile. Plasmapheresis hastens recovery when used in the first 4 weeks of symptom onset. Rehabilitation usually follows the acute phase treatment modalities.

39. **B)** Charcot-Marie-Tooth disease is a demyelinating hereditary disorder that affects peripheral nerves. Patients will complain of loss of sensation in bilateral feet, as well as painful muscle contractions. Patients may also have the classic "inverted champagne bottle" sign, which is caused by lower leg muscle wasting. Also commonly seen is bilateral high arched feet or pes cavus. Diagnosis is by nerve conduction testing, DNA testing, or nerve biopsy. If nerve biopsy is done, an "onion bulb" appearance may be seen, which is caused by constant nerve demyelination and remyelination. Treatment consists of physical therapy, braces (especially ankle-foot orthosis), and surgery for foot stabilization. Becker's muscular dystrophy (BMD) is an X-linked recessive disorder that is similar to Duchenne muscular dystrophy (DMD), but is usually milder. Patients usually present with symptoms later in life. Disease progression is slower when compared to DMD. Unlike DMD, the dystrophin gene is partially functional in BMD. Werdnig-Hoffmann disease is a severe type of spinal muscular atrophy that presents within a month after birth. Motor neuron death usually leads to respiratory arrest, and patients rarely live past 2 years of age. Amyotrophic lateral sclerosis (ALS) is a progressive motor neuron disease affecting voluntary muscles. Patients will exhibit both upper and lower motor neuron signs on physical exam. Treatment includes physical therapy and possibly riluzole, which has been proven to prolong time to ventilator dependence.

40. **C)** SMA type III (spinal muscular atrophy) is also known as Kugelberg-Welander disease. The disease onset is later than that of type I and type II, occurring between 2 and 15 years of age. Patients typically live a normal life expectancy. The progression is slower than the other two variants. Patients usually achieve independent standing/walking. This patient presents with Gower's sign, which can be seen in SMA type III patients because proximal weakness is greater than distal weakness. These patients typically have normal intelligence. Complications in SMA type III are less frequent, but may include hand tremor, tongue fasciculations (late onset), and areflexia. All forms of spinal muscle atrophy are classified as lower motor neuron diseases, and ALS is classified as both upper and lower motor neuron disease.

41. **A)** Myasthenia gravis patients may complain of proximal muscle fatigue and weakness exacerbated with exercise, heat, or time of day (evening). It is important to note that there can be facial or bulbar symptoms, including ptosis, diplopia, dysphagia, or dysarthria. This patient presents with ocular myasthenia gravis. Ocular involvement is an extremely common initial presentation in MG patients. Drooping of eyelids and intermittent diplopia result from levator palpebrae (extraocular muscles) involvement, which is seen in 90% of MG cases. The test here describes the edrophonium (Tensilon) test. An intravenous solution of edrophonium chloride is injected into a patient. A total of 10 mg of the cholinergic drug is prepared, and a 2-mg dose is injected. If there is no reaction in 30 seconds, the remaining 8 mg is administered. A brief improvement in muscle activity is regarded as a positive result. Edrophonium chloride is also used to distinguish between MG and a cholinergic crisis. Because edrophonium chloride can precipitate respiratory depression, the test should not be performed unless an anticholinergic antidote, such as atropine, and respiratory resuscitation equipment are available.

42. **C)** FSHD is a slowly progressive muscular dystrophic myopathy and involves the facial and shoulder girdle muscles. It is an autosomal dominant condition. Presentation is usually before the age of 20 years and usually presents with weakness of the facial (orbicularis oculi and orbicularis oris) or shoulder girdle muscles (scapular and humeral distribution). Prominent scapula winging and biceps/triceps weakness may be present. There is relative sparing of the deltoid. Patients can be described as having an expressionless face and have difficulty with pursing lips, smiling, drinking through a straw, or whistling. There is also asymmetry of muscle involvement, which is unlike most other muscular dystrophies. Patients with FSHD also have sensorineural hearing deficits, and therefore all should have screening audiometry.

43. **C)** PD involves a pathologic degenerative process of the brain stem nuclei. This is especially true of dopaminergic cells of the substantia nigra. In addition, there is an excess of cholinergic neurons in the caudate nuclei. This causes an imbalance between cholinergic and dopaminergic input in the striatum and is responsible for the symptoms seen in PD.

44. **C)** There are six different subtypes of multiple sclerosis (MS). Eighty-five percent of MS cases are the relapsing-remitting form of MS. This form is characterized by an acute exacerbation followed by a remission period. During the remission, patients can return to their baseline function or may have some form of disability after an exacerbation. The six subtypes of MS are as follows:
    1. Relapsing-remitting
    2. Secondary progressive
    3. Benign
    4. Progressive-relapsing
    5. Primary progressive
    6. Malignant

45. **B)** Medial medullary syndrome is caused by an infarction of the medial medulla secondary to occlusion of penetrating branches of vertebral arteries or anterior spinal artery. This syndrome is rare and happens far less than lateral medullary syndrome (1–2:10). Signs and symptoms can include ipsilateral hypoglossal palsy, contralateral hemiparesis, and contralateral lemniscal sensory loss.

46. **C)** All of the answer choices are symptoms of MS except for choice (C). Choice (A) is due to demyelination of the dorsal column tracts. Choice (B) is seen in Charcot's triad or advance stages of the disease where scanning speech, intention tremor, and nystagmus can manifest themselves. Scanning speech is characterized as being explosive speech that is broken into syllables. Bowel and bladder incontinence are symptoms seen because of demyelination of the spinal cord. Convergence is one of the optical features not seen in MS, whereas nystagmus, optic neuritis, diplopia, and internuclear ophthalmoplegia (a disorder of lateral conjugate gaze in which the affected eye has impaired adduction, causing diplopia) may be noted. However, convergence is generally intact.

47. **C)** In spina bifida, a congenital malformation of the vertebral columns and spinal cord exists. Only in myelomeningocele, where the protruding sac contains meninges, spinal cord, and spinal fluid, is there an associated finding of Arnold-Chiari malformation, which presents in approximately 80% to 90% of patients.

48. **D)** Prematurity is the most common antecedent of CP. This is due to immaturity, fragile brain vasculature, and the physical stresses of immaturity, which predispose to compromised blood flow. Infants born between 32 and 42 weeks gestation with a low birth weight (below the 10th percentile) had four to six times higher risk of CP.

49. **B)** The toxin is usually found in stool or blood. Myasthenia gravis and Lambert-Eaton myasthenic syndrome would require a muscle biopsy.

50. **A)** SMA is an autosomal recessive disorder of infancy that presents within the first 2 months of life with hypotonia and symmetric weakness of the lower extremities more than the upper extremities. This is due to degeneration of the anterior horn cell of the spinal cord and brain stem. All of the answer choices are presenting symptoms of SMA type I, which is the most severe. Death usually occurs by age 3 years.

51. **B)** GBS is believed to be caused by *Campylobacter jejuni* or a viral attack on the myelin and Schwann cells. Initial symptoms will include weakness and tingling sensation in the legs and can progress to almost total paralysis.

52. **B)** This patient has Duchenne muscular dystrophy, an X-linked recessive genetic disorder. The way the child "walks up" the floor is described as Gower's sign. Patients usually present at around 3 to 5 years of age, and have proximal muscle weakness (especially pelvic girdle), scoliosis, calf pseudohypertrophy (where the calf may appear enlarged, but it is mostly fat and fibrous tissue), and progressive difficulty ambulating. Patients usually develop cardiac and respiratory issues, and have a life expectancy of around 25 years. Definitive diagnosis can be made with muscle biopsy, which would show absent dystrophin (compared to Becker's muscular dystrophy which shows decreased dystrophin). DNA tests also can now be used, even in pregnancy, to make the diagnosis. NCV/EMG studies will show normal sensory nerve action potential (SNAP), early recruitment, and +/− small amplitude polyphasic potentials. Labs will show an elevated CPK and aldolase level.

53. **D)** Upper motor neuron signs include weakness, spasticity, hyperreflexia, and upgoing plantar response. Lower motor neuron signs include atrophy, flaccidity, hyporeflexia, and fasciculations. Werdnig-Hoffmann disease is also known as spinal muscular atrophy type I, or acute infantile-onset SMA. This severe disorder often results in death by the age of 2 years, and disease onset is at 3 to 6 months. Recent studies have shown that there is a reported increase in longevity, most likely a result of better overall medical management. However, SMA type I carries the worst prognosis of all the forms of SMA, as patients may never be able to reach the childhood milestone of sitting independently. The disease course is rapid and fatal secondary to respiratory failure. SMA types II and III have later onset, and progression is generally slower. Kugelberg-Welander disease is also called SMA type III. All forms of spinal muscular atrophy are classified as lower motor neuron diseases. PLS is an upper motor neuron disease, and ALS is classified as both upper and lower motor neuron disease.

54. **B)** LEMS is a disorder of neuromuscular transmission due to an autoimmune response against the active sites on the presynaptic membrane. Patients complain of proximal fatigue and weakness that affects mainly the lower limbs, such as the quadriceps. Symptoms are exacerbated with rest and improved with exercise. Rarely are there neck, facial, or bulbar muscle involvements. It is important to note that there is sparing of ocular muscles. There is also often an association with malignancy, most commonly oat-cell carcinoma of the lung. Onset occurs more in males than in females (2:1) and in those older than 40 years. Unlike MG, LEMS patients may experience an increase in strength after a series of muscle contractions. Answer choices (C) and (D) are incorrectly paired.

55. **A)** BMD is an X-linked muscular dystrophy with similar clinical pattern and gene locus to Duchenne, but with mild and slower progression. The patient in this question is 18 years old and is still able to ambulate. Patients with Duchenne are usually wheelchair users by the age of 10 years if not treated with corticosteroids. Ambulation past 14 years of age should raise suspicion for a milder muscular dystrophy such as Becker's or LGMD. LGMD is an autosomal recessive condition.

56. **A)** Of the signs/symptoms of Parkinson's disease, the ones that are most common are resting tremor, bradykinesia/hypokinesia, and "cogwheel" rigidity. The resting tremor (sometimes referred to as pill rolling tremor) is 3 to 5 Hz and is the most common symptom, affecting about 65% of patients. The tremor is suppressed by activity or sleep and worsened by fatigue or stress. Bradykinesia is slowing of movements. "Cogwheel rigidity" is tremor superimposed on muscular rigidity. Other symptoms include a shuffling gait, masked facies, and postural instability. Patients can have depression, dementia, and/or orthostatic hypotension.

57. **A)** Multiple sclerosis actually affects females more than males (2:1 female to male ratio). Answer choices (B), (C), and (D) are all true. The net effect of pregnancy on the course of MS is neutral. This is due to the fact that there is a decrease in relapse during pregnancy, but higher than normal relapse during the first 3 months postpartum. Therefore, women should not fear that pregnancy can worsen their MS.

58. **C)** Lateral medullary syndrome, also known as Wallenberg's syndrome, posterior inferior cerebellar artery (PICA) syndrome, or vertebral artery syndrome, has a presentation that is very memorable. Signs and symptoms include the following:
    - Ipsilateral side findings: Horner's syndrome, decrease in pain and temperature sensation on ipsilateral face, cerebellar signs (ataxia) that characteristically make the patient fall toward the side of the lesion.
    - Contralateral side findings: Decreased pain and temperature sensation on the contralateral side of the body.
    - Dysphagia, dysarthria, hoarseness, paralysis of vocal cord, vertigo, hiccups, nystagmus, and diplopia can be seen. There is no facial or motor weakness in this syndrome.

59. **C)** All of the features mentioned portend a poor prognosis except for choice (C)—sensory findings/optic neuritis at onset. Other good prognostic indicators include a sudden onset with a long remission, retained ability to ambulate, and low current disability.

60. **C)** Features in this vignette are suggestive of the diagnosis of facioscapulohumeral dystrophy. Initial weakness affects facial muscles, especially the orbicularis oculi, zygomaticus, and the orbicularis oris. Clinical features include facial weakness, scapular winging, shoulder girdle weakness, and lordosis due to pelvic girdle weakness. Choice (A) is a syndrome that includes hypotonia, early contractures, equinovarus deformities, knee flexion contractures, and delayed motor milestones. A child of 12 years would already have symptoms. Choice (B) is a dystrophy marked by the presence of early contractures of the elbow flexors (limited extension) and heel cord tightness with ankle dorsiflexion weakness (toe-walking may be present). Choice (D) refers to syndromes that are similar to Becker's or Duchenne muscular dystrophy but predominantly affect shoulder and girdle muscles, causing weakness.

61. **A)** The classic findings in the MFV of GBS are ophthalmoplegia, ataxia, and areflexia. MFV represents only 5% of GBS cases and presents in descending fashion as opposed to the conventional ascending paralysis seen in conventional GBS forms. Thus, the eye is usually affected first. Gait and trunk muscles are often affected with general sparing of the limb muscles. The other choices (B) and (C) are seen in another variant of GBS, acute panautonomic neuropathy (which is the most rare form and potentially fatal).

62. **A)** Lambert-Eaton myasthenic syndrome is associated with small-cell lung tumor. Myasthenia gravis is associated with thymic tumor. Botulism is associated with ingestion of contaminated raw meat, canned vegetables, honey, or fish.

63. **B)** This type of dystrophy primarily affects the face and shoulder girdle muscles. It is a lower motor neuron disorder, so there is no spasticity or sensory findings.

64. **A)** Pompe's disease is an acid maltase deficiency. The resultant accumulation of glycogen leads to irreversible damage of skeletal, respiratory, and cardiac muscle tissue resulting in permanent disability and death.

65. **C)** Riluzole is the only medication proven to help delay the progression of ALS. Although the exact mechanism of action is not known, it does seem to have an inhibitory effect on glutamate receptors and sodium channels. Common side effects include nausea and weakness. Pyridostigmine is a cholinesterase inhibitor commonly used in exacerbations of myasthenia gravis. Baclofen, although used in patients with ALS and spasticity, does not have an effect on disease progression. Baclofen works as a gamma-aminobutyric acid-B (GABA-B) agonist which in turn can decrease release of excitatory transmitters, and decrease spasticity. Modafinil is a medication commonly used to treat narcolepsy but is also used to treat fatigue in multiple sclerosis patients. It stimulates norepinephrine, serotonin, dopamine, and histamine receptors.

66. **B)** This is an antiglutamate agent that may be effective in slowing the disease, prolonging ventilator time, and improving survival in patients with bulbar onset disease. However, side effects can include asthenia, and the medication is expensive. Nonpharmacological management of ALS includes rehabilitation, preventing contractures, submaximal exercise, tracheostomy, and respiratory therapy. Rebif is a beta interferon that is used to modify the course in multiple sclerosis patients. Baclofen is a derivative of gamma-aminobutyric acid (GABA) and is primarily used to treat spasticity. Levodopa is a medicine used to control symptoms of Parkinson's disease. Levodopa does not slow the disease process, but it improves muscle movement and delays severe disability.

67. **D)** This decreases calcium entry into the cell, causing a decreased release of acetylcholine into the synaptic cleft. There is a strong association with malignancy, such as small-cell (oat-cell) carcinoma of the lung. Answer choice (A) describes botulism, and answer choice (C) describes myasthenia gravis.

68. **A)** Patients with DMD often have contractures by 13 years of age. The lower limb contractures have been strongly associated with wheelchair reliance. Contractures may mostly affect ankle plantar flexors, knee flexors, hip flexors, iliotibial band, elbow flexors, and wrist flexors. Scoliosis is prevalent in 33% to 100% of DMD patients and is strongly related to age. Fifty percent will acquire scoliosis by the age of 12 to 15 years. There is no causal relationship between wheelchair use and scoliosis. Cardiac abnormalities happen in DMD patients because of absence of dystrophin, which is also present in myocardium and Purkinje fibers. ECG abnormalities can be seen, such as Q-waves in lateral leads, elevated ST segments, poor R-wave progression, and resting tachycardia. Cardiomyopathy is seen in nearly all DMD patients older than 18 years.

69. **B)** Medications used to treat Parkinson's disease work by increasing dopamine action and/or decreasing the cholinergic effect. Bromocriptine is an ergot derivative that stimulates dopamine D2 receptors. Non-Ergot derivatives include ropinirole (Requip) and pramipexole (Mirapex).

70. **C)** MS is considered an autoimmune disease. The disease affects the central nervous system most likely by causing demyelination, leading to plaque formation. The plaque causes oligodendrocyte destruction, astrocyte proliferation, and glial scarring, making the propagation of action potential down a nerve impossible. Remission may occur during this disease process as remyelination occurs.

71. **A)** Lateral medullary syndrome, also known as Wallenberg's syndrome, posterior inferior cerebellar artery (PICA) syndrome, or vertebral artery syndrome, has a presentation that is very memorable. Signs and symptoms include the following:

- Ipsilateral side findings: Horner's syndrome, decrease in pain and temperature sensation on ipsilateral face, cerebellar signs (ataxia) that characteristically make the patient fall toward the side of the lesion.
- Contralateral findings: Decreased pain and temperature sensation on the contralateral side of the body.
- Dysphagia, dysarthria, hoarseness, paralysis of vocal cord, vertigo, hiccups, nystagmus, and diplopia can be seen. There is no facial or motor weakness in this syndrome.

72. **D)** All the answer choices are features of Huntington's disease except for choice (D), which is seen in Parkinson's disease.

73. **B)** Although seldom used for spasticity, dantrolene has the least amount of sedation and cognitive impairment of all the antispasticity medications. This is primarily because its mechanism of action takes place peripherally in the sarcoplasmic reticulum, decreasing calcium release. It is an agent that is considered in the treatment of spasticity for patients having brain injury.

74. **C)** Infants should never be given honey. Honey ingestion can lead to hypotonia ("floppy baby") syndrome in an infant because of botulinum toxins in the honey.

75. **D)** All of the answer choices are associated features of CMD. Patients with Werdnig-Hoffmann disease (spinal muscular atrophy type I) usually die before scoliosis can occur.

76. **D)** Spastic (pyramidal) CP comprises 75% of all CP cases.

77. **B)** The other choices are not myopathies and not inflammatory.

78. **A)** The overall median 50% survival rate is 2.5 years after diagnosis. Survival rate is largely dependent on a patient's decision to use mechanical ventilation and/or a feeding tube, but the 5-year survival rate is between 4% and 30%. Around 10% will live for 10 years.

79. **A)** Neuromuscular junction disorders can be classified into two categories: presynaptic or postsynaptic. LEMS and botulism are presynaptic disorders, and myasthenia gravis is a postsynaptic disorder. Myasthenia gravis is a disorder resulting in a decreased quantal response because of an autoimmune response against acetylcholine receptors on the postsynaptic membrane. LEMS is a disorder of neuromuscular transmission due to an autoimmune response against the active sites on the presynaptic membrane. Botulism is a disorder of neuromuscular transmission caused by *Clostridium botulinum* toxins blocking exocytosis of acetylcholine from the nerve terminal. ALS is a motor neuron disease that presents with both upper and lower motor neuron lesions that is caused by degeneration of the anterior horn cell.

80. **B)** The dystrophin isomer is present in the brain. As there is an absence of this dystrophin protein in DMD, there have been lower IQ levels seen in affected children. Mean IQ scores have been 1 to 1.5 standard deviations below the normal population. An increase in autism and obsessive-compulsive disorder is also seen in DMD patients.

81. **D)** IBM clinically presents with asymmetric, slowly progressive, painless weakness in proximal and distal muscles. It is associated with a polyneuropathy. It is not responsive to pharmacologic intervention, such as steroids and immunosuppressive agents. Treatment choices primarily involve appropriate rehabilitation interventions, which include provision of assistive devices. Childhood dermatomyositis is treated with only corticosteroids, which are effective in inducing a remission and preventing a recurrence. Also, treatment can be stopped over time. Adult dermatomyositis and polymyositis are treated with corticosteroids and supplemented by immunosuppressive medications. This is usually not discontinued.

82. **B)** Interferon beta is a U.S. Food and Drug Administration (FDA) category C drug for pregnancy and is therefore stopped before a woman decides to try to have a child. Interferon beta has been shown to increase the rate of miscarriage. The risk for relapse is lower overall during pregnancy, so the drug is discontinued before conceiving. Glatiramer acetate is FDA category B and may be a better option for those who want to continue medications during pregnancy. Breastfeeding is known to decrease relapse rate in the first few months postpartum, and it is recommended to restart medications when breastfeeding is stopped.

83. **B)** Immunomodulator agents include interferon beta-1a (Avonex and Rebif), interferon beta-1b (Betaseron), and glatiramer acetate (Copaxone). These have been shown to reduce relapse rates in MS patients. Immunosuppressive agents include cyclosporine, azathioprine, methotrexate, and mitoxantrone, and can reduce relapse rate but have a greater side-effect profile and are therefore used as a second-line agent. Intravenous immunoglobulin is also an immunosuppressive agent and is still being studied for use in this patient population. Steroids can hasten recovery, but do not prevent further attacks, or alter progression.

84. **D)** All the medications listed can cause Parkinson's-like features through their effects on the dopamine neurotransmitter except for amantadine, which is actually used in the treatment of Parkinson's. It has mild anticholinergic activity and dopamine reuptake inhibiting properties.

85. **C)** All the symptoms involved suggest cerebellar impairment, including the ataxia and dysarthria. Multiple system atrophy has more autonomic involvement, including orthostatic hypotension, thermoregulatory dysfunction, and impotence. Choice (D) is harder to differentiate from primary Parkinson's, but is noted to have dystonia, with general absence of tremor. Choice (B) is associated with Parkinson's along with vertical gaze palsy.

86. **D)** All of the answer choices are considered lacunar syndromes, along with sensorimotor stroke, ataxia, and leg paralysis. Lacunar strokes comprise 20% of all strokes and are seen often in the putamen, pons, thalamus, internal capsule, and caudate. They are due to small occlusive arteriolar disease and are often associated with hypertension.

87. **A)** Botulism is caused by *C. botulinum* toxin. The toxin blocks release of acetylcholine.

88. **A)** Heat can worsen symptoms in patients with MS. They should be encouraged to use air conditioning. If pool therapy is used, the water should be below 84°F (29°C). When exercising, these patients must avoid raising their body core temperature.

89. **B)** CP is the leading cause of childhood disability with 2 to 3 cases per 1,000 births.

90. **A)** RLS sensations are sometimes compared to an itching or tickling in the muscles, which temporarily subside with movement of the affected extremities.

91. **D)** Poor prognostic factors include predominance of lower motor neuron (LMN) findings at diagnosis, short period from symptom onset to diagnosis, and older age at time of onset. Bulbar and pulmonary dysfunction early in the disease course is also a poor prognostic factor. Women typically present with bulbar symptoms, as compared with men. It is important to note that electrodiagnostic indicators of poor prognosis include profuse spontaneous fibrillations, positive sharp waves, and low-amplitude compound muscle action potential.

92. **C)** Acute poliomyelitis is a disease that causes degeneration of the anterior horn cell, and is caused by the polio virus. The polio virus is a small RNA virus belonging to the enterovirus group of the picornavirus family. Picornavirus enters the body orally and spreads via lymphoid system leading to orphaned muscle fibers and potential central nervous system involvement. All other answer choices are DNA viruses.

93. **C)** The presence of cardiac abnormalities in FSHD is rare. It is important to note that cardiomyopathy is seen prominently in Becker's and Duchenne muscular dystrophy. These patients have abnormalities in the dystrophin protein that is also present in myocardium and Purkinje fibers. ECG abnormalities can be seen, such as Q-waves in lateral leads, elevated ST segments, poor R-wave progression, and resting tachycardia. Cardiomyopathy is seen in nearly all patients older than 18 years in Duchenne. Cardiomyopathy may also be seen in Limb-girdle muscular dystrophy.

94. **B)** Patients with primary idiopathic dermatomyositis typically present with proximal muscle weakness and a characteristic rash on the face (heliotrope rash). A rash may also be noted on the extensor surfaces of the knees, elbows, ankles, and the dorsum of the hands.

95. **D)** The incidence of MS in the offspring of patients with MS is only slightly increased (3% for girls and 1% for boys). The net effect of pregnancy on the course of MS is neutral. This is due to the fact that there is a decrease in relapse during pregnancy, but higher than normal relapse during the first 3 months postpartum. Therefore, women should not fear that pregnancy can worsen their MS.

96. **C)** Corticosteroids (methylprednisolone) are used in acute attacks in MS patients. Corticosteroids have anti-inflammatory and antiedema properties. The dose that is given is 500 to 1,000 mg/day IV for 3 to 5 days and can be given with or without an oral taper. Long-term use is not recommended, as hyperglycemia, hypertension, osteoporosis, and cataracts can occur with prolonged use. Cerebellar and sensory symptoms are least responsive to corticosteroids. Steroids can hasten recovery, but do not prevent further attacks, or alter progression.

97. **D)** Environmental manipulation might influence both morphological change and the functional outcome after a cortical injury. Research studies revealed that animals reared or housed as adults in complex environments led to enhanced dendritic growth that was correlated with enhanced behavioral abilities. Patient motivation is an important factor in the success of his or her rehabilitation program. An important component of the rehabilitation process is to assist the patient in avoiding development of negative compensatory strategies.

98. **D)** All the following are typical features of LES except for choice (D). Weakness involving the eye muscles is very uncommon in LES.

99. **B)** This question describes findings of classical left-sided neglect. This feature is commonly seen in a right-MCA lesion (nondominant parietal lobe). With a lesion in the right MCA, the patient may present with intact speech but hemiparesis with focal weakness more on the upper extremity than lower extremity. There may be signs of impulsiveness and deficits in spatial perception as well as constructional apraxia. A lesion in the left MCA would involve the patient's speech and right-sided hemiparesis.

100. **B)** There is an autoimmune response to acetylcholine receptors in myasthenia gravis.

101. **A)** Lhermitte's sign is most commonly seen in MS. The patient may experience an electric shock–like sensation radiating to the spine and extremities when the neck is flexed. This is thought to be due to increased myelin sensitivity to traction.

102. **A)** Cerebral blood flow may be compromised in premature babies because of fragile brain vasculature.

103. **A)** ALS most commonly affects people in the age group of 40 to 60 years, and the mean age of onset is around 60 years. Onset is usually insidious and painless. Asymmetric weakness is the

most common presentation. Dysphagia (oral, pharyngeal), dysarthria, drooling, and aspiration can occur and are signs and symptoms representing bulbar muscular weakness. Also, strained, strangled quality of speech, reduced rate, and low pitch indicate a spastic dysarthria. Bowel and bladder function is typically spared in ALS.

104. **B)** Answer choice (B) would be correct if it referred to stability for approximately 15 years. Post-polio syndrome is a diagnosis based on exclusion. It has been well defined by the Halstead and Rossi criteria (1987):
    1. Confirmed history of poliomyelitis
    2. Partial to fairly complete neurologic and functional recovery
    3. A period of neurologic and functional stability of at least 15 years in duration
    4. Onset of two or more of the following health problems since achieving a period of stability: unaccustomed fatigue, muscle and/or joint pain, new weakness in muscles previously affected and/or unaffected, functional loss, cold intolerance, new atrophy
    5. No other medical diagnosis to explain these health issues.

105. **D)** Becker's muscular dystrophy has an X-linked inheritance, but has a slower clinical progression than Duchenne. They both have the same gene location (Xp21), but patients with Becker's muscular dystrophy have 20% to 80%, or even normal quantities, of dystrophin.

106. **A)** The three primary types of inflammatory myopathy are polymyositis, dermatomyositis, and inclusion body myositis (IBM). All are thought to involve immune-mediated processes, possibly triggered by environmental factors in genetically susceptible individuals. The age of onset for idiopathic inflammatory myopathies is bimodal. Peaks occur between 10 and 15 years of age in children and between 45 and 60 years of age in adults.

107. **C)** Huntington's disease is a hereditary disease (autosomal dominant) that has been linked to a trinucleotide cytosine, adenine, and guanine (CAG) repeat gene. Gamma-aminobutyric acid (GABA) has been found in decreased levels in the basal ganglia, and there is a decrease in substance P and enkephalins. The onset is usually from the ages 30 to 50 years, although 10% have been found to have juvenile onset, which occurs before the age of 20 years. Unfortunately, many die from aspiration pneumonia about 15 to 20 years after the onset of symptoms. The classic symptoms are chorea or choreoathetosis, which are hyperkinetic, involuntary, jerky movements. The other classic symptoms are dementia and personality disorder. A family history is usually noted.

108. **D)** Although both answer choices (A) and (B) may be seen in patients with MS, there is no pathognomonic test for MS. These tests are nonspecific and have to be interpreted with the entire clinical picture.

109. **D)** Partial body weight–supported gait training allows the simulation of task-specific walking movements and enables therapists to assist patients in the components of gait rather than bearing body weight. Gait training is necessary for the restoration of self-ambulation after brain injury. The patient works at improving coordination of movement and gradually increasing muscle strength. The lack of sufficient strength and balance to maintain an erect posture typically prevents gait training. Partial body weight support gait training is postulated to result in earlier weight bearing, increased strength, and reduced spasticity. It helps to prevent development of compensatory strategies for ambulation that may develop while using a cane or walker and creates undesirable motor habits. It also reduces the demands of muscles.

110. **D)** Increased tone, Babinski sign, and spasticity are all signs of an upper motor neuron (UMN) syndrome, whereas fasciculations are a sign of lower motor neuron syndrome. ALS is a disease with progressive injury and death to both pyramidal (upper motor) neurons and anterior horn (lower motor) neurons.

111. **A)** Weber's syndrome is due to obstruction of the paramedian branches of the posterior cerebral artery. It causes ipsilateral cranial nerve (CN) III paralysis (hence the ptosis, and dilated, downward, and out pupil) and contralateral hemiplegia. Millard-Gubler syndrome is caused by lesions to the basilar artery and results in ipsilateral CN VI and CN VII palsies with contralateral hemiplegia (lateral rectus and facial muscles). Medial medullary syndrome is caused by medial medullary infarction usually by atherosclerosis to the branches of the vertebral arteries or anterior spinal artery. It results in CN XII palsy (with tongue deviated toward side of lesion) and contralateral weakness and sensory loss.

112. **A)** Myasthenia gravis is a postsynaptic disorder. The other disorders are presynaptic.

113. **D)** Pregnancy in MS decreases relapses. However, relapses may increase after the delivery.

114. **B)** This is usually present in patients with CMT type II because of muscle wasting of the anterior leg compartment and the calf.

115. **C)** Weakness may be due to upper or lower motor neuron loss. Upper motor neuron (UMN) signs include weakness, spasticity, hyperreflexia, and upgoing plantar response. Lower motor neuron (LMN) signs include weakness, atrophy, flaccidity, hyporeflexia, and fasciculations. ALS patients with UMN pathology will often have a loss of dexterity or feeling of stiffness in their limbs. Spasticity may further exacerbate weakness and loss of function. This is due to the involvement of the vestibulospinal and reticulospinal tracts. LMN symptoms in the ALS population include muscle weakness, with some muscle fasciculations, atrophy, and muscle cramping. Cramping of abdominal or other trunk muscles should prompt a clinician to strongly consider ALS as a possible diagnosis. PLS is classified as a UMN lesion. Spinal muscle atrophy type II (SMA II) and poliomyelitis are classified as LMN lesions.

116. **A)** ALS is also called Lou Gehrig's disease, as it was named after the New York Yankees' first baseman who passed away from this disorder. This is unfortunately still the most widely known motor neuron disease and is the most common presenting form. The incidence of ALS is approximately 1.6 to 2.4 cases per 100,000 population.

117. **B)** DMD is an X-linked disorder with an abnormality in the Xp21 gene locus. There is dystrophin deficiency that disrupts the membrane cytoskeleton and leads to membrane instability. Chronically, this will lead to fibrotic replacement of muscle and failure of regeneration with muscle fiber death. Absent dystrophin or less than 3% of normal is diagnostic of DMD. Becker's is also an X-linked disorder, but quantitative dystrophin analysis shows dystrophin levels of 20% to 80%. Answer choices (C) and (D) are not X-linked disorders.

118. **D)** Dermatomyositis is an inflammatory myopathy that appears to have an association with occult carcinoma in adults. The true incidence may be as high as 10% to 20%. Because of this, it is important to search for carcinoma in adult patients, especially males of 40 years of age and older. There is a higher correlation with dermatomyositis and carcinoma, than with polymyositis. Steroid myopathy is a toxic myopathy and is caused by long-standing administration of exogenous steroids.

119. **B)** Interferon beta-1a is used to treat the relapsing-remitting form of multiple sclerosis. Answer choices (A), (C), and (D) all may cause drug-induced parkinsonism.

120. **D)** Patients commonly present with upper motor neuron (UMN) signs. MS is an autoimmune disease of the central nervous system. UMN signs include hyperreflexia, Hoffmann's and Babinski's signs, and spasticity. Weakness and decreased sensation can also be noted. Lhermitte's sign is a classic finding in MS. Patients complain of an electrical sensation that runs down the back and into the limbs (shoulders). It is elicited by bending the head forward (neck flexion); this is caused by involvement of the posterior columns. There is increased sensitivity of the myelin to stretch or traction. A pill-rolling tremor is frequently seen in Parkinson's disease.

121. **B)** Restoration focuses on reengaging residual brain areas that are initially dysfunctional after an injury. Recruitment involves engaging new residual areas of the brain. Retraining involves training the residual brain to perform new functions. Redacting refers to editing or drafting a document for publication.

122. **C)** Choice (A) refers to Lhermitte's sign, and choice (B) refers to internuclear ophthalmoplegia (INO), all seen in multiple sclerosis. Choice (C) describes Uhthoff's phenomenon. This effect is thought to reflect areas of impaired but still functioning myelin that break down in transmitting electrical impulses when surrounding fluid is heated. Ptosis is usually seen in myasthenia gravis.

123. **B)** This vignette is a classical presentation for Wallenberg's syndrome, otherwise known as lateral medullary syndrome. Usually due to occlusion of the vertebral artery or posterior inferior cerebellar artery (PICA), this syndrome causes ipsilateral Horner's syndrome, decrease in pain and temperature of face, and cerebellar signs of ataxia (ipsilateral) with decrease in pain and temperature on contralateral side of body.

124. **C)** In conduction aphasia, there is a normal rate of speech, preserved comprehension, but impaired repetition. The lesion is noted to be in the arcuate fasciculus, a band of white matter that joins the Broca's and Wernicke's areas. Choice (A) describes patients who have fluent speech, good comprehension, but signs of difficulty finding words, along with alexia and agraphia. Choice (B) describes patients with fluent speech, without comprehension, but preserved repetition. Choice (D) describes patients with nonfluent speech but good comprehension and preserved repetition.

125. **A)** LMN lesions can present with flaccidity, atrophy, and fasciculations. Spasticity is a sign of an upper motor neuron lesion.

126. **B)** In neuromuscular disorders, scoliosis is uncommon in children who are able to stand and walk. Prevention of scoliosis is usually accomplished by early bracing. Surgical intervention is indicated prior to a patient's vital capacity falling below 35% and prior to a spinal curvature of 35°.

127. **D)** Locked-in syndrome is caused by lesion to the ventral pons with an intact reticular activating system. This can be seen with a lesion in the distribution of the midline basilar artery. Choices (A) and (B) are often seen in Wallenberg's syndrome, whereas choice (C) is seen in Benedikt's or Weber's syndrome.

# 6

# Brain Injury

## QUESTIONS

1. The following is **not** a phase of swallowing:
   A) Oral phase
   B) Lingual phase
   C) Esophageal phase
   D) Pharyngeal phase

2. All of the following are associated with poor performance behind the wheel for driving evaluation after a stroke **except**:
   A) Right hemisphere location of stroke
   B) Visual perceptual deficits
   C) Aphasia
   D) Poor judgment or impulsivity

3. Patients complaining of having "the worst headache" of their lives should raise suspicions of:
   A) A migraine headache
   B) A subdural hematoma
   C) A subarachnoid hemorrhage
   D) An epidural hematoma

4. Traumatic brain injuries (TBI) in elderly patients are most frequently due to:
   A) Falls
   B) Motor vehicle accidents
   C) Alcohol (ETOH) abuse
   D) Assault

5. Seizures in stroke patients are associated with:
   A) Large parietal or temporal hemorrhages
   B) Older age
   C) Confusion
   D) All of the above

6. A 54-year-old woman experiences a left-middle cerebral artery infarction. She presents with impaired comprehension, fluent speech, impaired naming, and the presence of a homonymous hemianopsia. The most likely diagnosis is:
   A) Broca's aphasia
   B) Conduction aphasia
   C) Anomic aphasia
   D) Wernicke's aphasia

7. All of the following functions have been shown to be important cognitive predictors of driving ability **except**:
   A) Attention
   B) Memory
   C) Language
   D) Executive functioning

8. Following a concussion, a player should:
   A) Be evaluated the same day and not return to play
   B) Return to play; he is fine
   C) Be evaluated and, if he is fine, be allowed to return to play the same day
   D) Be sent to the emergency room (ER) immediately for admission

9. Which of the following is **not** a clinical finding in Parkinson's disease?
   A) Resting tremor
   B) Hallucinations
   C) Festinating gait
   D) Hypophonia

10. Coup-contrecoup injuries due to acceleration-deceleration forces (as in motor vehicle collisions) are typically concentrated in:
    A) Frontal and parietal lobes
    B) Frontal and occipital lobes
    C) Occipital and parietal lobes
    D) Subcortical structures

11. Which of the following is **not** true with regard to the left hemisphere of the brain?
    A) Damage results in loss of details
    B) Damage results in left neglect
    C) It is the dominant hemisphere for language for right handers
    D) It is the dominant hemisphere for language for most left handers

12. Which of the following is **not** a description of a subdural hematoma (SDH)?
    A) Occurs primarily in younger patients
    B) Clinical findings may sometimes be delayed for weeks
    C) Caused by an injury to the bridging veins
    D) Lentiform in shape on imaging

13. How should a behaviorally agitated traumatic brain injury (TBI) patient be managed?
    A) Restrain them even if not a risk to self or others
    B) Administer lorazepam or haloperidol to calm them
    C) Call hospital security to restrain them
    D) Identify cause of agitation and reorient the patient

14. The gold standard for assessment of swallowing function is:
    A) Bedside swallow evaluation
    B) Videofluoroscopic swallowing study (VFSS)
    C) Fiberoptic endoscopic evaluation of swallowing (FEES)
    D) Esophagoscopy

15. Common medical complications after stroke include all of the following **except**:
    A) Infections
    B) Falls
    C) Thrombosis
    D) Anemia

16. A stroke affecting the right hemisphere of the brain will usually cause weakness on the:
    A) Ipsilateral side
    B) Contralateral side
    C) Bilaterally
    D) None of the above

17. Risk factors for disability after a stroke would include all of the following **except**:
    A) Bilateral lesions
    B) Severe neglect
    C) Young age
    D) Delay in rehabilitation

18. Risk factors for developing poststroke depression include:
    A) Lack of social support
    B) Cognitive impairment
    C) High severity of deficits
    D) All of the above

19. Which of the following is **not** a symptom of Gerstmann's syndrome?
    A) Agraphia
    B) Acalculia
    C) Alexia
    D) Finger agnosia

20. On testing, a 75-year-old former engineer currently has an IQ score that is 2.5 standard deviations below the mean. She is alert and not depressed. What is the most likely diagnosis?
    A) Delirium
    B) Dementia
    C) Amnestic disorder
    D) Mental retardation (MR)

21. Which of the following is **not** a recommendation to reduce agitation in traumatic brain injury patients?
    A) Reduce noise
    B) Stay calm
    C) Rest breaks
    D) Correct confabulations

22. A clinical feature of normal pressure hydrocephalus (NPH) is:
    A) Memory impairment
    B) Urinary incontinence
    C) Ataxic gait
    D) All of the above

23. Damage to the right hemisphere of the brain can cause all of the following **except**:
    A) Anosognosia
    B) Inability to recognize prosody
    C) Difficulty analyzing sequences of stimuli
    D) Difficulty analyzing the gestalt of stimuli

24. Pseudobulbar palsy is characterized by:
    A) Emotional lability
    B) Dysphagia
    C) Frontal damage
    D) All of the above

25. What type of bleeding does an injury to the medial meningeal artery cause?
    A) Subdural hematoma (SDH)
    B) Epidural hematoma (EDH)
    C) Subarachnoid hemorrhage (SAH)
    D) Intracranial hemorrhage (ICH)

26. What should be initially prescribed to a patient with a traumatic brain injury (TBI) who suffers from insomnia, poor attention, poor memory, depressed mood, and headaches?
    A) A stimulant to help with the attention
    B) A sleeping medication and sleep hygiene
    C) A headache medication
    D) An antidepressant

27. Which of the following cranial nerves is **not** involved in the swallowing function?
    A) Trigeminal nerve
    B) Spinal accessory nerve
    C) Glossopharyngeal nerve
    D) Hypoglossal nerve

28. Malnutrition and hypoalbuminemia have been associated with which of the following in acute rehabilitation of stroke patients?
    A) Better functional outcome
    B) Higher complication rate
    C) Shorter length stay
    D) Improved functional improvement rate

29. A patient diagnosed with alexia is unable to:
    A) Read
    B) Write
    C) Recognize
    D) Calculate

30. Techniques to prevent aspiration while eating in a patient with a stroke would include:
    A) Chin tuck
    B) Head rotation
    C) Mendelsohn maneuver
    D) All of the above

31. Dysarthria involves all of the following **except**:
    A) Chewing and swallowing difficulty
    B) Hoarseness

C)  Drooling
D)  Complete movement of the lip, tongue, and jaw

32.  You are most likely to see conduction aphasia following damage to:
A)  The arcuate fasciculus
B)  The angular gyrus
C)  Middle cerebral artery-posterior cerebral artery (MCA-PCA) watershed areas
D)  Middle cerebral artery-anterior cerebral artery (MCA-ACA) watershed areas

33.  Which type of memory would be most affected by Alzheimer's disease?
A)  Episodic memory
B)  Remote memory
C)  Implicit memory
D)  Procedural memory

34.  Children who sustain a brain injury early in life sometimes appear to have no residual sequelae. This is because:
A)  They are resilient and "bounce back" even after severe trauma
B)  The effects of brain injury sometimes take time to emerge
C)  Other parts of their brain immediately take over
D)  They do not really sustain true brain injury

35.  According to the Glasgow Coma Scale (GCS), a severe brain injury would be:
A)  13 to 15
B)  0 to 2
C)  9 to 12
D)  3 to 8

36.  Which of the following is **not** characteristic of a grand mal seizure?
A)  The seizure involves motor convulsions
B)  The seizure is preceded by an aura
C)  The seizure has a clonic phase
D)  The seizure has a spell of absence

37.  Alzheimer's disease patients are placed in nursing homes primarily because of:
A)  Wandering
B)  Memory impairment
C)  Incontinence
D)  Hallucinations

38.  What is the description of a Rancho Los Amigos level of IV?
A)  Localized response to stimuli
B)  Confusion with inappropriate behavior
C)  Confusion but appropriate behavior
D)  Confusion and agitated behavior

39.  What is the most common symptom described after a concussion?
A)  Dizziness
B)  Poor sleep
C)  Headache
D)  Fatigue

40. Unawareness of illness in patients with spatial neglect is called:
    A) Asomatognosia
    B) Anosodiaphoria
    C) Anosognosia
    D) Apraxia

41. Shoulder subluxation after stroke:
    A) Occurs late in the recovery phase
    B) Is always associated with pain
    C) Is associated with flaccid hemiplegia
    D) Will need radiological studies for diagnosis

42. In a transient ischemic attack (TIA), the symptoms last for:
    A) Greater than 24 hours
    B) Less than 24 hours
    C) Greater than 48 hours
    D) Greater than 1 week

43. Overall, the most common cause of severe traumatic brain injury (TBI) is:
    A) Alcohol (ETOH) intoxication
    B) Falls
    C) Motor vehicle accidents (MVA)
    D) Assault

44. Which of the following may be helpful for a traumatic brain injury (TBI) patient with bladder and bowel dysfunctions?
    A) Frequent toileting
    B) Anticholinergics
    C) Condom catheter for men and absorbent pads for women
    D) All of the above

45. A 63-year-old right-handed woman with hypertension suddenly had difficulty getting words out. Speech was sparse, halting, and labored. She was able to follow three-step commands and repeated words and sentences with 100% accuracy. Where is the most likely location of her lesion?
    A) Middle cerebral artery-anterior cerebral artery territory (extrasylvian, anterior)
    B) Middle cerebral artery-posterior cerebral artery territory (extrasylvian, posterior)
    C) Broca's area
    D) Wernicke's area

46. Which of the following is true?
    A) Dementia is necessarily progressive
    B) Dementia does not always impair memory
    C) Dementia cannot have acute onset
    D) Dementia is "global" impairment

47. Which of the following is **not** true with regard to frontal lobe damage and emotion/behavior?
    A) Orbitofrontal damage has been associated with disinhibition
    B) Orbitofrontal damage has been associated with impulsivity
    C) Right frontal damage has been associated with depression
    D) Medial frontal damage has been associated with lack of initiation (abulia)

48. Generalized seizures that involve only involuntary muscle jerking are called:
    A) Myoclonic
    B) Tonic
    C) Absence
    D) Tonic-clonic

49. Amnesia for events that occurred before the disturbance to the brain is called:
    A) Anterograde amnesia
    B) Retrograde amnesia
    C) Declarative amnesia
    D) Korsakoff's amnesia

50. Which is the best study for locating white matter plaque in multiple sclerosis or vascular infarcts?
    A) CT
    B) Electroencephalogram (EEG)
    C) MRI
    D) Lumbar puncture (LP)

51. What is the Glasgow Coma Scale (GCS) score for someone who withdraws from pain, is confused, and opens eyes to pain?
    A) 6
    B) 8
    C) 10
    D) 12

52. How is the severity of a concussion graded?
    A) Concussion grading scales, such as Cantu and Colorado Head Injury Scales
    B) Presence of loss of consciousness (LOC)
    C) Presence of posttraumatic amnesia (PTA)
    D) Severity of ongoing symptoms

53. Spatial neglect is more commonly seen in:
    A) Dominant hemisphere infarcts
    B) Nondominant hemisphere infarcts
    C) Brain stem strokes
    D) Cerebellar strokes

54. The goals of intrathecal baclofen therapy in patients with post-stroke spastic hypertonia include all of the following **except**:
    A) Improved positioning and hygiene
    B) Prevention of complications
    C) Ease caregiver burden and time
    D) Initiate ambulation

55. What is the most important modifiable risk factor for ischemic and hemorrhagic stroke?
    A) Hypertension (HTN)
    B) Gender
    C) Race
    D) Age

56. Good prognosis of recovery after stroke is associated with:
    A) Complete arm paralysis
    B) Prolonged flaccidity
    C) Severe proximal spasticity
    D) Some motor recovery of the hand by 4 weeks

57. A first-line intervention for posttraumatic agitation would be:
    A) Placing patient in a quiet room and limiting the number of visitors
    B) Restraining the patient
    C) Medicating the patient
    D) Getting a psychiatric evaluation

58. A 63-year-old right-handed woman with hypertension suddenly had difficulty getting words out. Speech was sparse, halting, and labored. She was able to follow three-step commands and repeated words and sentences with 100% accuracy. What kind of aphasia is present in this patient?
    A) Broca's aphasia
    B) Wernicke's aphasia
    C) Transcortical sensory aphasia
    D) Transcortical motor aphasia

59. A 55-year-old patient complains of some difficulty paying attention and episodic memory problems (such as forgetting what she ate yesterday for dinner). She is not depressed. What is the most likely diagnosis (although, of course, you would want to evaluate further)?
    A) Delirium
    B) Alzheimer's disease
    C) Amnestic disorder
    D) Normal aging

60. All of the following are common brain areas affected by traumatic brain injury (TBI) **except**:
    A) Parietal areas
    B) Orbitofrontal
    C) Anterior temporal
    D) Limbic areas

61. Seizures that involve only one region of the brain and do not impair consciousness are called:
    A) Generalized
    B) Complex partial
    C) Simple partial
    D) Simple generalized

62. Which cortical lobe contains the primary somatosensory cortex?
    A) Frontal lobe
    B) Temporal lobe
    C) Parietal lobe
    D) Occipital lobe

63. Severity of brain injury is most reliably indicated by:
    A) Presence of seizure
    B) Presence of vomiting
    C) Chronic neck pain
    D) Length of coma and amnesia

64. Which best describes someone who is in a vegetative state?
    A) Eyes are open, eyes are tracking, he or she has sleep-wake cycles
    B) Eyes are closed, eyes are not tracking, he or she has no sleep-wake cycles
    C) Eyes are closed, eyes are not tracking, he or she has sleep-wake cycles
    D) Eyes are open, eyes are not tracking, he or she has sleep-wake cycles

65. Which is the most commonly injured cranial nerve (CN)?
    A) CN I
    B) CN II
    C) CN VII
    D) CN VIII

66. Wernicke's aphasia is characterized by intact _____, and deficits such as aphasia or cognitive impairment.
    A) Naming
    B) Comprehension
    C) Repetition
    D) Fluency

67. Which of the following is a side effect of tizanidine, a medication used in spasticity?
    A) Abnormal renal function tests
    B) Somnolence
    C) Cardiac toxicity
    D) Electrolyte abnormalities

68. Physiological factors that account for stroke recovery include all the following **except**:
    A) Side of stroke
    B) Resolution of post-stroke edema
    C) Reperfusion of ischemic penumbra
    D) Cortical reorganization

69. In a patient with transcortical mixed aphasia, the patient will have:
    A) Fluent speech
    B) Good comprehension
    C) Preserved repetition (echolalia)
    D) None of the above

70. Uncal herniation would cause compression of:
    A) Cranial nerve (CN) III
    B) CN I
    C) CN VII
    D) CN X

71. Aphasia classification is based on which three parts of the language assessment?
    A) Fluency, repetition, prosody
    B) Fluency, comprehension, naming
    C) Fluency, comprehension, repetition
    D) Comprehension, reading, writing

72. Which of the following dementias is characterized by fluctuating course, extrapyramidal features, and occasionally visual hallucinations and delusions?
    A) Alzheimer's disease
    B) Frontotemporal dementia
    C) Lewy body disease
    D) Dementia pugilistica

73. All of the following are common secondary effects of closed head injury **except**:
    A) Hypoxia
    B) Meningeal/cerebral laceration
    C) Edema
    D) Intracranial bleeding (eg, subdural hematoma)

74. Disorientation and transient attentional difficulties due to infection, medications, electrolyte imbalance, or dehydration is likely to be:
    A) Delusional disorder
    B) Dementia
    C) Amnestic disorder
    D) Delirium

75. What part of the central nervous system (CNS) is affected in multiple sclerosis (MS)?
    A) Dendritic receptors
    B) Axon
    C) Terminal branches
    D) Myelin sheath

76. Compared with epidural hematomas, subdural hematomas:
    A) Originate from arterial bleeding
    B) May develop slowly
    C) Cause severe headaches
    D) Are often fatal

77. Which of the following is **not** true about diffuse axonal injury (DAI)?
    A) Primarily occurs at the gray matter
    B) Only seen in traumatic brain injury (TBI)
    C) Responsible for loss of consciousness (LOC)
    D) Occurs from acceleration-deceleration and rotational forces

78. What does **not** describe posttraumatic amnesia (PTA)?
    A) It is a predictor of recovery and outcome in traumatic brain injury (TBI)
    B) It measures retrograde amnesia
    C) It is an indication of the ability to retain ongoing new memories
    D) It can be assessed using the Galveston Orientation and Amnesia Test (GOAT)

79. Aphasia is an impairment in:
    A) Language
    B) Speech
    C) Phonation
    D) Swallowing

80. Baclofen is an antispasticity agent that is:
    A) A structural analogue of gamma-amino butyric acid (GABA)
    B) An alpha-2 adrenergic agonist

C) A hydantoin derivative

D) An imidazoline derivative

81. Which of the following statements regarding the National Institutes of Health (NIH) stroke scale is **incorrect**?

A) It requires training and certification

B) It is valuable in quantifying deficits after a stroke

C) It may help in predicting posthospital disposition

D) Elements of brain stem function are well reflected

82. The inclusion criterion for tissue plasminogen activator (tPA) is:

A) 18 years of age or older with informed consent

B) Head CT negative for blood

C) Well-established time of onset less than 3 hours before treatment initiation with moderate to severe stroke symptoms

D) All of the above

83. A Glasgow Coma Scale (GCS) score of 3 to 8 would indicate:

A) Death

B) Severe traumatic brain injury (TBI)

C) Mild TBI

D) Moderate TBI

84. In "locked-in" syndrome, the patient is:

A) Paralyzed with possible preserved vertical gaze and blinking

B) Unable to speak

C) Awake and sensate

D) All of the above

85. All of the following are associated with frontal-subcortical dementia **except**:

A) Normal pressure hydrocephalus

B) Frontotemporal dementia

C) Vascular dementia

D) Parkinson's dementia

86. Which of the following is **least** true regarding cognitive rehabilitation?

A) Cognitive rehabilitation is informed and guided by theoretical models

B) Cognitive rehabilitation's goal is to increase test scores

C) Cognitive rehabilitation focuses on both amelioration of and compensation for deficits

D) Cognitive rehabilitation has a large education component

87. Which of the following tests is most useful for evaluation of memory loss?

A) Mini Mental Status Examination (MMSE)

B) Galveston Orientation and Amnesia Test (GOAT)

C) Ranchos Los Amigos Scale

D) Glasgow Coma Scale (GCS)

88. Parkinson's disease has been linked to:

A) Loss of cholinergic neurons in the nucleus basalis of Meynert

B) Loss of dopaminergic neurons in the substantia nigra

C) Overproduction of gamma-amino butyric acid (GABA) in the caudate nucleus

D) Overproduction of dopamine in the basal ganglia

89. Which disorder is **least** associated with a higher incidence of depression?
    A) Alzheimer's disease (AD)
    B) Parkinson's disease
    C) Huntington's disease
    D) Stroke

90. Which are the most commonly injured areas of the brain after a traumatic brain injury (TBI)?
    A) Occipital and frontal
    B) Frontal and temporal
    C) Parietal and frontal
    D) Occipital and temporal

91. What is the best acute predictor of outcome after a traumatic brain injury (TBI)?
    A) Best motor response of the Glasgow Coma Scale (GCS)
    B) Best verbal response on the GCS
    C) Best eye-opening response on the GCS
    D) Initial GCS score

92. In a patient with symptoms of a stroke, which of the following is the first-line diagnostic radio-logical test?
    A) MRI of the brain
    B) Carotid Dopplers
    C) Magnetic resonance angiogram (MRA) of the head
    D) CT brain without contrast

93. What is the greatest predictor of community ambulation after a stroke?
    A) Use of an assistive device
    B) Walking speed
    C) Degree of lower extremity motor strength
    D) Type of stroke

94. Which of the following is a contraindication for administration of tissue plasminogen activator (tPA)?
    A) Stroke symptom onset less than 3 hours
    B) Platelet count greater than 100,000
    C) International normalized ratio (INR) less than 1.7
    D) History of recent myocardial infarction (MI) within 3 months

95. In a patient with a stroke, the intracranial pressure (ICP) should be kept at:
    A) Greater than 20 mmHg
    B) Greater than 40 mmHg
    C) Less than 20 mmHg
    D) Less than 80 mmHg

96. In decerebrate posturing, there is:
    A) Flexion of the upper and lower extremities
    B) Extension of the upper and flexion of the lower extremities
    C) Flexion of the upper and extension of the lower extremities
    D) Extension of the upper and lower extremities

97. Syndrome of inappropriate antidiuretic hormone (SIADH) is found in:
    A) Acute stroke
    B) Chronic traumatic brain injury (TBI)
    C) Acute TBI
    D) Chronic stroke

98. How long should phenytoin be administered for seizure prophylaxis after a traumatic brain injury (TBI)?
    A) 1 week
    B) 6 months
    C) 1 year
    D) Indefinitely

99. Which statement is correct about the Mini Mental Status Examination (MMSE)?
    A) The MMSE is unfortunately not available in many languages besides English
    B) The MMSE can be used with patients with at least a first-grade education
    C) The MMSE is a cognitive screening instrument, with a maximum of 20 points
    D) The MMSE is a cognitive screening instrument, but does not measure executive functioning

100. Which of the following syndromes means an inability to recognize or appreciate stimuli?
    A) Aphasia
    B) Amnesia
    C) Apraxia
    D) Agnosia

101. Ischemic strokes are caused by:
    A) Aneurysm tear
    B) Intracranial bleeding
    C) Thrombi or emboli
    D) All of the above

102. Which is the most common cause of falls in the elderly?
    A) Neuropathy
    B) Normal pressure hydrocephalus
    C) Medications, especially sedatives
    D) Transient ischemic attack (TIA)

103. Repeated concussions may result in:
    A) Parkinson's-like symptoms
    B) Alzheimer's-like neuropathology
    C) Second impact syndrome
    D) All of the above

104. Which is the most sensitive test used to identify early heterotopic ossification (HO)?
    A) X-ray
    B) Serum alkaline phosphatase
    C) CT scan
    D) Bone scan

**105.** The most common cause of hemorrhagic stroke is:
A) Ruptured aneurysm
B) Arteriovenous malformation
C) Hypertension
D) Amyloid angiopathy

**106.** Factors increasing the risk of urinary incontinence after a stroke include all of the following **except**:
A) Male sex
B) Advanced age
C) Greater stroke severity
D) Diabetes mellitus

**107.** All of the following are accepted options for initial therapy for patients with noncardioembolic ischemic stroke **except**:
A) Coumadin
B) Aspirin
C) Clopidogrel
D) Combination of aspirin and extended-release dipyridamole

**108.** A suspected intracranial hemorrhage would require a CT of the head:
A) With contrast
B) Without contrast
C) With and without contrast
D) Would not require a CT of the head

**109.** Of the following disorders of consciousness, which would have the best prognosis?
A) Coma
B) Vegetative state
C) Minimally conscious state
D) Brain death

**110.** A traumatic brain injury (TBI) patient who is confused and inappropriate would be considered a Ranchos level:
A) IV
B) V
C) VI
D) None of the above

**111.** What is considered the most effective method for the prevention of heterotopic ossification (HO)?
A) Radiation of bone tissue
B) Range of motion
C) Nonsteroidal anti-inflammatory drugs (NSAIDs)
D) Diphosphonates

**112.** Which of the following is **not** true with regard to assessing a patient's ability to return to work?
A) Assessment of emotional and behavioral functioning is important
B) Assessment of academic ability and IQ is not necessary
C) Much depends on the demands of the individual's specific job
D) Assessment of the patient's family circumstances is necessary

113. The inability to attend to a side of space, usually the left, is referred to as:
    A) Amnesia
    B) Neglect
    C) Disorientation
    D) Gerstmann's syndrome

114. Which of the following is a benign tumor arising from dural or arachnoid cells?
    A) Glioma
    B) Astrocytoma
    C) Meningioma
    D) Glioblastoma multiforme

115. Which of the following dementias features spongiform cerebral cortex?
    A) Alzheimer's dementia
    B) Creutzfeldt-Jakob disease
    C) AIDS dementia
    D) Wilson's disease

116. Significant amounts of pain are reported by 95% of _____ traumatic brain injury (TBI) patients, but by only 22% of _____ TBI patients.
    A) Severe; mild
    B) Mild; severe
    C) Moderate; mild
    D) All of the above

117. What is the most common location of heterotopic ossification (HO) after traumatic brain injury (TBI)?
    A) Shoulder
    B) Knee
    C) Hip
    D) Elbow

118. Which of the following is a nonmodifiable risk factor for stroke?
    A) Hypertension
    B) Atrial fibrillation
    C) Age
    D) Smoking

119. Predictors of aspiration on a bedside swallow exam include all of the following **except**:
    A) Tachycardia
    B) Cough
    C) Voice change after swallow
    D) Dysphonia

120. All of the following are features of lateral medullary syndrome **except**:
    A) Hemiplegia
    B) Dysphagia
    C) Ipsilateral facial hemisensory deficit
    D) Palate and vocal cord paralysis

121. On a CT scan, a hemorrhage would appear:
    A) Black
    B) White
    C) Gray
    D) None of the above

122. Epidural hematoma occurs most frequently from:
    A) Rupture of the middle meningeal artery
    B) Arteriovenous malformation
    C) Shearing of bridging veins between pia-arachnoid and the dura
    D) Brain tumors

123. Skin integrity is maintained in stroke patients by all of the following measures **except**:
    A) Protection from moisture
    B) Decrease in patient mobility
    C) Maintenance of adequate nutrition and hydration
    D) Frequent position changes

124. All of the following are reasons to refer for a neuropsychological evaluation or consult **except**:
    A) When impairment of cognitive functioning or behavior is suspected
    B) When medication is being considered for a patient's mood disorder or behavior
    C) When you want to track progress of rehabilitation after traumatic brain injury (TBI) or other neurological disorder
    D) To plan treatments which utilize cognitive strengths to compensate for weaknesses

125. Which test would be most useful as a predictor of driving ability?
    A) Boston naming test (BNT)
    B) Clock drawing
    C) Trailmaking Test
    D) Rorschach inkblot test

126. Asking a patient to count backward from 100 by 7 (or spell WORLD backward) is a test of:
    A) Orientation
    B) Abstraction
    C) Attention
    D) Memory

127. Pseudodementia is best characterized as:
    A) Malingering
    B) Delirium
    C) Normal aging
    D) Depression

128. Which is the most common dementia accompanied by a peripheral neuropathy?
    A) Alzheimer's disease
    B) Vascular dementia
    C) Traumatic brain injury dementia
    D) Wernicke-Korsakoff syndrome

129. Which behavioral problem, common after brain injury, is frequently confused with depression?
    A) Impulsivity
    B) Disinhibition

C) Abulia

D) Agitation

130. Which of the following is true about the Glasgow Coma Scale (GCS) in traumatic brain injury (TBI)?

A) A GCS of 2 is a severe injury

B) A GCS of 8 is a moderate injury

C) A GCS of 10 is a moderate injury

D) A GCS of 12 is a mild injury

131. What neurotransmitter should be enhanced to improve cognitive recovery in patients with a traumatic brain injury (TBI)?

A) Norepinephrine

B) Dopamine

C) Histamine

D) Acetylcholine

132. Which antiseizure medication is associated with disorders of the vestibular and cerebellar systems, such as nystagmus, ataxia, and vertigo, as well as gingival hyperplasia?

A) Phenobarbital

B) Valproic acid

C) Phenytoin

D) Gabapentin

133. A 28-year-old woman after a motor vehicle accident sustained a traumatic brain injury (TBI). The impact of injury was to the right side of her head and she now has visual changes consistent with an oculomotor cranial nerve (CN) dysfunction. What would the ocular exam demonstrate?

A) Dilation of the ipsilateral pupil

B) Constriction of the ipsilateral pupil

C) Dilation of the contralateral pupil

D) Constriction of the contralateral pupil

134. Which of the following statements is correct regarding epidural hematomas (EDH)?

A) Bleeding occurs between the dura and the arachnoid mater

B) Symptoms develop slowly, over hours or days after injury

C) Most commonly associated with venous bleeding

D) Patients classically have a lucid interval before the development of neurological symptoms

135. What is the best recommendation for return to play (RTP) in an adolescent who has sustained a concussion?

A) If the athlete has no symptoms after 24 hours, can RTP the next day

B) If the athlete has had loss of consciousness (LOC), RTP is delayed for a week

C) If the athlete has no symptoms at rest for 24 hours, can begin light aerobic activities

D) If the athlete has no symptoms at rest for 7 days, can RTP the next day

136. What is the initial management for a traumatic brain injury (TBI) patient who has a sodium (Na+) level of 132, is asymptomatic, and has no signs of dehydration?

A) Administer hypertonic saline

B) Prescribe demeclocycline

C) Give NaCl tablets

D) Restrict oral (PO) fluids

# *Brain Injury*

## ANSWERS

1. **B)** The phases of swallowing include the oral (oral preparatory and oral propulsive), pharyngeal, and esophageal phases. While the tongue is important in the oral phase of swallowing, there is no lingual phase of swallowing. The oral preparatory phase prepares the bolus for swallow. The oral propulsive phase involves food being transported posteriorly by the action of the tongue contacting the palate and propelling food into the pharynx. The pharyngeal phase is controlled centrally by the medulla, and allows for bolus to be propelled toward the esophagus. In the esophageal phase, a peristaltic wave propels the food into the stomach.

2. **C)** Aphasia may affect performance on written and road tests, but does not always interfere with self-directed driving. Right-hemisphere stroke may affect problem solving and memory, as well as potentially cause a left hemineglect, all of which would impair driving. Visual defects and poor judgment would also lead to poor performance during a driving evaluation.

3. **C)** A subarachnoid hemorrhage is usually caused by the rupture of an aneurysm. The blood irritates the meninges, causing a severe headache. A migraine headache can sometimes be severe and may be associated with an aura, nausea, vomiting, and sensitivity to light or other stimuli. Subdural hematoma and epidural hematoma usually result from head injury.

4. **A)** In the elderly population, gait and visual disturbances lead to falls, which cause most of the TBIs in the elderly. Motor vehicle accident is the most common cause of head injury in adolescents and adults. Violence and assault is the second most common cause of TBI in young adults. ETOH use is common in TBI patients at time of injury.

5. **D)** All of the answer choices are associated with seizures in stroke patients. Seizures can be classified as occurring at stroke onset, early after stroke (1 to 2 weeks) or late after stroke (later than 2 weeks). Seizures are associated with older age, confusion, and large parietal or temporal hemorrhages. The majority of seizures are generalized tonic-clonic.

6. **D)** Although both Wernicke's aphasia and conduction aphasia are characterized by fluent speech, only Wernicke's aphasia also includes impaired comprehension.

7. **C)** Driving is demanding on attention, memory, and executive functioning (sequencing, planning, and shifting), but less so language.

8. **A)** The 2011 update of the American College of Sports Medicine's consensus statement on concussion explicitly states no return to play same day.

9. **B)** Hallucinations may be seen in Lewy body disease, which has extrapyramidal features; the rest are findings in Parkinson's disease. Findings in Parkinson's disease include pill rolling tremor, bradykinesia, rigidity, postural instability, shuffling gait, cognitive impairment, and mood disorders.

10. **B)** The coup is the contusion directly beneath the impact; the contrecoup is the side opposite the impact. In an acceleration-deceleration situation, the brain moves forward anteriorly until it strikes the skull, and then recoils backward, hitting the back of the skull. Thus, in this type of injury, the frontal and occipital lobes are the most affected. This is different than striking the side of the head, in which the injuries would be to lateral opposite sides of the brain.

11. **B)** Ninety-five percent of right handers and 70% of left handers are left-dominant for language. The left hemisphere is involved in detail analysis, whereas the right hemisphere is involved in whole/gestalt analysis. Left neglect occurs from right-hemisphere damage.

12. **A)** Bridging veins connect the brain to the subdural venous sinuses. These bridging veins can be ruptured by acceleration-deceleration shearing stress. When the bridging veins are ruptured, blood can accumulate in the subdural space. An SDH appears as a crescent or lentiform shape on CT. Subdural hematoma can be acute, subacute, or chronic. The elderly are particularly at risk owing to atrophy which already stresses bridging veins, which can then rupture with even mild trauma. The SDH expands slowly, which can cause a delay in symptoms.

13. **D)** Agitation from a TBI is caused by confusion and inability to retain memory (posttraumatic amnesia). First, the inciting factor should be identified. Then, one person should speak with the patient in a calm manner and redirect the patient as to where he or she is and why they are in the hospital. The environment should be altered to minimize distractions, provide a structured program of therapies, and be safe. Restraints and medications, such as lorazepam, should only be used if there is a risk for the patient to injure himself or herself or others. Haloperidol should never be used because it has been shown to negatively impact recovery.

14. **B)** The VFSS, also known as a modified barium swallow study, is the gold standard in swallowing assessment. This evaluation involves using videofluorography and a radio opaque bolus to visualize the entire swallow. The consistency of a bolus that the patient is able to swallow safely can be assessed by observing the path of a swallowed bolus. FEES is a bedside procedure in which a nasally inserted flexible endoscope is used to directly view the nasopharynx and larynx during swallowing, and is an option when a patient cannot tolerate radiology or fluoroscopy. FEES does not visualize the esophagus. A bedside swallow examination is a screening examination and may miss silent aspiration. Esophagoscopy is useful in assessing anatomical abnormalities of the esophagus.

15. **D)** The common medical complications after a stroke include both urinary and chest infections, falls, deep vein thrombosis, decubitus ulcers, and pain. Anemia may be an associated finding, but is not reported as a common complication.

16. **B)** Owing to crossing of the corticospinal tract motor pathways, a stroke in either hemisphere will usually cause weakness on the contralateral side.

17. **C)** The prognosis for recovery is better in a younger individual. Severe neglect, bilateral lesions, and a delay in rehabilitation are risk factors for disability after a stroke.

18. **D)** All of the answer choices are risk factors for poststroke depression. Risk factors for poststroke depression include prior psychiatric history, significant impairment in activities of daily living, high severity of deficits, female gender, nonfluent aphasia, cognitive impairment, and lack of social supports. Persistent depression correlates with delayed recovery and poorer prognosis.

19. **C)** The four components of Gerstmann's syndrome are finger agnosia, acalculia, right-left disorientation, and agraphia. Alexia is a form of receptive aphasia in which there is inability to understand written language.

20. **B)** This was an acquired (and not congenital) disorder, so dementia rather than MR would be likely. Given that the patient had been an engineer, MR is unlikely, and as she is alert, delirium is unlikely. Given that other cognitive functions are involved in addition to memory, she does not meet criteria for an amnestic disorder.

21. **D)** Continually correcting patients may confuse or agitate them further; common recommendations are to "go with" their confabulations while they are acutely agitated. Patients should be maintained in a safe, structured, low-stimulus environment, which is frequently adequate to manage short-term behavior problems. Reducing the level of stimulation in the environment and protecting the patient from harming self or others will reduce the patient's cognitive confusion.

22. **D)** Sometimes called the "3 Ws" for wet, wobbly, and wacky, NPH is characterized by urinary incontinence, ataxic gait, and dementia.

23. **C)** The right hemisphere analyzes the gestalt and emotional prosody of speech and has to do with awareness; the left hemisphere is involved in speech and sequential or linear reasoning.

24. **D)** Pseudobulbar palsy (dysarthria, dysphagia, hyperactive gag reflex, and labile emotional responses) is due to damage to the bilateral upper motor neuron corticobulbar tract and can occur from frontal damage.

25. **B)** The middle meningeal artery is responsible for causing an EDH. An EDH has a biconvex shape and is rapidly evolving. SDH occurs from shearing of the bridging veins between the pia-arachnoid and dura maters. SAH is closely associated with ruptured cerebral aneurysms and arteriovenous malformations.

26. **B)** For a patient with a TBI, sleep is one of the most important aspects of medication management. If it is not addressed, lack of sleep may cause difficulty with attention, memory, headaches, poor mood, and overall poor general health.

27. **B)** The spinal accessory nerve does not have a role in the swallowing mechanism. The trigeminal, facial, glossopharyngeal, vagus, and hypoglossal nerves all have a role in the swallowing function. There are four phases of swallowing: oral preparatory, oral propulsive, pharyngeal, and esophageal. The oral preparatory phase prepares the bolus for swallow. The oral propulsive phase involves food being transported posteriorly by the action of the tongue contacting the palate and propelling food into the pharynx. The pharyngeal phase is controlled centrally by the medulla, and allows for bolus to be propelled toward the esophagus. In the esophageal phase, a peristaltic wave propels the food into the stomach. The trigeminal nerve, cranial nerve (CN) V, is involved in the oral preparatory phase because food stimulates mechanoreceptors, which produce contraction and relaxation of the muscles, allowing for chewing. The facial nerve (CN VII) also controls motor function of buccinator, which assists with mastication. The glossopharyngeal nerve (CN IX) innervates the stylopharyngeus, which helps accommodate a swallowed bolus. The hypoglossal nerve (CN XII) provides motor function of the tongue, which is involuntary and allows for swallow. The vagus nerve innervates the palatoglossus muscle.

28. **B)** Malnutrition and hypoalbuminemia have been associated with poorer functional outcomes, higher complication rates, longer length of stay, and reduced functional improvement rates in acute rehabilitation stroke patients.

29. **A)** Alexia is a neurologic inability to read (different from illiteracy). Agraphia is an inability to write. Agnosia is an inability to recognize objects, people, sounds, smells, or shapes. Acalculia is an inability to perform mathematical tasks.

30. **D)** All of the maneuvers mentioned prevent aspiration by providing airway protection. Tucking the chin helps prevent liquid from entering the larynx. Head rotation (turning the head toward the paretic side) helps force the bolus of food into the contralateral pharynx. The Mendelsohn maneuver involves having the patient voluntarily hold the larynx at its maximal height to increase the duration of the cricopharyngeal opening.

31. **D)** In dysarthria, there are limited lip, tongue, and jaw movements. Dysarthria is a motor-speech disorder. It results from impaired movement of the muscles used for speech production, including the lips, tongue, vocal folds, jaw, and/or diaphragm. Signs and symptoms of dysarthria include slurred or mumbled speech, slow rate of speech, abnormal pitch and rhythm when speaking, changes in voice quality, and/or drooling. Patients may also develop dysphagia, difficulty swallowing, due to the weakened muscles.

32. **A)** Conduction aphasia is considered a disconnection syndrome in which speech comprehension (Wernicke's area) is disconnected via a lesion in the arcuate fasciculus from the speech production area (Broca's area).

33. **A)** Alzheimer's disease affects episodic memory.

34. **B)** Cognitive or behavioral issues may not be evident until that time, developmentally, when the child would reach certain milestones; as the child grows and their brain develops, problems may emerge.

35. **D)** The GCS is from 3 to 15. A score of less than 8 indicates a severe brain injury. A score of 9 to 12 indicates moderate brain injury and a score of 13 or over indicates mild injury.

36. **D)** Grand mal, or tonic-clonic, seizures have both a tonic and clonic phase, involve convulsions, and are often preceded by an aura. Absence spells are characteristic of petit mal, or absence, seizures.

37. **A)** Wandering is one of the main reasons that Alzheimer's disease patients are placed in a nursing home. Six in ten people with dementia will wander. A person with Alzheimer's may not remember his or her name or address, and can become disoriented, even in familiar places.

38. **D)** The Ranchos Los Amigos scale is a scale used to assess patients after TBI. Level I (no response), level II (generalized response), level III (localized response), level IV (confused, agitated response), level V (confused, inappropriate, nonagitated response), level VI (confused, appropriate response), level VII (automatic, appropriate response), level VIII (purposeful, appropriate response). Level III is answer choice (A) (localized response to stimuli), level V is answer choice (B), and level VI is answer choice (C).

39. **C)** Headaches are the most common symptom experienced after a concussion. The others can also occur, but are not as frequent as headaches.

40. **C)** Unawareness of illness in patients with spatial neglect is called anosognosia. Asomatognosia is a condition where patients do not recognize that parts of their body belong to them. When patients with spatial neglect appear unconcerned or joke about their disability, it is called anosodiaphoria. Apraxia is a disorder of motor planning when strength, sensation, and coordination are intact.

41. **C)** Shoulder subluxation tends to occur early after a stroke in patients with flaccid hemiplegia. Although shoulder subluxation is listed as a common cause of shoulder pain, the relationship between the two remains controversial. The clinical diagnosis of shoulder subluxation can be made without imaging studies.

42. **B)** By definition, in a patient with TIA, the symptoms will resolve in less than 24 hours. On the other hand, in a stroke, the symptoms persist for over 24 hours and may never fully resolve.

43. **C)** MVA accounts for approximately 50% of all TBI cases. Assault is the second most common cause. However, the most common cause of TBI varies by age group. Falls and child abuse are more common in infants and toddlers. Older children have higher rates of accidental trauma and MVA. In adolescents, TBI is more commonly due to violence and risk-taking behavior. In patients over age 65 years, TBI is most commonly due to falls.

44. **D)** All of the answer choices are appropriate interventions for a TBI patient with bowel and bladder dysfunction. TBI patients are frequently incontinent. A time-void program is usually helpful, in which the patient is offered the urinal or commode at a regularly scheduled interval. Anticholinergic medications, which decrease detrusor tone and increase bladder capacity, may also be helpful. Condom catheter for men and absorbent pads for women are also helpful tools for TBI patients.

45. **A)** This reflects a lesion in the anterior cerebral artery territory (extrasylvian). Nonfluent (motor) aphasias affect anterior (pre-Rolandic) regions. With intact arcuate fasciculus, repetition is intact. In this example, the patient is able to repeat words, so the arcuate fasciculus is intact. Broca's and Wernicke's areas are in the arcuate fasciculus. Therefore, with injury to these areas, the patient is unable to repeat words.

46. **B)** Some dementias, such as HIV dementia and some of the frontotemporal dementias, actually may not impair memory. Dementias can be treatable (eg, normal pressure hydrocephalus), can be acute (eg, traumatic brain injury or stroke), and are not always global.

47. **C)** Left-frontal damage is typically associated with depression; the rest are true. The orbitofrontal cortex is concerned with response inhibition. Patients with orbitofrontal lesions tend to have difficulty with disinhibition, emotional lability, and memory disorders. Patients with such acquired sociopathy, or pseudopsychopathic disorder, are said to have an orbital personality. Personality changes from orbital damage include impulsiveness, puerility, a jocular attitude, sexual disinhibition, and complete lack of concern for others.

48. **A)** Tonic seizures involve "drop attacks" or abrupt falls; absence seizures involve staring or trance-like states; tonic-clonic seizures have both convulsions and stiffening of the body followed by involuntary muscle jerking.

49. **B)** Amnesia for events prior to a brain injury is retrograde amnesia. Anterograde amnesia is loss of the ability to create new memories subsequent to a brain injury. Declarative amnesia patients lose the recollection of facts. Korsakoff's syndrome is a chronic disorder of memory caused by thiamine deficiency (usually due to alcohol abuse).

50. **C)** MRI has better resolution of white matter and other soft tissue; CT is better for detecting blood, bone, or shrapnel; EEG measures brain waves, such as in seizure; an LP is used to assess for infectious material in cerebrospinal fluid.

**51. C)** The score for withdrawing from pain (without localizing) is 4, confused is 4, and eyes opening to pain is 2. The GCS is a scale to assess the depth of coma. Lower scores are associated with worse outcomes. The GCS is calculated by three items which are scored: best motor response (which is scored out of 6), best verbal response (which is scored out of 5), and eye opening (which is scored out of 4):

| Score | Best motor response (out of 6) | Best verbal response (out of 5) | Eye opening (out of 4) |
|---|---|---|---|
| 1 | None | None | None |
| 2 | Decerebrate posturing (extension) to pain | Mutters unintelligible sounds | Opens eyes to pain |
| 3 | Decorticate posturing (flexion) to pain | Says inappropriate words | Opens eyes to loud voice (verbal commands) |
| 4 | Withdraws limb from painful stimuli | Able to converse—confused | Opens eyes spontaneously |
| 5 | Localizes pain/pushes away noxious stimulus | Able to converse—alert and oriented | — |
| 6 | Obeys verbal commands | — | — |

**52. D)** A concussion is a mild traumatic brain injury and should never be graded with grading scales. The majority of concussions do not have LOC and therefore should not be used as an indication of severity. Concussion severity is determined by the number, severity, and length of symptoms present.

**53. B)** Lesions in the dominant hemisphere of the brain result in severe involvement of language comprehension. Lesions affecting the nondominant hemisphere more commonly result in neglect. Brain stem infarcts affect cranial nerves. Cerebellar strokes cause bilateral symptoms.

**54. D)** The goals of intrathecal baclofen therapy in patients with post-stroke hypertonia include improved positioning, facilitation of hygiene, prevention of complications, ease caregiver burden, orthotic fit and compliance, and decreased pain due to night time spasms.

**55. A)** HTN is the most important modifiable risk factor in both ischemic and hemorrhagic stroke. In fact, studies have shown that patients with blood pressure less than 120/80 have about half the lifetime risk of stroke as compared with those with high blood pressure. The other risk factors listed are nonmodifiable.

**56. D)** If there is some motor recovery of the hand by 4 weeks, there is up to a 70% chance of making a complete or almost complete recovery.

**57. A)** The first step would be to create a low-stimulus environment for the patient. Patients should be maintained in a safe, structured, low-stimulus environment. Floor beds can eliminate the need for restraints. Use physical restraints only if the patient is a danger to self or others. Restraints should be used cautiously and should not be a substitute for a floor bed, 1:1 supervision, or other environmental interventions. Pharmacotherapy is second-line intervention.

58. **D)** This aphasic syndrome resembles Broca's aphasia, but because it involves the extrasylvian region, and the arcuate fasciculus is intact, repetition is intact.

59. **D)** Normal aging is characterized by decreased processing speed and some decrease in attention and episodic memory. Her age would be more consistent with normal aging, as opposed to Alzheimer's disease, but may warrant further evaluation. Delirium is an acute confusional state with a fluctuating time course and impaired cognition, attention, and level of consciousness. Alzheimer's disease is a chronic neurodegenerative disease that usually starts slowly and gets worse over time. It is the cause of 60% to 70% of cases of dementia. Amnestic disorders are a group of disorders that involve loss of memories previously established, loss of the ability to create new memories, or loss of the ability to learn new information.

60. **A)** TBI commonly affects frontal, temporal, and limbic areas due to the proximity of these areas to bony protuberances of the skull. Parietal injury is less common.

61. **C)** Simple seizures do not impair consciousness; partial seizures are isolated. Simple partial seizures are localized to one area on one side of the brain, but may spread to other areas. Consciousness is not lost during a simple partial seizure. Simple generalized seizures may spread to other areas of the brain. Complex partial seizures originate in one area of the brain that affects consciousness. Generalized seizures, which are different from partial seizures start in all parts of the brain simultaneously and have no identifiable onset.

62. **C)** Specifically, the postcentral gyrus contains the primary somatosensory cortex (Brodmann's areas 3, 1, and 2). Damage to this area results in decreased sensory thresholds and an inability to discriminate the properties of tactile stimuli or to identify objects by touch.

63. **D)** Seizures, vomiting, and neck pain may not be present and do not reliably indicate the severity of a brain injury. Severity of brain injury can be assessed by using the Glasgow Coma Scale (GCS). The longer the duration of coma, the worse the outcome and prognosis.

64. **D)** Patient in a coma lacks a sleep-wake cycle on EEG, eyes remain closed, there is no eye tracking, and no spontaneous purposeful movement. A patient in a vegetative state has a sleep-wake cycle on EEG, eyes are open with either spontaneous or noxious stimuli, but there is no eye tracking. A patient in a minimally conscious state has a sleep-wake cycle, eyes remain open, and there is smooth pursuit tracking.

65. **A)** The olfactory nerve (CN I) is the most commonly injured cranial nerve. Injury to CN I can lead to anosmia and an altered, usually poor, appetite. The injury occurs because of the shearing forces that damage the small nerves on the cribriform plate.

66. **D)** Wernicke's aphasia is a fluent aphasia and is characterized by impaired naming, comprehension, and repetition. Fluency is intact.

67. **B)** One of the common side effects of tizanidine is drowsiness or somnolence. Other side effects may include hypotension, dizziness, weakness, dry mouth, and elevated liver functions.

68. **A)** The physiological factors that account for stroke recovery include resolution of post-stroke edema, reperfusion of ischemic penumbra, resolution of diaschisis, and cortical reorganization.

69. **C)** In a patient with transcortical mixed aphasia, speech is nonfluent and the patient is unable to comprehend, but repetition is still intact. The arcuate fasciculus is not affected in transcortical mixed aphasia. Therefore, repetition is not affected.

70. **A)** Uncal herniation causes compression of the CN III, which may lead to complete ipsilateral CN III palsy (fixed pupil dilation, ptosis, and ophthalmoplegia).

71. **C)** Fluent versus nonfluent speech localizes anterior from posterior aphasic syndromes; impairment in comprehension distinguishes Wernicke's from conduction aphasia. The ability to repeat implies that perisylvian language areas are intact.

72. **C)** Lewy body disease is characterized by these symptoms. Lewy body disease is a progressive neurodegenerative dementia closely associated with Parkinson's disease primarily affecting older adults. Its primary feature is a more rapid cognitive decline than Parkinson's, which may lead to hallucinations. Lewy body disease is characterized by markedly fluctuating cognition, alertness, wakefulness, and short-term memory. Persistent or recurring visual hallucinations with vivid and detailed imagery often are an early diagnostic symptom. Frontotemporal dementia occurs due to frontotemporal lobar degeneration, which is characterized by progressive neuronal loss predominantly involving the frontal and/or temporal lobes. Common signs and symptoms include significant changes in social and personal behavior, apathy, blunting of emotions, and deficits in both expressive and receptive language. Dementia pugilistica is a type of chronic traumatic encephalopathy, a neurodegenerative disease with features of dementia. It may affect amateur or professional boxers, wrestlers, as well as athletes in other sports who suffer concussions.

73. **B)** This is a primary effect; the others are secondary effects. Primary injury is direct disruption of the brain parenchyma from the shear forces of the impact. It occurs immediately after the impact. Primary injury includes meningeal/cerebral laceration, contusions, diffuse axonal injury, and impact depolarization (a massive surge in extracellular potassium and glutamate release leading to excitotoxicity). Secondary injury is a cascade of biochemical, cellular, and molecular events, which include both endogenous cerebral damage as well as extracerebral damage that comes from trauma. Secondary injury includes hypoxia, edema, ischemia, and intracranial bleeding.

74. **D)** By definition, delirium is a temporary state of mental confusion and fluctuating consciousness, with numerous causes; dementia requires significant decrease in (usually memory) at least two areas of cognitive functioning; amnestic disorder only involves memory. Delusional disorder is a mental illness with no effect of a drug, medication, or general medical condition. Dementia is usually long-term, progressive, and has gradual decrease in the ability to think and function. Amnestic disorders involve memory loss.

75. **D)** In MS, the fatty covering surrounding the axon (the myelin sheath) is attacked by the immune system. MS does not affect peripheral nerve myelin.

76. **B)** Subdural hematomas are common in the elderly, may occur after a fall or even spontaneously, are due to tearing of weak venous blood vessels, and are often asymptomatic, sometimes resolving on their own or coming to attention only after several days.

77. **A)** DAI is seen in the white matter, primarily in the corpus callosum, midbrain, pons, and central white matter. DAI is caused by disruption of the axons due to acceleration-deceleration and rotational forces that cause shearing upon impact. DAI primarily occurs in TBI cases and can result in LOC. Injury primarily occurs in the white matter, where petechial hemorrhages are characteristic.

78. **B)** PTA assesses anterograde amnesia, the ability to retain ongoing memories, from the time of the TBI to present. Retrograde amnesia is memory loss of events occurring prior to the injury. The GOAT is an objective assessment tool that tracks PTA, where a score of 75 or greater for 2 consecutive days is considered the end of PTA.

79. **A)** Aphasia is an impairment in language. Dysarthria is a motor-speech disorder characterized by slow, weak, or uncoordinated movements of speech musculature. Impairment in the ability to produce sounds is dysphonia. Impairment in swallowing is called dysphagia.

80. **A)** Baclofen is a structural analogue of GABA, which is one of the main inhibitory neurotransmitters in the central nervous system. An example of an alpha-2 adrenergic agonist is tizanidine. A hydantoin derivative, dantrolene, is a muscle relaxant used to treat malignant hyperthermia, neuroleptic malignant syndrome, spasticity, and ecstasy intoxication.

81. **D)** Some of the limitations of the NIH stroke scale are that elements of brain stem function are not well reflected, palatal weakness is not scored, it does not assess distal weakness, and it does not screen for neurocognitive dysfunction.

82. **D)** All of the answer choices are required before tPA is administered to a patient with acute stroke. For a patient to receive IV tPA the patient should have onset of symptoms between 3 and 4.5 hours before beginning treatment. Patients should have a diagnosis of ischemic stroke. A noncontrast head CT should not show hemorrhage. The patient should be 18 years of age or older. The potential risks and benefits of using IV tPA should be discussed with the patient and/or family with verbal understanding. There are also many exclusion criteria when it comes to administering IV tPA, such as acute or previous hemorrhagic stroke, recent intercranial or spinal surgery, elevated blood pressures (systolic higher than 185 or diastolic higher than 110), use of anticoagulants, and heparin within the last 48 hours.

83. **B)** A GCS score of 3 to 8 = severe TBI (coma). A GCS score of 9 to 12 = moderate TBI. A GCS score of 13 to 15 = mild TBI.

84. **D)** "Locked-in" syndrome is due to bilateral pontine infarcts or damage affecting the corticospinal and bulbar tracts and sparing the reticular activating system. The characteristics of the syndrome are quadriplegia and anarthria with preservation of consciousness. Patients retain vertical eye movement, facilitating nonverbal communication. Anarthria is due to bilateral facioglossopharyngolaryngeal paralysis, which also causes dysphagia and limits the use of facial expression in communication. Although medial and lateral gaze palsies are typical, patients usually retain upper eyelid control and vertical eye movement because of sparing of the midbrain tectum, which allows communication.

85. **B)** Frontotemporal dementia (FTD) is actually a cortical dementia. FTD, or frontotemporal degenerations, refer to a group of disorders caused by progressive nerve cell loss in the brain's frontal lobes or temporal lobes. FTD used to be called Pick's disease after Arnold Pick, a physician who in 1892 first described a patient with distinct symptoms affecting language.

86. **B)** Cognitive rehabilitation strives for statistical validity. It is informed by theory, focuses both on amelioration (through practice) and compensation, and involves much psychoeducation. It is a comprehensive, holistic approach that attempts to address multiple cognitive deficits and incorporates psychological interventions for emotional, motivational, and interpersonal aspects of the patient's functioning.

87. **B)** The GOAT is out of 100 points and is useful for assessing severity of posttraumatic amnesia. The MMSE is a cognitive screener, the Ranchos Los Amigos Scale stages recovery from traumatic brain injury (TBI), and the GCS measures coma and severity of TBI.

88. **B)** Parkinson's disease is associated with loss of dopaminergic neurons in the substantia nigra.

89. **A)** Alzheimer's disease typically results in apathy early on; the others characteristically, due to subcortical involvement, involve depression. Apathy describes loss of interest, motivation, and/or persistence. It is the most common neuropsychiatric symptom reported among individuals with Alzheimer's disease. Patients are indifferent and not social with others.

90. **B)** Regardless of site of impact, the frontal lobe is often affected directly in TBI because it is the largest lobe and given its location in the skull. The temporal lobes are also affected, owing to the bony protuberances surrounding the temporal region. Therefore, the orbitofrontal and anterior temporal lobes are the most commonly injured sites of the brain because of the close relation of the lobes to the bones. The brain hits the inner table of the skull, causing cerebral contusions.

91. **A)** The best motor GCS and the best overall GCS within the first 24 hours is considered to be the best acute predictor of outcome in TBI.

92. **D)** Noncontrast CT of the brain is the first-line diagnostic radiological test done in a patient with symptoms of stroke, and is done to rule out an intracranial bleed. CT of the head is the first test done because it may help determine treatment, as a patient with an intracranial bleed would not be a candidate for tissue plasminogen activator.

93. **B)** The greatest predictor of community ambulation after a stroke is walking speed.

94. **D)** A history of MI within 3 months is a contraindication for tPA. The other answers are requirements for giving tPA in the setting of an acute stroke. In 2016, the American Heart Association/American Stroke Association increased the recommended time between stroke symptoms and initiation of tPA from 3 hours to 4.5 hours. However, the U.S. Food and Drug Administration (FDA) has approved tPA for stroke only within 3 hours of stroke symptoms. The FDA considers giving tPA from 3 to 4.5 hours post stroke as "off label" use.

95. **C)** ICP of 15 or lower is considered normal. In a patient with a stroke, the goal is to keep the ICP as close to normal as possible. Increased ICP reduces cerebral blood perfusion. Central perfusion pressure (CPP) should remain higher than 60 mmHg.

96. **D)** In decerebrate posturing, the limbs will be stiff and extended with internal rotation of arms and ankles in plantar flexion. In patients with decorticate posturing, the legs are extended and the arms are flexed and adducted.

97. **C)** SIADH is common in the acute TBI period and is characterized by hyponatremia, euvolemia, low blood urea nitrogen (BUN), and decreased blood and increased urine osmolality. Treatment for mild cases includes fluid restriction, loop diuretics, and monitoring weight and serum sodium level. In patients with severe symptoms, intravenous hypertonic saline can be used.

98. **A)** Phenytoin has been shown to be effective for prophylaxis of seizures when administered for 1 week. Beyond 1 week, treatment conferred no benefit to seizure prevention. Long-term use of phenytoin has been associated with impaired neurologic recovery.

99. **D)** The MMSE is out of 30 points, requires at least an eighth-grade education, and is translated into many languages. It is only a screening tool, and does not measure executive function.

**100. D)** Agnosia is the inability to process sensory information; it is also a term used to describe the loss of the ability to recognize what objects are and what they are used for. Apraxia is a term used to describe the inability to carry out voluntary and purposeful movements despite the fact that muscular power, sensibility, and coordination are intact. Aphasia is a language disorder; it is the term used to describe a difficulty or loss of the ability to speak or understand spoken, written, or sign language. Amnesia is defined as loss of memory, or the inability to remember facts or events.

**101. C)** Thrombi or emboli involve blockage of blood vessels and therefore ischemia of the cerebral tissue, leading to infarction. The other answers are hemorrhagic causes of stroke.

**102. C)** Medications, especially sedatives, are the most common cause of falls in the elderly.

**103. D)** Repeated concussions can result in all of the answer choices. Second-impact syndrome results from inability to autoregulate blood pressure after repeated concussions.

**104. D)** Phase 1 and 2 of a bone scan can help detect HO within 2 to 4 weeks. To detect HO on x-ray requires bone maturation, which can take as long as 4 weeks. CT scan is not indicated for HO identification, and serum alkaline phosphatase is a nonspecific/nonsensitive test.

**105. C)** The most common cause of hemorrhagic stroke is uncontrolled hypertension. Intracerebral hemorrhage makes up approximately 11% of strokes. Hypertension is thought to be a risk factor due to rupture of microaneurysms that develop in hypertensive patients. Amyloid angiopathy is present in 5% to 20% of cases. Other causes of hemorrhagic stroke include trauma, vasculitis, bleeding into a tumor, and anticoagulation therapy.

**106. A)** Factors increasing the risk of urinary incontinence after stroke include advanced age, greater stroke severity, and diabetes. Premorbid voiding dysfunction, benign prostatic hypertrophy (BPH) in males, or stress incontinence in females, can become more significant problems after stroke due to decreased mobility and difficulty with communication. However, sex alone is not a risk factor for urinary incontinence. Incontinence due to disinhibition of the bladder detrusor muscle is common, and can be treated with anticholinergic medications.

**107. A)** Aspirin, clopidogrel, and combination of aspirin and extended release dipyridamole are accepted options for initial therapy for patients with noncardioembolic ischemic stroke. Anticoagulant therapy with Coumadin is recommended in the setting of embolic stroke, unless there are contraindications.

**108. B)** The head CT would usually be done without contrast as both contrast and blood would appear white on the scan, making diagnosis more difficult. Fresh intracranial hemorrhage coagulates almost immediately, becoming dense and therefore glowing brightly on CT scans. Eventually, the clot is broken down by the body, becoming the same density as the brain after about 1 week, and then appearing dark after 2 to 3 weeks.

**109. C)** In a minimally conscious state, the patient will be able to show some evidence of self or environmental awareness and will show evidence of purposeful behaviors. A vegetative state is a condition of wakeful unresponsiveness, in which the patient does not show evidence of purposeful behaviors but the patient does have spontaneous sleep-wake cycles. There is presence of verbal or auditory startle but no localization or tracking. Patients in a coma lack a normal sleep-wake cycle and do not demonstrate purposeful behavior. A patient's eyes remain closed and there is no ability to discretely localize noxious stimuli.

110. **B)** Ranchos Los Amigos scale is used to rate recovery from TBI. Ranchos level I is no response; level II is generalized response to painful stimulus; level III is localized response to painful stimulus; level IV is confused and agitated; level V is confused, inappropriate, nonagitated; level VI is confused and appropriate; level VII is automatic, appropriate response; level VIII is purposeful, appropriate response.

111. **B)** Range of motion is the best prophylaxis and treatment of HO. Radiation would have to be given to the whole body because HO development cannot be predicted. NSAIDs and diphosphonates have a role in treatment, but not significantly in prevention.

112. **B)** Some aspects of IQ are very good predictors (eg, mathematics and vocabulary); the other answers are all true.

113. **B)** Visuospatial neglect is often due to damage to the usually nondominant right hemisphere, specifically to the right parietal lobe. Amnesia is a deficit in memory. Disorientation is the cognitive disability to sense person, place, or time. Gerstmann's syndrome is destruction to the inferior parietal lobule of the dominant hemisphere. It is characterized by dysgraphia, dyscalculia, finger agnosia, and left-right disorientation

114. **C)** The dura and arachnoid (as well as the pia) are meninges; thus, tumors arising from the meninges are called *meningiomas*. These are benign tumors, but can grow large and cause mass effect. Glioma arises from glial cells. Astrocytomas originate from a particular type of glial cells called *astrocytes*. Glioblastoma multiforme is a malignant tumor, also known as grade 4 astrocytoma, which can develop from normal cells or a low-grade astrocytoma.

115. **B)** Caused by a prion, Creutzfeldt-Jakob disease (CJD) belongs to a family of human and animal diseases known as the *transmissible spongiform encephalopathies* (TSEs) and results in a spongiform cortex, dementia, and rapid progression to death.

116. **B)** The most pain is actually reported by patients with mild brain injury; postconcussive syndrome is thought to involve psychiatric as well as cognitive symptoms.

117. **C)** HO is the formation of bone in ectopic sites and occurs most frequently in the hips, followed by elbows, shoulders, and knees. The mechanism of HO is unknown, but it occurs in 11% to 20% of patients with severe injuries, and affects proximal joints more than distal joints.

118. **C)** Of the factors listed, age is the only nonmodifiable risk factor for a stroke. The other risk factors listed can be lowered with interventions. Antihypertensives can be used to treat hypertension. Risk from atrial fibrillation can be modified by starting anticoagulation. Smoking can be modified by smoking cessation.

119. **A)** Predictors of aspiration on bedside swallow exam include abnormal cough, cough after swallow, dysphonia, dysarthria, abnormal gag reflex, and wet vocal quality after swallow. Tachycardia is not a predictor of aspiration on bedside swallow exam.

120. **A)** As the corticospinal tract, a descending motor pathway, is a medial structure, lateral medullary syndrome, also known as *Wallenberg's syndrome*, does not cause motor paralysis. Lateral medullary syndrome is an infarct in the lateral wedge of the medulla, which causes impairment in contralateral pain and temperature. Symptoms also include ipsilateral Horner's syndrome (miosis, ptosis, and anhydrosis), dysphagia, dysarthria, dysphonia, nystagmus, vertigo, nausea and vomiting, and ipsilateral impaired sensation of the face due to involvement of the sensory nucleus of cranial nerve V, the trigeminal nerve.

121. **B)** On a CT scan, blood appears hyperdense (radiopaque) and will show up white. Unlike hemorrhage, ischemic strokes are not usually immediately detectable on a CT scan. After about 3 hours, subtle signs can be appreciated by skilled readers of CT scans, and after 6 to 12 hours, a more obvious hypodensity becomes apparent in the area of the stroke. This hypodensity will become even darker with time as brain tissue is resorbed and replaced by cerebrospinal fluid.

122. **A)** Epidural hematoma usually results from a skull fracture in the temporal bone crossing the vascular territory of the middle meningeal artery. Subdural hematomas result from shearing of the bridging veins between the arachnoid and the dura. Subarachnoid hemorrhage is associated with ruptured cerebral aneurysm and arteriovenous malformations.

123. **B)** Decreased patient mobility will lead to the development of decubitus ulcers. Stroke patients require frequent turning and repositioning. After experiencing a stroke, patients may be at risk for skin problems due to decreased movement and decreased sensation. Skin stays healthy with a balanced diet, good hygiene, regular skin checks, and pressure relief. Relieving pressure and checking skin ensures a good blood supply. Urine, sweat, or stool can cause skin breakdown as well.

124. **B)** Neuropsychologists do not prescribe medication, but do conduct cognitive evaluations and engage in cognitive remediation and psychotherapy.

125. **C)** The Trailmaking Test is a test for attention and set-shifting (executive functioning) and is therefore a useful predictor of driving ability; BNT is a language test, clock drawing is a good screen for Alzheimer's, and the Rorschach is a personality/psychopathology test.

126. **C)** Specifically, the test mentioned measures sustained attention and concentration. This is part of the Mini Mental Status Exam. To test orientation, you can ask for the date, location, season, etc. To test memory you can ask the patient to recall the name of three items you asked them to remember earlier.

127. **D)** Pseudodementia, or dementia of depression, often involves impairments in attention, memory, and processing speed, which may resemble dementia.

128. **D)** Owing to long-term alcohol abuse and thiamine deficiency, dementia and peripheral neuropathy often result.

129. **C)** Abulia, or lack of initiation, can look like depression and is more of a "negative" symptom, compared with the other "positive" symptoms, from frontal lobe injury.

130. **C)** A mild injury is a GCS of 13 to 15, a moderate injury is a GCS of 9 to 12, and a severe injury is a GCS of 3 to 8. The lowest score is a 3 on the GCS.

131. **B)** Medications such as amantadine, bromocriptine, and methylphenidate are dopaminergic, and assist in improving attention and cognitive function. Histamine has no role in cognitive recovery, except that histamine-2 blockers should be avoided because they cause sedation. Norepinephrine also has a limited role in the treatment of cognition in TBI.

132. **C)** Phenobarbital is often associated with dizziness, irritability, confusion, rash, and cerebellar signs. These side effects usually occur at very high doses. Phenobarbital is not recommended for treatment or prophylaxis of seizures as a result of traumatic brain injury, as it can contribute to poor recovery. Valproic acid commonly causes gastrointestinal dysfunction. Sedation, tremor, and ataxia can also occur. Gabapentin primarily causes fatigue, somnolence, ataxia, and dizziness.

133. **A)** An injury to CN III would cause ipsilateral dilation of the pupil. Normally, CN III constricts the ipsilateral pupil with light exposure.

134. **D)** An epidural hematoma occurs between the skull and the dura. It often develops quickly because it is usually secondary to an arterial bleed, such as the middle meningeal artery. Often, patients may have an initial headache with no other complaints. Within hours, patients may develop significant neurological deficits related to the expansion of the epidural hematoma, such as midline shift and brain stem herniation.

135. **C)** RTP is a very important decision to maintain safety of athletes. RTP should be based on the graduated RTP protocol. There are six stages, and to progress through each stage, the athlete must be asymptomatic for 24 hours. If the athlete experiences any postconcussive symptoms at any stage, he or she must return to the previous stage of activity. Symptoms in relation to physical activity must be assessed, and no player should RTP if he or she has only been asymptomatic at rest. LOC is not relevant for deciding whether a patient should RTP.

136. **D)** Syndrome of inappropriate antidiuretic hormone secretion (SIADH) is hyponatremia in the setting of normal hydration, whereas cerebral salt wasting (CSW) is hyponatremia with physical signs of dehydration. Initial management for SIADH is fluid restriction, between 1 and 1.5 L/day. If fluid restriction does not improve Na+ and there is significant symptomatology, then hypertonic saline should be considered. However, the hypertonic saline should be administered slowly so as to prevent pontine myelinolysis or cardiac dysfunction. If chronic SIADH is diagnosed, demeclocycline should be prescribed for continued management.

# 7

# Spinal Cord Medicine

## QUESTIONS

1. What is the recommended duration for anticoagulant prophylaxis for an uncomplicated complete spinal cord injury?
   A) 6 weeks
   B) 8 weeks
   C) 12 weeks
   D) Until discharge from rehabilitation

2. In a patient with a spinal cord injury, which of the following is **not** an effective evacuation technique in a bowel program?
   A) Push-ups
   B) Abdominal massage
   C) Supine position
   D) Deep breathing exercises

3. Which of the following is true of calcium metabolism in spinal cord injury (SCI)?
   A) Hypercalcemia occurs more commonly in females, incomplete paraplegia, and chronic injury
   B) The risk of fractures is comparable to the able-bodied population
   C) Passive weight bearing (standing with the use of adaptive equipment) results in improved bone mineral density
   D) All of the above

4. In the American Spinal Injury Association (ASIA) examination, the nipple line is the key dermatome for what level?
   A) T4
   B) T10
   C) T6
   D) L4

5. A patient with neurogenic bowel lower motor neuron injury affecting his bowels complains of constipation. Which of these medications is a promotility agent that can aid in treatment?
   A) Docusate
   B) Polyethylene glycol
   C) Lactulose
   D) Senna glycoside

6. Which of the following is an antispasticity medication with the **least** sedating side effects?
   A) Baclofen
   B) Dantrolene

ANSWERS TO THIS SECTION CAN BE FOUND ON PAGE 203

C) Valium

D) Tizanidine

7. Which of the following is the most common cause of spinal cord injuries in the general public?

A) Falls

B) Gunshot wounds

C) Motor vehicle accidents

D) Athletic injuries

8. At what level of the vertebral body does the spinal cord normally terminate?

A) T11/T12

B) L1/L2

C) L3/L4

D) L4/L5

9. Brown-Séquard syndrome presents with which of the following?

A) Contralateral decreased sensation to temperature and pain, with ipsilateral motor weakness and proprioception

B) Ipsilateral decreased sensation to temperature and pain, with contralateral motor weakness and proprioception

C) Contralateral decreased proprioception, with ipsilateral motor weakness and decreased sensation to temperature and pain

D) Ipsilateral decreased proprioception, with contralateral weakness and decreased sensation to temperature and pain

10. Which of the following is true of the recommendations regarding prevention of upper limb pain and injury in spinal cord injury (SCI) patients?

A) Minimize frequency of repetitive upper limb tasks

B) Minimize the force used to perform upper limb tasks

C) Minimize extreme positions of the joints

D) All of the above

11. Which of the following is a risk factor for developing depression post–spinal cord injury (SCI)?

A) Male gender

B) Age of onset above 40 years

C) Prior history of depression

D) Supportive social structure

12. Which of the following is a risk factor for the development of heterotopic ossification (HO) in spinal cord injury (SCI)?

A) Gender

B) Level of lesion

C) Spasticity

D) Race

13. In the American Spinal Injury Association (ASIA) examination, the C7 myotome correlates with which muscle group?

A) Elbow flexors

B) Long finger flexors

C) Elbow extensors

D) Wrist extensors

14. An 85-year-old male presents to your clinic after a fall. On manual motor testing, the patient is noted to have strength of 3/5 in shoulder abduction; 2/5 in elbow flexion; 2/5 in wrist extension; 2/5 in elbow extension; and 1/5 in finger flexion and abduction. Lower extremities bilaterally show 5/5 hip flexion; 4/5 knee extension; and 4/5 with ankle dorsiflexion, plantarflexion, and hallux extension. Shortly after his injury, he noted difficulty with initiating urination. What can be said about the most likely mechanism of this patient's injury?
   A) Excessive rotation
   B) Hyperextension
   C) Hyperflexion
   D) Vascular injury to bilateral vertebral arteries within the foramen transversarii

15. Of the following, which is the most common intramedullary neoplasm of the spinal cord?
   A) Ependymoma
   B) Astrocytoma
   C) Meningioma
   D) Schwannoma

16. Which of the following is the most common cause of death in paraplegic patients?
   A) Suicide
   B) Sepsis
   C) Cardiovascular complications
   D) Respiratory complications

17. Falls are a leading cause of spinal cord injury (SCI) in:
   A) Children
   B) Teenagers
   C) Elderly
   D) Women

18. Which of the following would **not** likely be due to cauda equina syndrome?
   A) Groin paresthesia
   B) Areflexic bowel or bladder
   C) Increased tone of lower extremities
   D) Weakness of lower extremities

19. What is the typical presentation of an individual with Brown-Séquard syndrome?
   A) Ipsilateral motor loss at the level of the lesion, and contralateral loss of position sense, pain, and temperature below the level of the lesion
   B) Contralateral proprioceptive and motor loss at the level of the lesion, with ipsilateral loss of pain and temperature below the level of the lesion
   C) Ipsilateral motor and proprioceptive loss at and below the level of the lesion, with contralateral loss of pain and temperature below the lesion
   D) Contralateral motor loss at the level of the lesion, ipsilateral proprioceptive loss at the level of the lesion, and contralateral loss of pain and temperature below the lesion

20. Individuals with an injury of which of the following can be expected to transfer on level surface without the use of a board?
   A) C4
   B) C5
   C) C6
   D) C7

21. What is the most common location of heterotopic ossification (HO) in spinal cord injury (SCI) patients?
    A) Hip
    B) Knee
    C) Shoulder
    D) Elbow

22. In the American Spinal Injury Association (ASIA) examination, the C5 myotome correlates with which muscle group?
    A) Elbow extensors
    B) Finger abductors
    C) Wrist extensors
    D) Elbow flexors

23. Which of the following spinal tracts are involved in subacute combined degeneration?
    A) Ventral spinothalamic tract + lateral corticospinal tract
    B) Lateral corticospinal tract + spinocerebellar tract
    C) Lateral corticospinal tract + dorsal columns
    D) Dorsal columns + ventral spinothalamic tract

24. Which of the following classifications of spinal cord injury is second most common?
    A) Complete tetraplegia
    B) Incomplete tetraplegia
    C) Complete paraplegia
    D) Incomplete paraplegia

25. Which of the following may be utilized in the treatment of a lower motor neuron injured bowel?
    A) Gastrocolic reflex
    B) Digital rectal stimulation
    C) Manual digital evacuation of stool
    D) A warm beverage taken daily at the same time prior to desired bowel movement

26. Which of the following is the most common cause of spinal cord injuries (SCI)?
    A) Sports
    B) Falls
    C) Violence
    D) Vehicular crashes

27. Which of the following is a symptom of a lower motor neuron lesion?
    A) Spasticity
    B) Hypertrophy of muscles
    C) Fasciculations
    D) Increased reflexes

28. A hyperextension injury that occurs in low-velocity trauma that affects the upper (greater than the lower) extremities is called?
    A) Central cord syndrome
    B) Brown-Séquard syndrome
    C) Anterior cord syndrome
    D) Cauda equina syndrome

29. Which of the following statements is true regarding prognosis and spinal cord injury (SCI)?
    A) Preserved sacral sensation has a better prognosis for lower extremity recovery
    B) Individuals older than 50 years have a better prognosis for recovery
    C) A sensory incomplete injury has a less than 10% chance for ambulation
    D) Muscles with antigravity strength can recover two grades in the first year

30. The external urethral sphincter is innervated by the:
    A) Hypogastric nerve
    B) Pelvic nerve
    C) Vagus nerve
    D) Pudendal nerve

31. Which of the following is the most common cause of death for persons with a spinal cord injury (SCI)?
    A) Heart disease
    B) Disease of the respiratory system
    C) Cancer
    D) Stroke

32. A 17-year-old female is stabbed in the back and presents as follows: Loss of sensation, paralysis, and loss of vibration below T5 on the left; loss of pain and temperature below T5 on the right. What syndrome does she have?
    A) Brown-Séquard
    B) Central cord
    C) Anterior cord
    D) Cauda equine

33. What is the highest possible level of complete injury following which a patient can still live independently?
    A) C5
    B) C6
    C) C7
    D) T1

34. The non–key muscle groups in the ASIA Impairment Scale (AIS) grading system have what significance?
    A) They can be used to distinguish between AIS C and AIS D
    B) They can be used to distinguish between AIS B and AIS C
    C) Reflexes in all non–key muscle groups can be used to track recovery from spinal shock
    D) They are used to assess for recovery of the specific peripheral nerves innervating each muscle

35. More than 80% of all spinal cord injuries (SCI) occur in:
    A) Children
    B) Males
    C) Females
    D) Elderly

36. Which of the following is an upper motor neuron symptom?
    A) Flaccidity
    B) Increased reflexes

    C) Decreased tone

    D) Atrophy of muscles

37. Which of the following is true regarding the zone of partial preservation (ZPP)?

    A) Classified only in incomplete injuries

    B) The most rostral segment below the assigned level that has sensory or motor function

    C) The motor ZPP does not follow the sensory ZPP

    D) All of the above

38. An individual with T4 American Spinal Injury Association (ASIA) Impairment Scale (AIS) C in your office begins to get flushed. You check the individual's blood pressure and find that it is elevated with a decreased pulse. What should you do next?

    A) Sit the person up and loosen any clothing

    B) Catheterize the individual

    C) Perform fecal disimpaction

    D) Administer nifedipine

39. Which statement is true regarding the use of alpha blockers in the treatment of detrusor sphincter dyssynergia?

    A) Urethral resistance is increased with the use of alpha blockers

    B) Phosphodiesterase inhibitors should be used with caution in patients on alpha blockers

    C) Alpha blockers should be taken in the morning in the upright position

    D) All of the above

40. The lateral spinothalamic tracts:

    A) Control voluntary muscle activity

    B) Transmit proprioception only

    C) Transmit pain and temperature

    D) Transmit proprioception, fine touch, and vibration

41. An 82-year-old man trips and falls. On presentation, he has an ecchymosis on his chin. On physical examination, bilateral upper extremities were found to have 2/5 strength with elbow flexion and wrist extension; 3/5 strength with elbow extension, finger flexion, and finger abduction; and 4/5 strength in bilateral lower extremities. He has intact sensation. What is this spinal cord injury (SCI) syndrome?

    A) Brown-Séquard

    B) Central cord

    C) Anterior cord

    D) Cauda equina

42. A 34-year-old male has a traumatic spinal cord injury and is diagnosed according to American Spinal Injury Association (ASIA) classification as C6 ASIA Impairment Scale (AIS) B. He has no other bony injuries or prior medical history. Given his classification, what regimen of deep vein thrombosis (DVT) prophylaxis would you initiate?

    A) Sequential compressive devices for 2 weeks along with 6 weeks of unfractionated heparin

    B) Sequential compressive devices for 2 weeks along with 6 weeks of enoxaparin

    C) Sequential compressive devices for 2 weeks along with 8 to 12 weeks of unfractionated heparin

    D) Sequential compressive devices for 2 weeks along with 8 to 12 weeks of enoxaparin

43. Which of the following criteria seen on urinalysis in a spinal cord injury patient would be an indication for antibiotic therapy?
    A) An inability to sense the genitourinary tract/perineal region
    B) Qualitative grading of any more than "moderate" leukocyte esterase and/or nitrate
    C) Thirteen leukocytes visible per square millimeter of high-powered field
    D) A urine pH level above 7.5

44. According to recent research, the highest incidence for spinal cord injuries (SCI) involves what age group:
    A) 10 to 15 years
    B) 16 to 30 years
    C) 30 to 35 years
    D) 35 to 40 years

45. Ischemic damage to the anterior spinal artery leads to which of the following syndromes?
    A) Central cord syndrome
    B) Anterior cord syndrome
    C) Posterior cord syndrome
    D) Brown-Séquard syndrome

46. Which of the following are key muscles tested in the scoring of the American Spinal Injury Association (ASIA) exam?
    A) C5-biceps, C7-triceps, T1-adductor digiti minimi, L5-quadriceps, S1-flexor hallucis longus
    B) C5-biceps, C6-flexor carpi ulnaris, C8-flexor digitorum profundus, L3-quadriceps, L4-adductor magnus
    C) C5-biceps, C8-flexor digitorum superficialis, L2-sartorius, L3-quadriceps, L5-biceps femoris
    D) C5-biceps, C8-flexor digitorum profundus, T1-abductor digiti minimi, L4-tibialis anterior, S1-gastrocnemius

47. What is the most common cause of autonomic dysreflexia?
    A) Pressure injury
    B) Fractures or other trauma
    C) Restrictive clothing
    D) Bladder distention

48. In patients with spinal cord injury (SCI), what are the long-term complications of an indwelling catheter?
    A) Bladder and kidney stones
    B) Hydronephrosis
    C) Pyelonephritis
    D) All of the above

49. What is the most common level of spinal cord injury (SCI)?
    A) T10
    B) T6
    C) L5
    D) C5

50. A 78-year-old female comes into your office complaining that whenever she laughs hard, coughs, sneezes, or gets up from her chair, she has "accidents" with an inability to hold her urine. These are the only times when she has these accidents. Which of the following therapies might you consider for her?
   A) A trial of oxybutynin
   B) Flomax to relax the bladder
   C) Kegel exercises
   D) Trial of imipramine

51. Which of the following pulmonary function test parameters is expected to increase following a T1 ASIA Impairment Scale (AIS) A spinal cord injury?
   A) Minute ventilation
   B) Peak inspiratory flow
   C) Residual volume
   D) Tidal volume

52. Which of the following nerves is responsible for the feeling of bladder fullness?
   A) Hypogastric nerve
   B) Pudendal nerve
   C) Pelvic splanchnic nerves
   D) Genitofemoral nerve

53. Which of the following vessels does not supply blood to the spinal cord?
   A) Radicular artery
   B) Artery of Adamkiewicz
   C) Basilar artery
   D) Anterior spinal artery

54. A spinal cord–injured patient was noted to have the following on physical examination: motor preservation greater than 3 levels below the neurologic level, and greater than half the key muscles below the single neurologic level were less than 3. This would be classified as an American Spinal Injury Association (ASIA) level:
   A) AIS A
   B) AIS B
   C) AIS C
   D) AIS D

55. What level spinal cord injury leads one to be concerned about the risk of developing autonomic dysreflexia?
   A) T4 and above
   B) T6 and above
   C) T8 and above
   D) T10 and above

56. In a patient with spinal cord injury (SCI), suprapubic catheterization should be considered for which of the following?
   A) Sacral pressure injury
   B) Urethral abnormalities or obstruction
   C) Improved body image
   D) All of the above

57. Which of the following is the most common cause of traumatic spinal cord injury (SCI)?
    A) Motor vehicle crash
    B) Sports
    C) Violence
    D) Falls

58. Which of the following pairs is accurate regarding bladder neurophysiology?
    A) Somatic innervation to the external urethral sphincter is provided by the hypogastric nerve.
    B) Sympathetic innervation to the external sphincter is provided by the pudendal nerve
    C) Visceral afferents from the bladder are carried centrally by the hypogastric nerve
    D) Parasympathetic innervation to the detrusor muscle is provided by the pelvic nerve.

59. Which of the following is **not** a component of the Braden scale?
    A) Activity
    B) Body mass/frequent turning
    C) Friction and shear forces
    D) Nutrition

60. Which of these diseases present with **both** upper and lower motor neuron signs?
    A) Subacute combined degeneration
    B) Cauda equina syndrome
    C) Amyotrophic lateral sclerosis
    D) Poliomyelitis

61. Which of the following symptoms would not be representative of cauda equina syndrome?
    A) Areflexic bladder
    B) Areflexic bowel
    C) Weakness of lower limbs
    D) Intact sexual sensation

62. According to the International Standards for the Neurologic Classification of Spinal Cord Injury (ISNCSCI), American Spinal Injury Association (ASIA) Impairment Score B is defined as?
    A) Motor preservation greater than 3 levels below neurologic level, and greater than half the key muscles below the single neurologic level are less than 3
    B) No motor function more than 3 levels below the motor level with sensory preservation including sacral sparing
    C) Motor preservation greater than 3 levels below the neurologic level, and greater than half the key muscles below the single neurologic level are graded greater than or equal to 3
    D) Complete injury with no sensory or voluntary anal sphincter contraction

63. In the treatment of erectile dysfunction in spinal cord–injured males, the physiatrist should discuss which of the following options?
    A) Phosphodiesterase type 5 (PDE-5) inhibitors
    B) Intracavernosal injections
    C) Vacuum devices
    D) All of the above

64. In a patient with spinal cord injury (SCI), intermittent catheterization should be considered in which of the following?
    A) Small bladder capacity (less than 200 mL)
    B) Cognitive impairment

    C) Adequate hand function

    D) Prone to autonomic dysreflexia -

65. The C6 nerve root exits:
    A) Above the C5 vertebra
    B) Above the C6 vertebra
    C) Below the C7 vertebra
    D) Above the C4 vertebra

66. Which of the following spinal cord injury syndromes carries the best overall prognosis for independent ambulation following rehabilitation?
    A) Central cord syndrome
    B) Brown-Séquard syndrome
    C) Posterior cord syndrome
    D) Anterior cord syndrome

67. A 9-year-old male is diagnosed with C5 ASIA Impairment Scale (AIS) A traumatic spinal cord injury. What is the most common site for development of a pressure injury in his age category?
    A) Occiput
    B) Greater trochanter
    C) Sacrum
    D) Ischial tuberosity

68. A patient with multiple sclerosis presents with new onset weakness in left upper extremity. MRI shows enhancing lesions in the upper cervical and brainstem area. The patient also complains of electrical shocks down his spine whenever he touches his chin to his chest. Which clinical sign is evident in this presentation?
    A) Lhermitte's sign
    B) Apley's compression sign
    C) Adson's sign
    D) Thoracic outlet sign

69. In a cross-sectional view of the spinal cord, the gray matter is divided into two horns, the ventral or anterior horns and the posterior or dorsal horns. The dorsal horns contain cell bodies for:
    A) Motor
    B) Temperature
    C) Proprioception
    D) Motor and temperature

70. What is the leading cause of death in chronic spinal cord injury (SCI)?
    A) Heart disease
    B) Respiratory disease
    C) Genitourinary disease
    D) Suicide

71. Which of the following is a true statement regarding spinal cord injury (SCI) in women and pregnancy?
    A) The likelihood of pregnancy is reduced as amenorrhea is common
    B) The risk of complications during pregnancy is equivalent to that in the able-bodied population
    C) A cesarian section is the preferred method of delivery
    D) Autonomic dysreflexia may be the only presentation of labor in injuries above the T6 level

72. What is the classification of a pressure injury with full thickness skin loss involving subcutaneous tissue and extending into but not through fascia?
    A) Stage 1
    B) Stage 2
    C) Stage 3
    D) Stage 4

73. How many cervical nerve roots are there?
    A) 5
    B) 6
    C) 7
    D) 8

74. Poliomyelitis and Werdnig-Hoffmann disease affect which portion of the spinal cord?
    A) Fasciculus cuneatus + ventral horns
    B) Fasciculus gracilis + dorsal horns
    C) Dorsal horns only
    D) Ventral horns only

75. Which of the following marks the American Spinal Injury Association (ASIA) Impairment Scale (AIS) neurological examination sensory point for L4?
    A) Lateral malleolus
    B) Over the dorsum of the foot at the third metatarsal phalangeal (MTP) joint
    C) Medial malleolus
    D) Over the ischial tuberosity

76. A patient comes in complaining of sudden onset back pain while bending over to pick up a fallen piece of paper. The patient's neurological exam is significant for weakness in his left L5 nerve root. Which of the following disk herniations is most likely?
    A) Paracentral/posterolateral at L3/L4
    B) Paracentral/posterolateral at L5/S1
    C) Foraminal at L4/L5
    D) Foraminal at L5/S1

77. Regarding epidemiology, which of the following is the most common cause of spinal cord injury (SCI)?
    A) Falls
    B) Violence
    C) Motor vehicle accidents
    D) Sports/recreation

78. Vena cava filter placement should be considered for spinal cord–injured patients with which of the following?
    A) High cervical cord injury with poor cardiopulmonary reserve
    B) As a substitute for prophylaxis in a complete injury
    C) Older than 70 years
    D) All of the above

79. In a spinal cord–injured (SCI) patient, which of the following is **not** true when establishing a bowel program?
    A) Schedule a routine the same time of the day after a meal
    B) In areflexic bowel, the goal is firm-formed stool that can be manually evacuated

C) Fiber should be uniformly started in each patient

D) A mini-enema can trigger reflexic bowel by acting as mucosal stimulus

80. The most caudal end of the spinal cord is at which level?
    A) The 12th thoracic vertebra
    B) The 10th thoracic vertebra
    C) The 4th lumbar vertebra
    D) The 2nd lumbar vertebra

81. In the American Spinal Injury Association (ASIA) examination, the umbilicus is the key dermatome for what level?
    A) T6
    B) T4
    C) T10
    D) L4

82. Which of the following conditions may lead to anterior spinal artery (ASA) syndrome?
    A) Bilateral occlusion of vertebral arteries at their origins
    B) Basilar artery occlusion
    C) Occlusion of bilateral posterior spinal arteries
    D) Occlusion of distal right vertebral artery

83. What is significant about the T6 level with regard to autonomic dysreflexia?
    A) Injuries above T6 will sever connection to more than half of the sympathetic chain, thereby causing an overall imbalance in sympathetic function
    B) T6 through T12 mark the sympathetic outflow to pelvic splanchnic vessels, and injuries above this level will particularly disrupt supraspinal modulation of this sympathetic outflow.
    C) There is nothing significant about the T6 level
    D) All spinal cord injury patients experience autonomic dysreflexia. Epidemiologically it has been found that T6 is the most significant level above which cord injury leads to dysreflexia.

84. Which of the following vertebral levels is the most common level to find a chance fracture?
    A) C5
    B) T2
    C) T12
    D) L5

85. Spasticity is defined as:
    A) Velocity-dependent increased resistance to passive motion
    B) Time-dependent increase in resistance
    C) Length-dependent increase in resistance
    D) Tightening of muscles

86. Pressure injuries are of concern in spinal cord injury (SCI) patients because of their decreased mobility and sensation. At what stage of a pressure injury do you see full thickness tissue loss with exposed bone, tendon, or muscle?
    A) Stage 1
    B) Stage 2
    C) Stage 3
    D) Stage 4

87. Heterotopic ossification is increased bone deposition outside of the skeleton and can develop in patients after spinal cord injuries (SCI). Heterotopic ossification often develops around what location on the body in SCI patients?
    A) Hips
    B) Shoulders
    C) Knees
    D) Elbows

88. Flexion contractures at the wrist and fingers can interfere with performance of self-care; however, mild tightening of finger flexors in patients with C6 tetraplegia can permit a weak grasp during wrist extension. This mechanism is known as:
    A) Flexor effect
    B) Tenodesis effect
    C) Contracture effect
    D) Extensor effect

89. Which of the following is not an effective treatment for male erectile dysfunction resulting from a spinal cord injury?
    A) Oral medications
    B) Vacuum tumescence devices
    C) Penile injections
    D) Psychological counseling

90. Which of the following injuries would not result in a lower motor neuron (LMN) bowel?
    A) Cauda equina
    B) Injury to the pudendal nerve
    C) Destruction of the S2 through S4 anterior horn cells
    D) Transection of spine at S1

91. A 56-year-old female is admitted to your service after having a spinal cord injury (SCI) and complains of dizziness and light-headedness that occurs whenever she changes position from supine to sitting. Which of the following are management strategies for this condition?
    A) Administration of midodrine
    B) Administration of propranolol
    C) Restrict fluids
    D) Remain in the supine position

92. Autonomic dysreflexia is a syndrome that affects people with spinal cord injuries (SCI) usually at what level and above?
    A) T3
    B) T4
    C) T5
    D) T6

93. Immediately after a spinal cord injury (SCI), sympathetic tone is completely lost, resulting in "spinal shock" whereby hypotension, bradycardia, and hypothermia occur. Which of the following is not considered a factor leading to hypotension?
    A) Systemic loss of vascular resistance
    B) Loss of the ability to ambulate
    C) Accumulation of blood within the venous system
    D) Decreased cardiac output

94. At what level of injury can a patient with a spinal cord injury breathe without mechanical ventilation?
    A) C2
    B) C3
    C) C4
    D) C5

95. Which of the following is the most common respiratory complication in people with spinal cord injury (SCI)?
    A) Pneumonia
    B) Atelectasis
    C) Pulmonary embolism
    D) Pleural effusions

96. Which of the following complications is the leading cause of death for persons with spinal cord injuries (SCI)?
    A) Cardiac
    B) Pulmonary
    C) Gastrointestinal
    D) Renal

97. The International Standards of Neurological Classification of Spinal Cord Injury (ISNCSCI) includes a scale of impairment called the American Spinal Injury Association (ASIA) Impairment Scale (AIS), which classifies spinal cord injury (SCI) in five categories of severity, labeled A to E. Which of the categories represents a sensory incomplete classification?
    A) A
    B) B
    C) C
    D) D

98. The American Spinal Injury Association (ASIA) exam is a test to classify spinal cord injuries. What tests are required in order to classify patients under the ASIA exam?
    A) Sensory testing via dermatomes and strength testing via 10 myotomes
    B) Strength testing via 10 myotomes and reflex testing of upper and lower extremities
    C) Sensory testing via dermatomes and reflex testing of upper and lower extremities
    D) None of the above

99. To evaluate for stability, the spine can be divided into three columns: the anterior, middle, and posterior. In order for the spine to be considered unstable, which of the following must be true?
    A) The anterior column is damaged
    B) The anterior and middle column is damaged
    C) The posterior column is damaged
    D) The anterior and posterior column is damaged

100. Fractures and dislocations in the thoracic and lumbar spine most commonly involve which of the following?
    A) T11 and L1
    B) T11 and L2
    C) T12 and L1
    D) T12 and L2

**101.** Which of the following would you initially order to evaluate for vertebral stability?
- A) MRI of spine
- B) Anterior-posterior (AP) x-ray of spine
- C) CT of spine
- D) Flexion and extension x-ray views of spine

**102.** A complete spinal cord injury is defined as:
- A) A transection of the spinal cord
- B) No motor or sensory function preserved in the sacral segments S4 to S5
- C) No motor sparing, but sensory sparing below the level of injury
- D) Strength less than antigravity below the level of injury

**103.** A patient sustains a spinal cord injury with the following motor examination:
C5—5/5 bilateral
C6—5/5 bilateral
C7—3/5 bilateral
C8—2/5 bilateral
T1—2/5 bilateral
L1—1/5 bilateral
L2—1/5 bilateral
L3—1/5 bilateral
L4—0/5 bilateral
L5—0/5 bilateral
*Sensation*—Intact to pinprick and light touch to the armpit; impaired (1/2) from armpit to rectum with pinprick and light touch sparing at S4 to S5 and rectal tone.
What is the motor level of injury for this individual?
- A) C6
- B) T1
- C) L3
- D) C7

**104.** A patient sustains a spinal cord injury with the following motor examination:
C5—5/5 bilateral
C6—5/5 bilateral
C7—3/5 bilateral
C8—2/5 bilateral
T1—2/5 bilateral
L1—1/5 bilateral
L2—1/5 bilateral
L3—1/5 bilateral
L4—0/5 bilateral
L5—0/5 bilateral
*Sensation*—Intact to pinprick and light touch to the armpit; impaired (1/2) from armpit to rectum with pinprick and light touch sparing at S4 to S5 and rectal tone.
What is the sensory level of injury?
- A) T1
- B) T4
- C) S5
- D) C7

**105.** A patient sustains a spinal cord injury with the following motor examination:

C5—5/5 bilateral
C6—5/5 bilateral
C7—3/5 bilateral
C8—2/5 bilateral
T1—2/5 bilateral
L1—1/5 bilateral
L2—1/5 bilateral
L3—1/5 bilateral
L4—0/5 bilateral
L5—0/5 bilateral

*Sensation*—Intact to pinprick and light touch to the armpit; impaired (1/2) from armpit to rectum with pinprick and light touch sparing at S4 to S5 and rectal tone.

What is the American Spinal Injury Association (ASIA) classification for this patient?

A) AIS A
B) AIS B
C) AIS C
D) AIS D

# Spinal Cord Medicine

## ANSWERS

1. **B)** Anticoagulation with either low–molecular weight heparin or adjusted dose unfractionated heparin should be initiated within 72 hours of injury if there is no contraindication. It should be continued for 8 weeks in an uncomplicated case and 12 weeks or until discharge from rehabilitation for those individuals with other risk factors, such as lower limb fracture, history of cancer/thrombosis, age over 70 years, heart failure, or obesity even in those with inferior vena cava filters.

2. **C)** The use of certain maneuvers may aid in evacuation, including push-ups, abdominal massage, a forward-leaning position, breathing exercises, and drinking warm fluids. In addition, the upright position can also stimulate motility more effectively than attempting a bowel program while in bed.

3. **C)** In SCI, there is a disparity between bone formation and resorption. This results in a greater risk of fractures from osteoporosis, hypercalcemia, and hypercalciuria. Hypercalcemia is seen most often with recent injury, male gender, complete injury, tetraplegia, dehydration, and immobilization. Chronic SCI patients may develop vitamin D deficiency, which requires supplementation. Restricting calcium intake is not recommended. Treatment includes bisphosphonates, intravenous fluids, or calcitonin. Functional electrical stimulation and weight bearing may decrease bone loss.

4. **A)** The T4 dermatome includes the nipple. The T6 level is the xiphoid, L4 is the medial malleolus, and T10 is the umbilicus.

5. **D)** It is important to know the mechanism of action of the medications used in bowel management of patients with spinal cord injury. As the injury to bowel may be classified typically into upper motor neuron or lower motor neuron, the physiatrist must utilize particular medications to make up for corresponding physiological deficits. Of the medications listed, senna glycoside acts via stimulation of Auerbach's/myenteric plexus producing a promotility effect. Although a relatively small and local effect, over time, this can propel stool over a great distance in the colon.

6. **B)** Of the medications listed, dantrolene has the least sedating side effects. The mechanism of action of dantrolene lies within the sarcomere at the level of the sarcoplasmic reticulum, preventing calcium release, while all the other medications are centrally acting and sedating. Theoretically, given dantrolene's peripheral site of action, there should be no sedative side effects. One must be careful to monitor for pregnancy (category C) and intermittently monitor hepatic function tests while a patient is on dantrolene.

7. **C)** The overall most common cause of spinal cord injuries is motor vehicle accidents. When narrowing the population to the elderly, the most common cause is falls.

8. **B)** The bony vertebral column elongates more than the spinal cord during development. The normal level of spinal cord termination is at the L1 to L2 level. Owing to natural variation, the spinal cord termination can be as low as L3 and as high as T12.

9. **A)** A Brown-Séquard syndrome refers to an injury of the spinal cord in which one side is damaged more than the other, resulting in relatively greater ipsilateral weakness and position sense loss, but with contralateral pain and temperature sensation loss.

10. **D)** Task frequency can be modified by limiting the number of transfers or switching to power mobility in high-risk patients. Minimizing force can be achieved by using a lighter wheelchair, improving propulsion techniques, and maintaining an optimal weight. Individuals are encouraged to avoid extreme positions of the wrist, avoid positioning above the shoulder by implementing assistive devices/technology, and avoid extreme shoulder internal rotation and abduction to prevent mechanical impingement.

11. **C)** Screening for depression should be performed on the initial visit and subsequent follow-up appointments. Owing to limited research, the number of those having depression after their injuries may be underrepresented. The following are general risk factors: prior or family history of depression, age of onset below 40 years, chronic pain, female gender, poor support system, multiple comorbidities, substance abuse, and other major stresses. An individual with a previous depressive episode has a 50% probability of a second event. In the SCI population, the completeness and associated medical issues, such as a brain injury, heighten the risk of developing depression.

12. **C)** The risk of HO is greater in complete spinal cord injuries, older individuals, in the presence of spasticity, and in patients with pressure injuries. No relationship has been shown with gender, race, level, or cause of injury.

13. **C)** The key muscle groups in the ASIA examination for the upper extremities are as follows:
C5 = Elbow flexors
C6 = Wrist extensors
C7 = Elbow extensors
C8 = Long finger flexors
T1 = Finger abductors

14. **B)** This patient has central cord syndrome. This syndrome includes a characteristic motor weakness of upper extremities greater than lower extremities with or without disturbance in sensation and bowel and bladder function. It is thought that the corticospinal tract lamination represents the upper extremities medially and the lower extremities laterally. With such a representation, a centrally located lesion would affect medial fibers to a greater extent. The typical mechanism of injury is hyperextension of the cervical spine, typically in the setting of preexisting osteophytes and spondylosis.

15. **A)** Spinal cord tumors are one cause of nontraumatic spinal cord injury. Ependymomas are the most common intramedullary neoplasms of the spinal cord, followed by astrocytomas. Meningiomas and schwannomas are intradural tumors. To review, tumors outside the dura mater are considered extradural. Those within the dura mater are intradural and can be subclassified as being extramedullary or intramedullary. Those within the pia mater and/or arising from the spinal cord parenchyma are intramedullary. Those outside of the pia are extramedullary.

16. **C)** The top three causes of death in spinal cord–injured patients classified as paraplegic patients are cardiovascular disease, sepsis, and suicide. Routine follow-up with primary care physicians, bowel and bladder management, and depression screening using tools such as the Beck Depression Inventory are paramount in these patients.

17. **C)** Falls are the most common cause of SCI among the elderly, whereas violence is the most common cause of SCI in African Americans. Women rarely sustain SCI from gunshots, motorcycle crashes, or diving.

18. **C)** The cauda equina syndrome refers to an injury to the lumbosacral roots within the spinal canal, resulting in an areflexic bladder, bowel, and lower limbs. Additional symptoms include loss or altered sensation between the legs, over the buttocks, the inner thighs and the back of the legs (saddle paresthesia). It is a lower motor neuron lesion.

19. **C)** The neurological findings seen in Brown-Séquard are based on where various pathways travel and cross over in relation to the brain stem and spinal cord. As it is a hemisection of the cord, the following are seen:
    - Ipsilateral motor and proprioceptive loss at and below the level of lesion
    - Ipsilateral sensory loss at the level of the lesion
    - Contralateral loss of pain and temperature below the level of the lesion

20. **D)** Expected functional outcomes are important to discuss with an acutely injured patient and his or her family. For transfers, patients with a lesion at C4/C5 usually require total assistance with a board or a mechanical lift, C6 patients require minimal assistance with the use of a board or lift or may be independent, and C7 patients are usually independent with or without the board on level surfaces (and some assistance to independence on uneven terrain). An individual should gain complete independence in transfers at C8 to T1, which was not listed as a choice.

21. **A)** HO is the formation of true bone in ectopic sites that restricts range of motion. HO can present with swelling, fever, limited mobility, or pain. Ninety percent of the time, in spinal cord–injured patients, it occurs in the hips. Serum alkaline phosphatase will be elevated, but is not a specific measure and levels gradually diminish with maturation. HO may not be visible on plain films in the acute phase, but will be seen on bone scan. Treatment includes gentle ranging exercises, etidronate, and rarely radiation therapy. Surgical resection can be considered in severe cases after maturation.

22. **D)** The key muscle groups in the ASIA examination for the upper extremities are as follows:
    C5 = Elbow flexors
    C6 = Wrist extensors
    C7 = Elbow extensors
    C8 = Long finger flexors
    T1 = Finger abductors

23. **C)** Subacute combined degeneration describes a progressive loss of the posterior and lateral columns of the spinal cord. Deficits in patients include loss in vibratory, proprioceptive, and light touch sense (dorsal column), as well as weakness involving upper and lower limbs and the trunk (lateral corticospinal tract). Common etiologies include vitamin $B_{12}$ deficiency, nitrous oxide exposure, and vitamin E deficiency, among others. This may occur in patients with $B_{12}$ absorption diseases including Crohn's disease, patients with terminal ileum resection, pernicious anemia, recent anesthesia exposure, and strict longstanding vegetarian diets.

24. **C)** In order of prevalence, spinal cord injuries are most frequently classified as incomplete tetraplegia, complete paraplegia, incomplete paraplegia, and finally complete tetraplegia.

25. **C)** Patients with lower motor neuron injury only have the intrinsic myenteric plexus propelling stool through the colon. As such, the gastrocolic reflex, digital rectal stimulation, and warm beverage taken daily prior to desired bowel movement (gastrocolic reflex) will be of minimal to no use in a lower motor neuron–injured bowel.

26. **D)** In descending order, the incidence of SCI are as follows: Vehicular crashes (42%), falls (26.7%), violence (15.1%), and sports (7.6%). In recent years there has been a slight decrease of incidence of SCI from vehicular crashes and sports, with slight increase from falls.

27. **C)** Lower motor neuron injuries occur either in the ventral horn of the spinal cord or anterior nerve roots. These injuries can lead to muscle atrophy, decreased strength and reflexes, fasciculations, and paralysis.

28. **A)** Central cord syndrome is an incomplete injury that results in lower motor neuron weakness at the level of injury and upper motor neuron spasticity below the injury. It typically occurs in the elderly who have a preexisting spondylosis. Brown-Séquard is a hemisection of the cord that results in ipsilateral motor and proprioceptive loss with contralateral loss of pain and temperature. Anterior cord syndrome occurs with a vascular injury that results in loss of motor and pain/temperature sensation with preservation of light touch and position sense. Cauda equina occurs with burst fractures or central disc herniations, resulting in lower motor neuron flaccid paralysis with loss of sensation in the lower lumbar and sacral segments.

29. **A)** The recovery is faster and more favorable in incomplete injuries and in younger patients. To achieve antigravity strength, it can take an average of 2 months in a complete injury compared with 2 weeks in an incomplete injury. Muscles with a grade of 1 or 2 have a greater probability of improving one grade by 1 year compared with muscles with no activity. American Spinal Injury Association (ASIA) grade D has the best prognosis for ambulation. Of those persons with ASIA C, 75% will regain the ability to ambulate and 50% in ASIA B. The most significant predictor is the preservation of sacral sensation.

30. **D)** The external urethral sphincter is innervated by the pudendal nerve (S2–S4). The internal urethral sphincter is innervated by the hypogastric nerve (T11–L2) and allows for the storage of urine. The parasympathetic system, through the pelvic splanchnic nerve (S2–S4), promotes bladder contraction and voiding.

31. **B)** Twenty-two percent of deaths for persons with SCI treated at a model systems site were due to diseases of the respiratory system. The next most common cause is heart disease (11.8%), followed by infectious diseases (10.4%).

32. **A)** Brown-Séquard syndrome involves an injury to the transverse section of the spinal cord (relative hemisection). The resultant injury involves ipsilateral motor and proprioception loss with contralateral loss of pain and temperature.

33. **B)** Taking advantage of tenodesis grasp (where intact wrist extension causes a passive hand-grasp mechanism), a C6 complete injury is the highest level following which a patient can be modified-independent with activities of self-care, transfers, bowel/bladder management, and mobility.

34. **B)** By definition in the AIS grading, key muscle groups were added in 2012 to distinguish between AIS B and C.

35. **B)** More than 80% of all SCI occurs in males, a figure that has been consistent in the last 30 years. This gender difference is similar in other countries.

36. **B)** Upper motor neuron injuries occur along the neural or corticospinal pathway above the anterior horn cell. Symptoms associated with upper motor neuron injury are loss of voluntary movement, spasticity, hyperreflexia, clonus, and Babinski sign.

37. **C)** The ZPP is defined as the most caudal dermatomes and myotomes below the sensory and motor levels that remain partially innervated. It is classified only in complete injuries. The motor ZPP does not follow the sensory ZPP. In the scoring sheet, enter the motor or sensory level if there are no segments below and "N/A" for incomplete injuries. To calculate the length, count the number of levels from the sensory or motor level to the ZPP level.

38. **A)** There are several causes for autonomic dysreflexia, but the first action should be to sit the person up and loosen any restrictive clothing, which will lower blood pressure by pooling blood in the lower extremities. Then, it is important to determine the stimulus causing the autonomic dysreflexia. For instance, the most common cause is bladder distention—check for kinks or flush the catheter. Pharmacologic management may be necessary if symptoms persist.

39. **B)** Detrusor sphincter dyssynergia is a common bladder condition seen in spinal cord injury patients. The detrusor is overactive and spastic, and the internal sphincter is also hyperactive. It results in a small bladder that is unable to empty. This increases the risk of high voiding pressures and vesicoureteral reflux. Alpha receptors are found in the proximal urethra and bladder neck, and therefore alpha blockers can lower urethral resistance. One of the complications of using this medication is orthostatic hypotension. The medication should be taken at night while in the supine position. Patients taking alpha blockers should be cautioned to avoid phosphodiesterase inhibitors to prevent an abrupt drop in blood pressure.

40. **C)** Spinocerebellar tracts transmit unconscious proprioception from the ipsilateral side of the body. Lateral corticospinal tracts control voluntary muscle activity. Dorsal columns transmit proprioception, fine touch, and vibration sense from the ipsilateral side of the body.

41. **B)** Central cord syndrome is the most common of the incomplete spinal cord lesions. It produces motor weakness greater in the arms than in the legs and variable sensory loss. There is sacral sensory sparing. This syndrome is due to an injury to the central part of the cervical spinal cord.

42. **D)** According to the Consortium for Spinal Cord Medicine Clinical Practice Guidelines, patients with limited mobility (AIS A and B motor complete diagnoses) should be treated with 2 weeks of mechanical DVT prophylaxis, such as sequential compression devices, as well as a total of at least 8 weeks of DVT chemoprophylaxis. If a patient has complications or comorbidities such as hypercoagulable state, cancer, lower extremity fracture, or prior DVT/pulmonary embolism (PE), the chemoprophylaxis is recommended to be at least 12 weeks. Studies have also shown superiority of low–molecular weight heparin (LMWH) (enoxaparin) over unfractionated heparin.

43. **C)** Bacteriuria and urinary tract infections are common in spinal cord injury patients. Treatment of bacteriuria is not warranted except in certain circumstances. One of these circumstances is the presence of pyuria of anything greater than 10 white blood cells (WBC) per square millimeter high powered field. Another indication is colonization of urease-producing organisms including *Proteus mirabilis*, *Morganella morganii*, *Providencia rettgeri* and *stuartii*, which may lead to struvite stone production.

44. **B)** The incidence of SCI is lowest for persons under 15 years and highest for persons 16 to 30 years. After the age of 30 years, there is a decline in incidence.

45. **B)** Ischemic damage often affects the anterior spinal cord more so than the posterior portion, because the posterior portion has two posterior spinal arteries as opposed to the ventral region, which only has one anterior spinal artery. In anterior cord syndrome, the corticospinal and spinothalamic tracts are affected while the dorsal columns are relatively spared. The anterior cord syndrome can lead to paraplegia with loss of pain and temperature sensation.

46. **D)** There are 10 key muscles tested, which include the following:
    - C5 = biceps brachialis; elbow flexors
    - C6 = extensor carpi radialis; wrist extensors
    - C7 = triceps; elbow extensors
    - C8 = flexor digitorum profundus; finger flexor of middle finger
    - T1 = abductor digiti minimi; small finger abductor
    - L2 = iliopsoas; hip flexors
    - L3 = quadriceps; knee extensors
    - L4 = tibialis anterior; ankle dorsiflexors
    - L5 = extensor hallucis longus; long toe extensors
    - S1 = gastrocnemius; ankle plantar flexors

47. **D)** The most common causes of autonomic dysreflexia involve the bladder and bowel. There are a number of causes, all of which involve noxious stimuli below the level of the spinal cord injury. All of the answer choices are potential causes, as well as infection, pregnancy, sexual intercourse, diagnostic medical procedures, deep venous thrombosis, and ingrown toenails.

48. **D)** Indwelling catheters may be an option for a higher level of injury (such as complete tetraplegia). Although reports have shown that the risk of urinary tract infections is greater with an indwelling catheter compared with intermittent catheterization, there are studies that have shown that the risk may be analogous. It should be considered in individuals with elevated detrusor pressures who are at risk for upper tract complications. It is associated with an increased risk of bladder/kidney stones, epididymitis, urinary tract infections, incontinence, pyelonephritis, hydronephrosis, and cancer. Therefore, more frequent cystoscopic evaluation is warranted in these patients.

49. **D)** C5 is the most common level of spinal cord injury. For patients with paraplegia, T12 and L1 are the most common levels.

50. **C)** This patient likely has weakness of her pelvic floor musculature and external urethral sphincter. This is the most likely of the listed options, given her inability to hold in urine only in circumstances where increased intra-abdominal pressure applies a pressure to the bladder that exceeds the internal and external urethral sphincter pressures, thus, causing her accidents. A trial of oxybutynin and imipramine may lead to urinary retention, which may exacerbate the patient's symptoms as bladder volumes will tend to be even higher with the retained urine, and on valsalva may be even easier to leak out. Flomax would also exacerbate her problem, lowering the applied pressure by the internal urethral sphincter. Kegel exercises would strengthen the pelvic floor musculature and external urethral sphincter, allowing a greater ability to retain urine voluntarily.

51. **C)** Owing to loss of function in musculature involved in respiratory function (for example the intercostals and abdominal muscles), patients with high thoracic and cervical injuries often have impaired respiratory function. Sequelae include impaired cough, a decreased ability to clear secretions, and decreased lung function parameters. An inability to maximally inspire due to loss of inspiratory muscle function leads to an increase in residual volume.

52. **C)** Visceral afferents to the bladder travel via the pelvic splanchnic nerve fibers.

53. **C)** The posterior spinal artery, anterior spinal artery, radicular arteries, and artery of Adamkiewicz supply blood to the spinal cord. The posterior spinal arteries branch from the vertebral arteries and travel along the posterior surface of the spinal cord to supply the posterior 1/3 of the spinal

cord. Two anterior spinal arteries that also branch from the vertebral arteries unite to travel along the anterior surface supplying the anterior 2/3 of the spinal cord. The artery of Adamkiewicz normally travels on the left side of the spinal cord and divides into a small ascending and larger descending branch. The artery of Adamkiewicz normally ends around L2.

54. **C)** • A = Complete. No sensory or motor preservation in sacral segments, S4 to S5.
    - B = Sensory incomplete. Sensory preservation below the neurologic level with sacral sparing. No motor function more than 3 levels below the motor level.
    - C = Motor incomplete. Motor preservation below the neurologic level (greater than 3 levels) and greater than half key muscles below the single neurologic level graded less than 3.
    - D = Motor incomplete. Motor preservation below neurologic level (greater than 3 levels) and greater than half key muscles below the single neurologic level graded greater than or equal to 3.
    - E = Sensory and motor exams are normal.

55. **B)** Autonomic dysreflexia occurs as a result of unopposed sympathetic discharge above the major splanchnic outflow (which occurs at T6 through L2). It occurs after spinal shock, when reflexes return. The patient may present with flushing and diaphoresis above the level of the lesion, hypertension, bradycardia, piloerection, skin pallor, and/or headache.

56. **D)** Suprapubic catheterization is an alternative to those individuals who cannot perform intermittent catheterization because of the following reasons: urethral stricture or obstruction, perineal skin breakdown, prostatitis, urethritis, or epididymo-orchitis. It can be considered to improve body image and sexual function. It is the preferred method in the acute phase in patients with urethral trauma.

57. **A)** Motor vehicle crashes account for 47% of traumatic SCIs.

58. **D)** Somatic innervation to the external sphincter is via the pudendal nerve. Sympathetic innervation is not provided to the external sphincter, rather it is provided to the **internal** sphincter via the hypogastric nerve. Visceral afferents are carried via parasympathetic fibers by the pelvic nerve.

59. **B)** The Braden scale, developed in 1987, is a tool for measuring the risk of pressure injury. It measures six components: activity, mobility, sensory perception, nutrition, friction and shear, and moisture. Each component carries a minimum of 1 point and maximum of 4 points except for friction and shear which carry a minimum of 1 point and maximum of 3 points. The greater the level of impairment (decreased sensation, activity, mobility, or nutrition, and the increased moisture and level of friction and shear forces), the lower the score in each category. The overall grading is from 6 to 23 points, with a score of 18 or less indicating increased risk, as stratified below:
19 to 23: no risk
15 to 18: mild risk
13 to 14: moderate risk
10 to 12: high risk
9 or less: very high risk

60. **C)** Subacute combined degeneration presents with upper motor neuron signs. Cauda equine syndrome and poliomyelitis both present with lower motor neuron signs. Amyotrophic lateral sclerosis presents commonly with upper and lower motor neuron signs due to involvement of anterior horns of the gray matter as well as the lateral corticospinal tracts.

61. **D)** The cauda equina syndrome refers to injury to the lumbosacral roots within the spinal canal, resulting in areflexic bladder, bowel, weakness of lower limbs, and loss of sexual sensation. Cauda equina syndrome occurs when the nerve roots in the lumbar spine are compressed, cutting off sensation and movement. Nerve roots that control the function of the bladder and bowel are especially vulnerable to damage.

62. **B)** • A = Complete. No sensory or motor preservation in sacral segments, S4 to S5.
    • B = Sensory incomplete. Sensory preservation below the neurologic level with sacral sparing. No motor function more than 3 levels below the motor level.
    • C = Motor incomplete. Motor preservation below the neurologic level (greater than 3 levels) and greater than half key muscles below the single neurologic level graded less than 3.
    • D = Motor incomplete. Motor preservation below the neurologic level (greater than 3 levels) and greater than half key muscles below the single neurologic level graded greater than or equal to 3.
    • E = Sensory and motor exams are normal.

63. **D)** The physiatrist should begin the discussion of sexual function early and be respectful of this sensitive subject. PDE-5 inhibitors have been successful and well tolerated. Its use is contraindicated with the concurrent use of nitrates. When oral medications are ineffective, an injection of alprostadil can be given, but priapism can occur. A vacuum device requires manual dexterity and is contraindicated in those on blood thinners or with a history of sickle cell. Other options include intraurethral medications (which are not as widely available) and implantable penile prostheses (which are not preferred because they can lead to corporal tissue destruction).

64. **C)** Intermittent catheterization is a treatment option for neurogenic bladder. It should be avoided in individuals who are unable to catheterize because of poor hand strength, a caregiver who is unwilling to assist, urethral abnormalities, small bladder capacity, high fluid intake, and the tendency to develop autonomic dysreflexia. Intermittent catheterization can lead to the development of urinary tract infections, stones, incontinence, urethral trauma, and autonomic dysreflexia. Routine urologic follow-up is crucial.

65. **B)** In the cervical region, nerves exit the intervertebral foramina just rostral to the vertebra of the same name with the exception of the C8 nerve root, which has no corresponding vertebral body. It resides below C7 and above T1.

66. **B)** Brown-Séquard syndrome carries the best prognosis for independent ambulation following rehabilitation. While central cord syndrome may be a tempting choice, the prognosis for ambulation particularly in the elderly is dismal, on the order of 30% to 40%. While there is no corticospinal involvement in posterior cord syndrome, the proprioceptive deficits make ambulation overall quite difficult for patients, so the prognosis is poor for independent ambulation.

67. **A)** A more up-to-date term, rather than pressure ulcer, is pressure injury. The reason behind this, following the 2016 National Pressure Ulcer Advisory Panel meeting, is that not all pressure injuries have true "ulceration," for example, stage 1 injury. The most common site of a pressure injury in children with spinal cord injury, especially those under the age of 13 years, is the occiput. For adults, the most common site is the sacrum.

68. **A)** Patients with electric shock–like pain down the spine or into the upper extremities following forward flexion of the neck are said to have a positive *Lhermitte's sign*, named after neurologist Jean Lhermitte. While there are many pathologies that may lead to cervical and brain stem area lesions that might clinically manifest with Lhermitte's sign, multiple sclerosis and transverse myelitis are two common ones.

69. **C)** The dorsal horns contain cell bodies for sensory neurons: proprioception and vibration. The ventral horns contain cell bodies for motor control as well as pain and temperature sensation.

70. **B)** The leading cause of death in spinal cord injury patients is respiratory diseases, with pneumonia as the most common cause.

71. **D)** Amenorrhea may occur after injury, but most often menstruation returns 6 months after injury. Reproductive function and fertility is unaffected once menstruation returns. These women should be educated about the issues related to pregnancy and SCI, including complications, such as increased risk of urinary tract infections, changes in respiratory function, and biomechanical effects of being in a wheelchair. As uterine innervations arise from T10 to T12, these individuals may not present with the typical symptoms of labor and must be aware of autonomic dysreflexia. Although caesarian sections may be more common in this population, it is not the preferred plan for delivery.

72. **C)** It is vital to learn the classification of pressure injuries. Stage 1 involves changes in skin temperature, tissue consistency, and sensation. The skin appears red or pigmented but is intact. Stage 2 is a partial thickness skin loss with exposed dermis. Stage 3 involves full thickness tissue loss, but muscle, bone, and tendon are not affected. Stage 4 is similar to Stage 3, in that there is full thickness involvement but it extends to muscle, bone, tendon, and joint capsule. If eschar is present, then it cannot be staged and is labeled unstageable.

73. **D)** There are eight pairs of cervical nerve roots. The first seven exit above the corresponding vertebrae and the eighth cervical nerve root exits below the seventh cervical vertebra. Thereafter, all nerve roots are named by the vertebra above the root (ie, T7 exits between the T7 and T8 vertebrae).

74. **D)** Poliomyelitis and Werdnig-Hoffmann disease (progressive infantile muscular atrophy) affect the ventral horns of the spinal cord, causing a lower motor neuron injury. These injuries result in flaccid paralysis, areflexia, atrophy, fasciculations, and fibrillations.

75. **C)** Knowledge of all key sensory points is paramount in the AIS neurological assessment. The key point for the L4 dermatome is at the medial malleolus. It is also helpful to know the overall distribution of the dermatomes.

76. **D)** Paracentral herniations typically affect the nerve root of the lower vertebral level, for example, L4/L5 will affect L5 nerve root. Foraminal herniations will typically affect the nerve root of the higher vertebral level (eg, L4/L5 will affect the L4 nerve root).

77. **C)** Automobile accidents are the leading cause of SCI. However, there are differences among age groups. Falls are reported as the most common cause in the elderly, and violence is the leading cause in African Americans.

78. **A)** Vena cava placement is indicated in those who have failed prophylaxis, have a contraindication to anticoagulation, or have high cervical cord injury lesions with poor cardiopulmonary reserve. It is not a substitute for prophylaxis and may increase the risk of complications in the future, such as cava thrombosis or filter migration.

79. **C)** The establishment of a regular and predictable bowel routine is a crucial part of postinjury management. The type of program may depend on whether the bowels are reflexic or areflexic. The bowel program should be scheduled at the same time daily—usually a half hour after a meal to stimulate the gastrocolic reflexes. For the reflexic bowel, the goal is to use a water-soluble

lubricant along with suppository to create soft-formed stool that can be evacuated with digital stimulation. For areflexic bowel, the goal is firm-formed stool that can be manually evacuated. A mini-enema, which is docusate, glycerin, and polyethylene glycol, has been shown to minimize the time from medication insertion to evacuation. The decision to incorporate fiber in the diet should take into consideration the individual bowel pattern and is not recommended to be automatically started in every SCI patient.

80. **D)** In adults, the most caudal end of the spinal cord is at the L2 level. Up through the third month of fetal life, the spinal cord occupies the whole length of the vertebral canal. After the third month, the rate of lengthening of the spinal cord is slower than the lengthening of the vertebral column.

81. **C)** The T10 dermatome includes the umbilicus. The T6 level is the xiphoid, L4 is the medial malleolus, and T4 is the nipple.

82. **A)** ASA syndrome (also known as anterior cord syndrome) describes vascular disruption of the ASA, which supplies the anterior 2/3 of the spinal cord. While occlusion of the ASA is not listed as a choice, a disruption of the arteries which give rise to the ASA, namely the vertebral arteries, may also result in such a syndrome. While bilateral occlusion of vertebral arteries is improbable, this question tests your knowledge of the vascular anatomy and blood supply to the spinal cord.

83. **B)** T6 through T12 marks the sympathetic outflow to pelvic splanchnic nerves. In autonomic dysreflexia, a noxious stimulus below the level of the lesion causes hypersympathetic output to the pelvic splanchnic vessels causing widespread vasoconstriction and increasing blood pressure to dangerous levels. Baroreceptors within the carotid or aorta facilitate reflex bradycardia via descending parasympathetic output, bringing about the textbook picture of autonomic dysreflexia.

84. **C)** The most common levels for chance fractures to occur are T12 to L1 to L2. Chance fractures (sometimes referred to as *seatbelt fractures*) involve all three spinal columns and are therefore unstable fractures. They are flexion-distraction injuries and there is an increased association with intra-abdominal injuries.

85. **A)** Spasticity is defined as velocity-dependent increased resistance to passive motion, involuntary muscle contractions or spasms, and hyperreflexia. Spasticity can lead to difficulty with positioning and mobility; however, it can be helpful during ambulation. Assessment of spasticity includes the Ashworth scale, the Spasm Frequency Score and the Penn Spasm Frequency Score.

86. **D)** Stage 1—Intact skin with nonblanchable redness of a localized area. The area may be painful, soft, and warmer compared to the adjacent tissue. Stage 2—partial thickness loss of the dermis presenting as a shallow open ulcer with a red-pink wound; may also present as an intact or open/ruptured serum-filled blister. Stage 3—full thickness tissue loss where subcutaneous fat may be visible, but bone tendon and muscle are not exposed. Stage 4—full thickness tissue loss with exposed bone, muscle, or tendon. Unstageable—a full thickness tissue loss in which the base of the ulcer is covered by slough or eschar, therefore the true depth and stage cannot be determined.

87. **A)** Heterotopic ossification (HO) usually presents clinically as a warm local swelling around the affected joint. HO most often develops around the hips (90%) in patients with spinal cord injuries. It has been reported to occur in 20% to 30% of patients with SCI.

88. **B)** Tenodesis is a passive hand-grasp mechanism where extension of the wrist leads to flexion of the digits. Patients with C6 tetraplegia can use this tenodesis effect to hold objects without true finger function.

89.  **D)** Erectile dysfunction can be treated with oral medications, vacuum tumescence devices, intracavernous (penile) injections, and penile implants.

90.  **D)** An LMN bowel results from disruption of the parasympathetic innervation to the rectum and descending colon. The parasympathetic innervation to the descending colon and rectum is provided by the pelvic nerve, which exits from the spinal cord at S2 through S4 segments. The pudendal nerve, also originating from segments S2 through S4, innervates the external anal sphincter and pelvic floor. Cauda equina can also produce an areflexic or LMN bowel in which there is no reflex-mediated colonic peristalsis. The anal sphincter of an LMN bowel is typically atonic and prone to leaking.

91.  **A)** The patient has orthostatic hypotension. After SCI, sympathetic tone is lost resulting in hypotension, bradycardia, and hypothermia. Over the course of time, the sympathetic reflex activity returns and blood pressure becomes normalized. However, as the supraspinal control continues to be absent in patients with high-level SCI, they continue to be prone to orthostatic hypotension. Some treatment options for orthostatic hypotension are elastic stockings, abdominal binders, hydration, gradually progressive daily head-up tilt, and administration of midodrine or fludrocortisone.

92.  **D)** Autonomic dysreflexia usually affects persons with an SCI at the T6 level or above. Autonomic dysreflexia occurs when a noxious stimulus below the level of injury elicits a sudden reflex sympathetic activity (which is uninhibited by the supraspinal centers) leading to profound vasoconstriction and autonomic responses. Some symptoms are: pounding headache, hypertension, bradycardia, flushing of face and neck, and pupillary dilation.

93.  **B)** The hypotension occurs as a result of systemic loss of vascular resistance, accumulation of blood within the venous system, reduced venous return to the heart, and decreased cardiac output. Over the course of time, the sympathetic reflex activity returns, with normalization of blood pressure.

94.  **D)** Persons with a neurologic level of C2 or above with a complete SCI usually have no diaphragmatic function and require mechanical ventilation or diaphragmatic or phrenic pacing. Persons with a complete C3 SCI have severe diaphragmatic weakness and commonly require mechanical ventilation, at least temporarily. Persons with a complete C4 SCI often also have severe diaphragmatic weakness and can also require mechanical ventilation, at least temporarily. Persons with a complete C5 through C8 SCI usually are able to maintain independent breathing, but because of the loss of innervation to the intercostal and abdominal muscles, they remain at high risk for pulmonary complications.

95.  **B)** Atelectasis is the most common respiratory complication in people with SCI and can predispose to pneumonia, pleural effusion, and empyema. Pneumonia commonly occurs in areas of atelectasis. Pleural effusions often develop in close proximity to areas of atelectasis. Treatment of atelectasis includes lung expansion, secretion mobilization, and secretion clearance.

96.  **B)** Pulmonary complications, including atelectasis, pneumonia, respiratory failure, pleural complications, and pulmonary embolism, are the leading causes of death for persons with SCI in all years after SCI.

97.  **B)** An SCI that results in the absence of any sensory or motor function in the sacral segments S4 to S5 would have an AIS category of A and be designated as complete. For an SCI where sensation is preserved in the sacral segments S4 to S5, but there is no motor function caudal to three

segments below the neurological level of injury (NLI) the AIS is B, sensory incomplete. For an SCI where sensation is preserved in the sacral segments S4 to S5, but more than half the key muscles below the NLI have a muscle grade less than 3/5, the AIS is C. For an SCI where sensation is preserved in the sacral segments S4 to S5, but at least half the key muscles below the NLI have a muscle grade greater than or equal to 3/5, the AIS is D. When sensory and motor function is normal, the AIS is E. AIS categories B through E designate incomplete injuries.

98. **A)** The International Standards for Neurological Classification of Spinal Cord Injury (ISNCSCI) provides a procedure for classifying a spinal cord injury (SCI). The procedure includes a systematic evaluation of all the dermatomes and extremity myotomes. Because SCI usually affects the spinal cord at a discrete site, determining the last intact sensory and motor level can reliably and accurately determine the neurologic level of injury.

99. **B)** The anterior column is composed of the anterior longitudinal ligament, the anterior 2/3 of the vertebral body, and the anterior 2/3 of the annulus fibrosus or disk. The middle column is composed of the posterior 1/3 of the vertebral body, the posterior 1/3 of the annulus fibrosus, and the posterior longitudinal ligament. The posterior column is composed of the pedicles, facet joints, laminae, supraspinous ligament, interspinous ligament, facet joint capsule, and ligamentum flavum. When the integrity of the middle and either the anterior or the posterior column is affected, the spine is likely to be unstable. The columns can be compromised by either fracture or ligamentous disruption. *(P.261 #169 explanation says middle OR any 2+ columns)*

100. **C)** Fractures or dislocations in the thoracic and lumbar spine most commonly involve the T12 and the L1 vertebrae, respectively. Common mechanisms include compression-flexion, distraction-flexion, translation, and torsion-flexion.

101. **D)** Flexion and extension views of the spine are good initial imaging modalities to look for vertebral instability.

102. **B)** (ASIA A classification)
The ASIA Classification System is as follows:
A = Motor and sensory complete—no sacral sparing including pin prick (PP) or light touch (LT) at any of the S4-5 dermatomes
B = Sensory incomplete
C = Motor incomplete—defined as
  1) Sacral sparing of motor function (anal contraction)
  2) Sacral sparing of sensation with motor function present in more than three levels below the motor level on either side (may include non–key muscles)
  Less than half of muscles 3/5 or greater below the motor level of injury
D = Motor incomplete—as ASIA C with more than half 3/5 or greater
E = Neurologically intact

103. **D)** The motor level of injury is defined as the lowest key muscle that has a grade of at least 3, provided the key muscles above that level are graded as 5.
   The sensory level of injury is the most caudal dermatome to have normal (score of 2) sensation for both pinprick and light touch.
   The ASIA classification system is as follows (please see the ASIA Drawing and Chart information on page 216):
A = Motor and sensory complete—no sacral sparing including pin prick (PP) or light touch (LT) at any of the S4-5 dermatomes
B = Sensory incomplete

C = Motor incomplete—defined as
   1) Sacral sparing of motor function (anal contraction)
   2) Sacral sparing of sensation with motor function present in more than three levels below the motor level on either side (may include non–key muscles)
   Less than half of muscles 3/5 or greater below the motor level of injury
D = Motor incomplete—as ASIA C with more than half 3/5 or greater
E = Neurologically intact

104. **A)** The motor level of injury is defined as the lowest key muscle that has a grade of at least 3, provided the key muscles above that level are graded as 5.

The sensory level of injury is the most caudal dermatome to have normal (score of 2) sensation for both pinprick and light touch.

The ASIA Classification System is as follows (please see the ASIA Drawing and Chart information on page 216):

A = Motor and sensory complete—no sacral sparing including pin prick (PP) or light touch (LT) at any of the S4-5 dermatomes
B = Sensory incomplete
C = Motor incomplete—defined as
   1) Sacral sparing of motor function (anal contraction)
   2) Sacral sparing of sensation with motor function present in more than three levels below the motor level on either side (may include non–key muscles)
   Less than half of muscles 3/5 or greater below the motor level of injury
D = Motor incomplete—as ASIA C with more than half 3/5 of greater
E = Neurologically intact

105. **C)** The motor level of injury is defined as the lowest key muscle that has a grade of at least 3, provided the key muscles above that level are graded as 5.

The sensory level of injury is the most caudal dermatome to have normal (score of 2) sensation for both pinprick and light touch.

The ASIA Classification System is as follows (please see the ASIA Drawing and Chart information on page 216):

A = Motor and sensory complete—no sacral sparing including pin prick (PP) or light touch (LT) at any of the S4-5 dermatomes
B = Sensory incomplete
C = Motor incomplete—defined as
   1) Sacral sparing of motor function (anal contraction)
   2) Sacral sparing of sensation with motor function present in more than three levels below the motor level on either side (may include non–key muscles)
   Less than half of muscles 3/5 or greater below the motor level of injury
D = Motor incomplete—as ASIA C with more than half 3/5 of greater
E = Neurologically intact

Patient Name _____   Date/Time of Exam _____

Examiner Name _____   Signature _____

**ASIA**
AMERICAN SPINAL INJURY ASSOCIATION

**INTERNATIONAL STANDARDS FOR NEUROLOGICAL CLASSIFICATION OF SPINAL CORD INJURY (ISNCSCI)**

**ISCOS**
INTERNATIONAL SPINAL CORD SOCIETY

**RIGHT**

**MOTOR**
KEY MUSCLES

**UER**
(Upper Extremity Right)
Elbow flexors C5
Wrist extensors C6
Elbow extensors C7
Finger flexors C8
Finger abductors (little finger) T1

**SENSORY**
KEY SENSORY POINTS
Light Touch (LTR)   Pin Prick (PPR)

C2
C3
C4
T2
T3
T4
T5
T6
T7
T8
T9
T10
T11
T12
L1
S2
S3
S4-5 (56)  (56)

Comments (Non-key Muscle? Reason for NT? Pain?):

**LER**
(Lower Extremity Right)
Hip flexors L2
Knee extensors L3
Ankle dorsiflexors L4
Long toe extensors L5
Ankle plantar flexors S1

(VAC) Voluntary Anal Contraction [ ] (Yes/No)

RIGHT TOTALS (MAXIMUM) (50)

**LEFT**

**MOTOR**
KEY MUSCLES

C2
C3
C4

C5 Elbow flexors
C6 Wrist extensors
C7 Elbow extensors
C8 Finger flexors
T1 Finger abductors (little finger)

**UEL**
(Upper Extremity Left)

**MOTOR**
(SCORING ON REVERSE SIDE)
0 = total paralysis
1 = palpable or visible contraction
2 = active movement, gravity eliminated
3 = active movement, against gravity
4 = active movement, against some resistance
5 = active movement, against full resistance
5* = normal corrected for pain/disuse
NT = not testable

**SENSORY**
KEY SENSORY POINTS
Light Touch (LTL)   Pin Prick (PPL)

T2
T3
T4
T5
T6
T7
T8
T9
T10
T11
T12
L1

**SENSORY**
(SCORING ON REVERSE SIDE)
0 = absent       2 = normal
1 = altered      NT = not testable

L2 Hip flexors
L3 Knee extensors
L4 Ankle dorsiflexors
L5 Long toe extensors
S1 Ankle plantar flexors

**LEL**
(Lower Extremity Left)

S2
S3
S4-5  (56)  (56)

(DAP) Deep Anal Pressure [ ] (Yes/No)

LEFT TOTALS (MAXIMUM) (50)

● Key Sensory Points

**MOTOR SUBSCORES**

UER [ ] + UEL [ ] = UEMS TOTAL [ ]
MAX (25)    (25)    (50)

LER [ ] + LEL [ ] = LEMS TOTAL [ ]
MAX (25)    (25)    (50)

**SENSORY SUBSCORES**

LTR [ ] + LTL [ ] = LT TOTAL [ ]
MAX (56)    (56)    (112)

PPR [ ] + PPL [ ] = PP TOTAL [ ]
MAX (56)    (56)    (112)

**NEUROLOGICAL LEVELS**
Steps 1-5 for classification as on reverse

                    R    L
1. SENSORY        [ ]  [ ]
2. MOTOR          [ ]  [ ]

3. NEUROLOGICAL LEVEL OF INJURY (NLI) [ ]

4. COMPLETE OR INCOMPLETE?
Incomplete = Any sensory or motor function in S4-5 [ ]

5. ASIA IMPAIRMENT SCALE (AIS) [ ]

(In complete injuries only)
ZONE OF PARTIAL PRESERVATION
Most caudal level with any innervation

              R    L
SENSORY     [ ]  [ ]
MOTOR       [ ]  [ ]

This form may be copied freely but should not be altered without permission from the American Spinal Injury Association.

REV 11/15

## Muscle Function Grading

**0** = total paralysis

**1** = palpable or visible contraction

**2** = active movement, full range of motion (ROM) with gravity eliminated

**3** = active movement, full ROM against gravity

**4** = active movement, full ROM against gravity and moderate resistance in a muscle specific position

**5** = (normal) active movement, full ROM against gravity and full resistance in a functional muscle position expected from an otherwise unimpaired person

**5*** = (normal) active movement, full ROM against gravity and sufficient resistance to be considered normal if identified inhibiting factors (i.e. pain, disuse) were not present

**NT** = not testable (i.e. due to immobilization, severe pain such that the patient cannot be graded, amputation of limb, or contracture of > 50% of the normal ROM)

## Sensory Grading

**0** = Absent

**1** = Altered, either decreased/impaired sensation or hypersensitivity

**2** = Normal

**NT** = Not testable

## When to Test Non-Key Muscles:

In a patient with an apparent AIS B classification, non-key muscle functions more than 3 levels below the motor level on each side should be tested to most accurately classify the injury (differentiate between AIS B and C).

| Movement | Root level |
|---|---|
| **Shoulder:** Flexion, extension, abduction, adduction, internal and external rotation **Elbow:** Supination | C5 |
| **Elbow:** Pronation **Wrist:** Flexion | C6 |
| **Finger:** Flexion at proximal joint, extension. **Thumb:** Flexion, extension and abduction in plane of thumb | C7 |
| **Finger:** Flexion at MCP joint **Thumb:** Opposition, adduction and abduction perpendicular to palm | C8 |
| **Finger:** Abduction of the index finger | T1 |
| **Hip:** Adduction | L2 |
| **Hip:** External rotation | L3 |
| **Hip:** Extension, abduction, internal rotation **Knee:** Flexion **Ankle:** Inversion and eversion **Toe:** MP and IP extension | L4 |
| **Hallux and Toe:** DIP and PIP Flexion and abduction | L5 |
| **Hallux:** Adduction | S1 |

## ASIA Impairment Scale (AIS)

**A = Complete.** No sensory or motor function is preserved in the sacral segments S4-5.

**B = Sensory Incomplete.** Sensory but not motor function is preserved below the neurological level and includes the sacral segments S4-5 (light touch or pin prick at S4-5 or deep anal pressure) AND no motor function is preserved more than three levels below the motor level on either side of the body.

**C = Motor Incomplete.** Motor function is preserved at the most caudal sacral segments for voluntary anal contraction (VAC) OR the patient meets the criteria for sensory incomplete status (sensory function preserved at the most caudal sacral segments (S4-S5) by LT, PP or DAP), and has some sparing of motor function more than three levels below the ipsilateral motor level on either side of the body.

(This includes key or non-key muscle functions to determine motor incomplete status.) For AIS C – less than half of key muscle functions below the single NLI have a muscle grade ≥ 3.

**D = Motor Incomplete.** Motor incomplete status as defined above, with at least half (half or more) of key muscle functions below the single NLI having a muscle grade ≥ 3.

**E = Normal.** If sensation and motor function as tested with the ISNCSCI are graded as normal in all segments, and the patient had prior deficits, then the AIS grade is E. Someone without an initial SCI does not receive an AIS grade.

**Using ND:** To document the sensory, motor and NLI levels, the ASIA Impairment Scale grade, and/or the zone of partial preservation (ZPP) when they are unable to be determined based on the examination results.

## Steps in Classification

The following order is recommended for determining the classification of individuals with SCI.

**1. Determine sensory levels for right and left sides.**
*The sensory level is the most caudal, intact dermatome for both pin prick and light touch sensation.*

**2. Determine motor levels for right and left sides.**
*Defined by the lowest key muscle function that has a grade of at least 3 (on supine testing), providing the key muscle functions represented by segments above that level are judged to be intact (graded as a 5).*
*Note: in regions where there is no myotome to test, the motor level is presumed to be the same as the sensory level, if testable motor function above that level is also normal.*

**3. Determine the neurological level of injury (NLI).**
*This refers to the most caudal segment of the cord with intact sensation and antigravity (3 or more) muscle function strength, provided that there is normal (intact) sensory and motor function rostrally respectively.*
*The NLI is the most cephalad of the sensory and motor levels determined in steps 1 and 2.*

**4. Determine whether the injury is Complete or Incomplete.**
*(i.e. absence or presence of sacral sparing)*
If voluntary anal contraction = **No** AND all S4-5 sensory scores = **0** AND deep anal pressure = **No**, then injury is **Complete**.
Otherwise, injury is **Incomplete**.

**5. Determine ASIA Impairment Scale (AIS) Grade:**

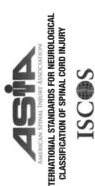

Is injury Complete?   If YES, AIS = A and can record
            ZPP (lowest dermatome or myotome
NO           on each side with some preservation)

Is injury Motor Complete?  If YES, AIS = B

          (No = voluntary anal contraction OR motor function
NO      more than three levels below the motor level on a
          given side, if the patient has sensory incomplete
          classification)

**Are at least half (half or more) of the key muscles below the neurological level of injury graded 3 or better?**

NO          YES

AIS = C       AIS = D

If sensation and motor function is normal in all segments, AIS = E
*Note: AIS E is used in follow-up testing when an individual with a documented SCI has recovered normal function. If at initial testing no deficits are found, the individual is neurologically intact; the ASIA Impairment Scale does not apply.*

*Source: American Spinal Injury Association: International Standards for Neurological Classification of Spinal Cord Injury, Revised 2011; Atlanta, GA, Revised 2011, updated, 2015. Used with permission.*

# Medical Rehabilitation (Cardiac, Pulmonary, Cancer, Burn, and Wound)

# 8

1. What does the TheraBite do?
   A) Acts as a temporary, unfitted set of dentures
   B) Prevents microstomia in patients with facial burns
   C) Allows the clinician to pry the patient's mouth open for feeding
   D) Assists burn patients in chewing

2. Which of the following is a benefit of strengthening exercises in the physical therapy regimen of a burn patient?
   A) Maintaining functional strength in the uninvolved limbs
   B) Improving cardiovascular function, which is lost during bed rest
   C) Recovering some strength in the involved extremity
   D) All of the above

3. Which of the following contributes to flame burns in pediatric patients?
   A) Playing with firecrackers
   B) Playing with matches
   C) Playing with inflammable aerosols
   D) All of the above

4. Which of the following is included in the goals of cardiac rehabilitation?
   A) Greater exercise tolerance
   B) Long-term exercise plan
   C) Smoking cessation
   D) All of the above

5. How would postsurgical cardiac rehabilitation be different for a patient with intermittent vascular claudication?
   A) Interspersed rest periods between exercises
   B) Target heart rate to be set at 90% of maximum heart rate
   C) Higher dosage of anticoagulation
   D) Patient is not a candidate for cardiac rehabilitation

6. What is the most prevalent lung disease in adults living in the United States?
   A) Asthma
   B) Chronic obstructive pulmonary disease (COPD)
   C) Cystic fibrosis
   D) Sarcoidosis

7. Pathologic dilation of the distal airways with destruction of alveolar walls best describes which condition?
   A) Asthma
   B) Cystic fibrosis
   C) Emphysema
   D) Bronchitis

8. Which test is used to diagnose central and obstructive sleep apnea?
   A) Polysomnography
   B) Spirometry with pulmonary function testing
   C) Diffusion capacity testing
   D) Pulse oximetry

9. During an acute episode of dyspnea in chronic obstructive pulmonary disease (COPD) patients, which breathing technique may help to reduce symptoms and the work of breathing?
   A) Controlled cough
   B) Huffing
   C) Pursed-lip breathing
   D) Breath holds

10. Which invasive treatment is used in severe, advanced emphysema?
    A) Diaphragmatic pacing
    B) Mouth intermittent positive pressure ventilation
    C) Lung-volume reduction surgery
    D) Tracheostomy

11. What is "air shifting"?
    A) A technique to decrease microatelectasis
    B) A technique to promote secretion drainage
    C) A technique to ventilate the apical lung fields
    D) A technique to reduce respiratory rate in patients with dyspnea

12. Methylphenidate (Concerta, Ritalin), a drug used frequently to increase arousal in patients with brain tumors, works by:
    A) Blocking the reuptake of norepinephrine and dopamine
    B) Blocking the reuptake of serotonin
    C) Gamma-aminobutyric acid analogue
    D) None of the above

13. Most neoplastic spinal cord compression is:
    A) Extramedullary
    B) Intramedullary
    C) The incidence of intramedullary and extramedullary involvement is about equal
    D) Supramedullary

**14.** Which joint is the most common site for heterotopic ossification in burn patients?
   A) Hip
   B) Shoulder
   C) Knee
   D) Elbow

**15.** The initial therapeutic exercise regimen for a burn patient (who has not undergone a skin graft) should include which of the following?
   A) Active range of motion against the contractile force of the healing scar
   B) Passive range of motion against the contractile force of the scar
   C) Active range of motion toward the contractile force of the scar
   D) Passive range of motion toward the contractile force of the scar

**16.** What type of shock is seen in patients' systemic response to burn?
   A) Neurogenic shock
   B) Cardiogenic shock
   C) Hypovolemic shock
   D) None of the above

**17.** In which of the following diseases should target heart rate **not** be used as a guide for exercise tolerance?
   A) Heart transplant
   B) Diabetes
   C) Post–myocardial infarction
   D) Traumatic brain injury

**18.** What is the target heart rate for a patient with stable arrhythmias during cardiac rehabilitation?
   A) Maximum heart rate
   B) Heart rate below the rate where arrhythmias are noted
   C) Heart rate 10 to 20 beats above the rate where arrhythmias are noted
   D) Patient is not a candidate for cardiac rehabilitation

**19.** On the basis of metabolic equivalent of a task, a patient having which of the following metabolic equivalent (MET) levels should **not** return to employment after cardiac rehabilitation?
   A) MET 6 to 7
   B) MET 5 to 6
   C) MET 4 to 5
   D) MET 2 to 3

**20.** Which test best assesses the magnitude of functional impairment in pulmonary disease?
   A) Pulmonary function tests (PFT)
   B) Arterial blood gas measurements (ABG)
   C) Chest radiography
   D) Ventilation perfusion (V/Q) lung scan

**21.** When would a mechanical insufflator-exsufflator be contraindicated?
   A) High spinal cord injury
   B) Bullous emphysema
   C) Cerebral palsy
   D) Neuromuscular disease

22. What intervention minimizes the reduction in vital capacity of tetraplegic patients when they are sitting?
    A) Use of an abdominal binder
    B) Supplemental oxygen
    C) Glossopharyngeal breathing
    D) Compressive leg stockings

23. What describes "Ondine's curse"?
    A) Acquired central hypoventilation syndrome
    B) Congenital central hypoventilation syndrome
    C) High cervical spinal cord injury resulting in severe diaphragmatic impairment
    D) Polio syndrome affecting the upper trunk more than the lower trunk and legs

24. What is the most cost-saving and clinically effective way to prevent chronic obstructive pulmonary disease (COPD)?
    A) Pulmonary rehabilitation
    B) Supplemental oxygen therapy
    C) Smoking cessation
    D) Daily aerobic training

25. What is a potential benefit of home oxygen use in patients with chronic obstructive pulmonary disease (COPD)?
    A) Reduction in polycythemia
    B) Reversal of disease process
    C) Provision of respiratory muscle rest
    D) Prevention of obstructive sleep apnea

26. Spinal cord injury (SCI) in a cancer patient occurs most commonly from:
    A) Spinal cord tumors
    B) Spinal metastases
    C) Radiation
    D) Chemotherapy

27. Debridement of burn wounds is performed for what purpose?
    A) To expose viable tissue and prepare the wound for coverage
    B) To remove unsightly parts of the wound
    C) For no actual clinical purpose, but rather because the placebo effect gives the impression that an intervention will help
    D) To determine the depth of the wound

28. How many hours per day should a pressure garment be worn to minimize hypertrophic scarring while a scar is maturing?
    A) 1 hour
    B) 12 hours
    C) 23 hours
    D) At the patient's leisure according to comfort

29. Decreased blood flow contributes to the tissue damage in which of the following types of burns?
    A) Heat burns
    B) Cold burns (frostbite)
    C) Both
    D) Neither

30. Which of the following is a useful tool in measuring exertion during a physical activity?
    A) Wong-Baker scale
    B) Borg scale
    C) Ranchos Los Amigos scale
    D) Disability rating scale

31. Which of the following exercise phases is important to prevent syncope?
    A) Aerobic phase
    B) Anaerobic phase
    C) Cooldown phase
    D) Stretching phase

32. Which of the following changes would **not** be noted during exercise therapy for a patient with congestive heart failure?
    A) Drop in ejection fraction
    B) Decrease in stroke volume
    C) Exertional hypotension
    D) Decrease in heart rate

33. What nerve supplies the diaphragm?
    A) Long thoracic nerve
    B) Thoracodorsal nerve
    C) Lateral pectoral nerve
    D) Phrenic nerve

34. Which device aids in secretion clearance by applying a positive pressure to the airways followed by a negative pressure?
    A) Mechanical insufflator-exsufflator
    B) Yankauer suction wall unit
    C) Bilevel positive airway pressure (BiPAP)
    D) Chest percussion

35. What is the normal rate of decline of forced expiratory volume at 1 second ($FEV_1$) with age?
    A) 5 mL/year
    B) 30 mL/year
    C) 50 mL/year
    D) 75 mL/year

36. What is an example of aerobic exercise?
    A) Upper extremity free-weight exercises
    B) Leg press
    C) Treadmill walking
    D) Isometric quadriceps exercises

37. Central chemoreceptors of respiratory regulation are sensitive to which of the following levels?
    A) Hydrogen ions
    B) $PO_2$
    C) $PCO_2$
    D) Both (A) and (C)

38. When should a vibratory flutter valve be used?
    A) When a patient is experiencing acute respiratory failure
    B) In a cooperative cystic fibrosis patient requiring assistance with mucous mobilization
    C) When tracking an asthmatic patient's response to therapy
    D) When a tracheostomy patient is ready to use a speaking valve

39. An example of a nonprogressive tumor often cured by surgical resection is:
    A) Meningioma
    B) Glioblastoma multiforme
    C) Astrocytoma
    D) Oligodendroglioma

40. A pediatric patient with burns in a bilateral stocking distribution should alert clinicians to the possibility of_____.
    A) Complex regional pain syndrome
    B) Child abuse
    C) Food allergy
    D) Malnourishment

41. Blood and pus under a graft are:
    A) A sign that the graft is taking and that healing is occurring under the graft
    B) A barrier to diffusion of nutrients before new capillaries have been formed, leading to failure to take of the graft
    C) An incidental finding when some grafts that fail to take are reexamined
    D) An indication for immediate and more radical surgical intervention

42. Which of the following body parts is considered a major burn in all cases?
    A) Face
    B) Hand
    C) Perineum
    D) (A) and (C)

43. Which of the following is the medically acute inpatient cardiac rehabilitation phase?
    A) Phase 1
    B) Phase 2
    C) Phase 3
    D) Phase 4

44. Which of the following components shows an increase in response to exercise training?
    A) Heart rate
    B) Myocardial oxygen capacity
    C) Stroke volume
    D) Peripheral resistance

45. If the patient is unable to undergo exercise echocardiography because of deconditioning, which of the following tests can be used to guide further rehabilitation goals?
    A) Restrained exercise tolerance testing
    B) Forced ambulation
    C) Exercise nuclear imaging
    D) Pharmacologic stress testing

46. Which of the following is an autosomal recessive disease of chloride ion channels in exocrine glands?
    A) Emphysema
    B) Asthma
    C) Cystic fibrosis
    D) Chronic obstructive pulmonary disease (COPD)

47. The maximum volume of air that a patient can hold with a closed glottis is called:
    A) Vital capacity (VC)
    B) Glossopharyngeal breathing (GPB)
    C) Maximum insufflation capacity (MIC)
    D) Intermittent positive pressure ventilation (IPPV)

48. Which respiratory disease causes a restrictive, parenchymal pattern of illness?
    A) Myasthenia gravis
    B) Asthma
    C) Sarcoidosis
    D) Ankylosing spondylitis

49. According to the Global Initiative for Chronic Obstructive Lung Disease (GOLD) classification of chronic obstructive pulmonary disease (COPD), what class is designated for patients who have a forced expiratory volume at 1 second ($FEV_1$) level of lesser than 30% of predicted?
    A) Stage 1
    B) Stage 2
    C) Stage 3
    D) Stage 4

50. Where are the central respiratory control centers located?
    A) Thalamus
    B) Hippocampus
    C) Cortex
    D) Medulla

51. How can respiratory muscles be rested in patients with chronic obstructive pulmonary disease (COPD)?
    A) By encouraging daytime napping
    B) By nasal piece or mouthpiece intermittent positive pressure ventilation at bedtime
    C) By diaphragmatic breathing exercises
    D) By prescribing muscle relaxants

52. The most common posterior fossa tumor in children is:
    A) Cerebellar astrocytoma
    B) Meningioma
    C) Glioblastoma multiforme
    D) None of the above

53. Which of the following is the most common cause of burns in the pediatric population?
    A) Chemical
    B) Flame
    C) Scald
    D) Electrical

54. What theoretical risk causes many physiatrists to prefer hydrotherapy on burn patients using a spraying system, rather than in a Hubbard tank?
    A) Infection caused by bacterial contamination of the tank or associated pipes and hoses
    B) Bleeding from wounds
    C) Drowning secondary to loss of consciousness
    D) Mechanical damage to any skin grafts present because of the flow of water caused by the jets in the tank

55. Superficial burns of the epidermis will potentially require which analgesic regimen?
    A) Oral opioid analgesics
    B) Acetaminophen and/or ibuprofen
    C) Oral corticosteroids
    D) Patient-controlled anesthesia pump

56. Which of the following is **not** a proven therapeutic benefit of cardiac rehabilitation after a myocardial infarction (MI)?
    A) Increased resting cardiac output
    B) Decreased rate of recurrent MI
    C) Improved left ventricular (LV) function
    D) Decreased mortality

57. In which of the following patients is target heart rate **not** used in cardiac rehabilitation?
    A) Patient taking a statin
    B) Patient taking a beta-blocker
    C) Patient undergoing anticoagulation therapy
    D) Patient taking a diuretic

58. The coronary arteries mostly perfuse the myocardium during which heart phase?
    A) Systole
    B) Diastole
    C) Mid-systole
    D) End-systole

59. The amount of gas moving in and out of the lungs during resting respiration is called:
    A) Vital capacity (VC)
    B) Total lung capacity (TLC)
    C) Tidal volume
    D) Forced vital capacity (FVC)

60. Which condition will most likely cause restrictive impairment of ventilation?
    A) Chronic bronchitis
    B) Asthma
    C) Cystic fibrosis
    D) Guillain-Barré syndrome

61. In the three-zone model of the lung, which zone has the highest pulmonary arterial pressure (PAP) when upright?
    A) Zone 1
    B) Zone 2
    C) Zone 3
    D) None, they all have equivalent hydrostatic pressure

62. What technique uses gravity to assist in the ultimate clearance of secretions from specific lung areas?
    A) Abdominal binder uses
    B) Manual suction through tracheostomy
    C) Postural drainage
    D) Abdominal thrust

63. Which test is useful in evaluating the phrenic nerve?
    A) Electrodiagnostic studies (electromyography [EMG]/nerve conduction studies [NCS])
    B) CT
    C) MRI
    D) Ultrasound

64. What causes airflow limitation in emphysema?
    A) Narrowed airway caliber
    B) Neuromuscular weakness of the chest wall
    C) Loss of elastic recoil and decreased air tethering
    D) Upper airway obstruction

65. The most common type of brain cancer is:
    A) Meningioma
    B) Glioblastoma multiforme
    C) Metastasis
    D) Astrocytoma

66. In treating burn patients, what is the "rule of nines"?
    A) The percentage of body surface area of each body part used to calculate the percentage body surface area burned
    B) The minimum age of family members allowed to visit burn patients in acute rehab units because of risk of infection
    C) The number of physical therapy sessions administered in a standard rehabilitation regimen for burns
    D) The number of minutes required for a burn injury to develop when a limb at room temperature is exposed to a source of heat

67. Why should clinicians and patients **not** pop the blister that develops over second-degree burns?
    A) In fact, the blister should be popped immediately upon forming to facilitate proper treatment
    B) The blister acts as a natural dressing with sterile fluid under it
    C) Popping the blister is an extremely painful procedure
    D) Popping or not popping the blister is purely a matter of consensus between the patient and the clinician treating the burn

68. Burned fat cells do not regenerate. Which of the following is a potential negative consequence of this?
    A) A disfigured appearance due to later development of obesity in nonburned areas
    B) Future difficulty losing weight
    C) Future difficulty gaining weight
    D) Anorexia

69. Which of the following is a physiologic measure expressing the energy cost of physical activities?
    A) Metabolic oxygen consumption
    B) Mean exercise training
    C) Measure of exercise tolerance
    D) Metabolic equivalent (MET) of task

70. How can cardiac rehabilitation benefit a patient with angina pectoris?
    A) Increase myocardial oxygen consumption
    B) Decrease the maximum heart rate
    C) Change angina threshold
    D) Improve efficiency

71. Which of the following is **not** an absolute contraindication for cardiac rehabilitation?
    A) Hypertrophic cardiomyopathy
    B) Active pericarditis
    C) Resting systolic blood pressure greater than 200
    D) Third-degree heart block without pacemaker

72. The volume of gas in the lungs at the end of normal expiration is called:
    A) Functional residual capacity (FRC)
    B) Vital capacity (VC)
    C) Residual volume (RV)
    D) Expiratory reserve volume (ERV)

73. Which oxygen delivery system provides close to 90% oxygen?
    A) Nasal cannula
    B) Non-rebreathing mask
    C) Venturi face mask
    D) Blow-by oxygen

74. Which lung volume increases in cervical spinal cord injury (SCI)?
    A) Residual volume
    B) Total lung capacity
    C) Vital capacity
    D) Tidal volume

75. During normal inspiration, what is the action of the vocal cords?
    A) The vocal cords should open
    B) The vocal cords should close
    C) The vocal cords should close then open
    D) The vocal cords remain inactive during inspiration

76. What is the leading cause of mortality in chronic tetraplegic spinal cord injury (SCI) patients?
    A) Decubitus ulcers
    B) Urinary complications
    C) Deep vein thrombosis (DVT)
    D) Pneumonia

77. What is the peak cough flow (PCF)?
    A) The maximum volume of air a patient can hold with a closed glottis
    B) A breathing technique that can be taught to patients with neuromuscular weakness

    C) A method to check for intact gag reflex prior to extubation
    D) The velocity of air expelled from the airways during a cough maneuver

78. Dexamethasone, a medication used frequently in patients with brain tumors, can cause:
    A) Sensory neuropathy
    B) Myopathy
    C) Motor neuropathy
    D) All of the above

79. Patients with electrical burns should always be admitted to the hospital for monitoring. Why?
    A) Psychiatric disturbances
    B) Visual field defects
    C) Potential cardiac arrhythmias
    D) Acute onset peripheral neuropathy

80. What are the objectives in the treatment of first- and second-degree burns?
    A) Minimizing cosmetic effects and diminished self-esteem due to these burns
    B) Preventing long-term disability and resource use in patients with these burns
    C) Immediate enrollment in a work-hardening program
    D) Pain relief and protection from further injury while epithelialization occurs

81. Which of the following psychological problems can develop after burn injury?
    A) Depression
    B) Posttraumatic stress disorder
    C) Both
    D) Neither

82. Cardiac output is defined as a product of which of the following components?
    A) Heart rate and stroke volume
    B) Stroke volume and oxygen consumption
    C) Ejection fraction and aerobic capacity
    D) Myocardial oxygen capacity and heart rate

83. Which of the following populations of patients has a higher energy expenditure during ambulation?
    A) Prosthetic lower extremity patients
    B) Peripheral vascular disease patients
    C) Smoker patients
    D) Diabetic patients

84. Which of the following positions would have the highest stroke volume?
    A) Exercising in supine position
    B) At rest in supine position
    C) Exercising in prone position
    D) At rest while standing

85. What is the term for the volume of gas in the lungs at maximal inspiration?
    A) Functional residual capacity (FRC)
    B) Vital capacity (VC)
    C) Residual volume (RV)
    D) Total lung capacity (TLC)

86. For an adult with a low oxygen requirement, delivery of supplemental oxygen is best achieved by using what interface?
    A) Nasal cannula
    B) Endotracheal intubation
    C) Continuous positive airway pressure (CPAP)
    D) Venturi face mask

87. Which is a reasonable treatment modality for moderate to severe obstructive sleep apnea (OSA)?
    A) Tracheal intubation
    B) Diaphragmatic pacing
    C) Nocturnal pulse oximetry
    D) Continuous positive airway pressure (CPAP)

88. What is the only genetic abnormality linked to chronic obstructive pulmonary disease (COPD)?
    A) Absence or abnormality of cystic fibrosis transmembrane receptor (CFTR) protein
    B) Dystrophin gene mutation
    C) Alpha1-antitrypsin (A1AT) protein deficiency
    D) G6PD deficiency

89. What is positive end-expiratory pressure (PEEP)?
    A) Fraction of inspired oxygen
    B) The patient's respiratory rate at a given tidal volume
    C) Pressure above atmospheric pressure at the end of expiration
    D) Adjunct to conventional modes of mechanical ventilation to decrease work of breathing

90. What is $VO_{2max}$?
    A) Maximal oxygen uptake and use by the body during exercise
    B) Fraction of inspired oxygen necessary to maintain $SpO_2$ at higher than 90%
    C) Maximum volume of oxygen necessary to carry out a designated activity
    D) Represents the arteriovenous oxygen difference

91. The American College of Rheumatology (ACR) recommends the following to prevent osteoporosis in patients receiving steroids for a prolonged amount of time:
    A) Calcium 1,500 mg/Vitamin D 800 IU per day
    B) Bisphosphonates
    C) Weight-bearing exercises
    D) All of the above

92. If a patient presents with a burn with damage to the epidermis, but only partial damage to the dermis, and has blistering, how is the burn classified?
    A) First degree or superficial
    B) Second degree or partial thickness
    C) Third degree or full thickness
    D) Unstageable

93. What is **true** of burn mortality in the adult population?
    A) Burn mortality is higher in older adults than in younger adults
    B) Burn mortality is higher in younger adults than in older adults
    C) Burn mortality is higher in women than in men
    D) Burn mortality is exactly the same across all subpopulations above the age of majority in their respective societies

94. Which of the following strategies would best control pain during dressing changes in a burn patient?
    A) Opioid analgesics on an as-needed basis with no attention paid to the environment in which wound care occurs
    B) Scheduled opioid analgesic prior to wound care with no attention paid to environment in which wound care occurs
    C) Scheduled opioid analgesic prior to wound care in a calm, soothing environment
    D) No opioids are indicated, but nonopioid analgesics are provided on a prn basis and wound care occurs in a calm, soothing environment

95. Which of the following organs has the highest percentage of oxygen extraction?
    A) Kidney
    B) Skin
    C) Heart
    D) Intestine

96. Which of the following exercises are allowed during phase 1 of cardiac rehabilitation?
    A) Isometric exercises
    B) Valsalva maneuvers
    C) Raising legs above the heart
    D) Dangle legs off bed

97. Which of the following phases of cardiac rehabilitation focuses on determining the maximum exertion to be performed by the patient?
    A) Phase 1
    B) Phase 2
    C) Phase 3
    D) Phase 4

98. Among the following, which represents primary respiratory muscle(s) during quiet respiration?
    A) Diaphragm
    B) External intercostal muscles
    C) Abdominal muscles
    D) Trapezius

99. A monophasic, high-pitched sound usually caused by partial obstruction in the upper airway is called:
    A) Wheezing
    B) Ronchi
    C) Crepitus
    D) Stridor

100. In cystic fibrosis (CF), which measure is the best predictor of survival?
    A) Age at onset of diagnosis
    B) Respiratory rate
    C) Forced expiratory volume at 1 second ($FEV_1$)
    D) Tidal volume

101. What is a consequence when caloric intake fails to meet the metabolic demands of increased work of breathing in chronic obstructive pulmonary disease (COPD)?
    A) Death
    B) Cachexia

    C) Osteoporosis

    D) Acute exacerbation

102. Which ventilator setting coordinates delivery of the ventilator-driven breath with the respiratory cycle of the patient?
    A) Assist-control ventilation (ACV)
    B) Intermittent mandatory ventilation (IMV)
    C) Pressure support ventilation (PSV)
    D) Synchronized intermittent mandatory ventilation (SIMV)

103. When should supplemental oxygen be prescribed with exercise?
    A) When the patient's heart rate (HR) is higher than 110 beats/minute
    B) When the $PaCO_2$ level is higher than 50 mmHg
    C) When the exercise-induced $SpO_2$ level is lower than 90%
    D) When the patient is in atrial fibrillation

104. Side effects of medications used to prevent seizures in patients with brain tumors include:
    A) Rash
    B) Cognitive dysfunction
    C) Drowsiness
    D) All of the above

105. If a burn patient is splinted in a comfortable position for grafted burns to heal, the patient is at risk for which of the following complications?
    A) Tendon rupture
    B) Skin breakdown
    C) Mechanical falls
    D) Wound contracture

106. What has happened to the mortality rate from burns in the last several decades?
    A) The burn mortality rate has increased because people get burned doing progressively more foolish things as time passes
    B) The burn mortality rate varies seasonally
    C) Improvements in medical and surgical treatment of burns have allowed patients with larger total body surface area burns to survive than previously lived through their burns
    D) Nothing, burn mortality has been the same since humans started recording their history

107. Which of the following complications can occur in lower extremity burns?
    A) Achilles tendon shortening
    B) Metatarsophalangeal joint hyperextension
    C) Foot drop
    D) All of the above

108. Which of the following is **not** a reversible risk factor for coronary artery disease?
    A) Hypertension
    B) Male gender
    C) Smoking
    D) Hyperlipidemia

109. Which of the following phases of cardiac rehabilitation is considered a structured outpatient program?
    A) Phase 1
    B) Phase 2
    C) Phase 3
    D) Phase 4

110. Which of the following is considered to be the greatest single modifiable risk factor for cardiac disease?
    A) Obesity
    B) Hypertension
    C) Hyperlipidemia
    D) Smoking

111. Which therapy has been shown to decrease mortality in chronic obstructive pulmonary disease (COPD)?
    A) Chest physiotherapy
    B) Pulmonary rehabilitation program
    C) Supplemental oxygen therapy
    D) Noninvasive ventilation

112. Which of the following is most useful in diagnosing obstructive lung disease?
    A) Maximal static expiratory pressure (PE max)
    B) Diffusing capacity for carbon dioxide
    C) Forced vital capacity (FVC)
    D) Ratio of the forced expiratory volume in 1 second to FVC ($FEV_1$/FVC)

113. Temporary bronchial narrowing induced typically by 15 minutes of strenuous activity is likely:
    A) Pneumonia
    B) Exercise-induced asthma (EIA)
    C) Duchenne muscular dystrophy
    D) Chronic obstructive pulmonary disease (COPD)

114. Which tracheostomy tube is appropriate for patients who are able to speak and who only require intermittent ventilator assistance?
    A) Cuffed tracheostomy tube
    B) Nonfenestrated tube
    C) Passy-Muir valve
    D) Fenestrated tube

115. Which device provides visual feedback for patients to practice deep inspiration during the post-operative period?
    A) Pulse oximeter
    B) Heart rate monitor
    C) Incentive spirometry
    D) Mirror

116. What is an intermittent abdominal pressure ventilator (IAPV)?
    A) A method of introducing air into the abdomen to manually raise the diaphragm
    B) A treatment for obstructive sleep apnea
    C) A cough-assist device that exerts abdominal thrusts
    D) A daytime inspiratory muscle aid worn underneath the clothing

117. A clinician needs to have a high index of suspicion for dysphagia when treating patients with:
   A) Breast cancer
   B) Bony metastases
   C) Brain tumors
   D) Lung cancer

118. Large body surface area burns put the body into a state of:
   A) Catabolism
   B) Anabolism
   C) Hypothermia
   D) Hyperthermia

119. What physical property allows split thickness skin grafts to heal spontaneously?
   A) The presence of dermal appendages, such as hair follicles and glands, provides growth centers that seed healing of skin
   B) The thinness of split thickness skin grafts allows them to heal because there is less tissue to heal
   C) Split thickness skin grafts require less blood supply than full thickness skin grafts
   D) None, split thickness skin grafts do not heal spontaneously

120. Which of the following is a consequence of bed rest in patients with hip and torso burns?
   A) Cardiovascular deconditioning
   B) Scoliosis
   C) Hip contracture
   D) All of the above

121. Destruction of which component of the skin leads to hypopigmentation in burn patients?
   A) Keratinocytes
   B) Melanocytes
   C) Basement membrane
   D) Hair follicles

122. How does the heart physiologically compensate for increased end-diastolic volume?
   A) Increased peripheral resistance
   B) Increased respiratory rate
   C) Increased systolic contractility
   D) Decreased systolic contractility

123. Which of the following phases begins when the patient has plateaued in exercise endurance?
   A) Phase 1
   B) Phase 2
   C) Phase 3
   D) Phase 4

124. What risk factor is associated with most cases of chronic obstructive pulmonary disease (COPD) in the United States?
   A) Chronic asthma
   B) Pneumonia
   C) Smoking
   D) Occupational exposure to irritants

**125.** Which nerve roots contribute to the phrenic nerve?
   A) C1-3
   B) C5-7
   C) C3-5
   D) C7-T1

**126.** In chronic obstructive pulmonary disease (COPD), which of the following is a potential benefit of pulmonary rehabilitation?
   A) Decreased anxiety
   B) Improved cognitive function
   C) Increased exercise tolerance
   D) Improved life expectancy

**127.** What is a contraindication for chest percussion therapy?
   A) Anticoagulation therapy
   B) Increased intracranial pressure
   C) Flail chest
   D) Severe osteoporosis

**128.** Which functional test is commonly used to measure outcomes before and after pulmonary rehabilitation and is thought to better reflect activities of daily living?
   A) 30-minute walk test
   B) 6-minute walk test
   C) 2-minute walk test
   D) Shuttle walk test

**129.** What is glossopharyngeal breathing (GPB)?
   A) Breathing through a tracheostomy
   B) Functional electrical stimulation technique used on the pharyngeal muscles
   C) Breathing technique used when off the ventilator where a patient takes in several boluses of air
   D) Airway secretion clearance technique

**130.** A side effect of radiation therapy in the treatment of brain tumors is:
   A) Cognitive dysfunction
   B) Nausea
   C) Fatigue
   D) All of the above

**131.** What is the best modality for detecting spinal metastases?
   A) MRI
   B) CT
   C) X-ray
   D) Bone scan

**132.** When prescribing physical therapy for a patient with bony metastases, it is prudent to avoid:
   A) Resistive exercises in that limb
   B) Active range of motion in that limb
   C) Bracing
   D) Cold therapy

133. The most common presenting symptom of metastatic bone disease is:
    A) Pain
    B) Pathologic fracture
    C) Weakness
    D) Bowel/bladder abnormality

134. Secondary lymphedema:
    A) Can be caused by lymph node dissection
    B) Is usually familial
    C) Is seen with arterial insufficiency
    D) Primarily involves the face

135. Which is usually the initial therapy for bone pain in cancer patients?
    A) Opioids
    B) Nonsteroidal anti-inflammatory drugs (NSAIDs)
    C) Calcium supplements
    D) Bisphosphonates

136. The most common site of skeletal metastases is the:
    A) Axial skeleton
    B) Femur
    C) Humerus
    D) Radius

137. According to multiple studies, cardiac rehabilitation can reduce mortality by __ % following myocardial infarction.
    A) 10
    B) 25
    C) 40
    D) 65

138. The most common site of metastasis in the spine is:
    A) V body
    B) Vertebral foramen
    C) Pedicle
    D) Lamina

139. Bisphosphonates prevent fractures by:
    A) Inhibiting osteoclasts
    B) Promoting osteoblasts
    C) Remodeling bone
    D) All of the above

140. Ototoxicity is commonly associated with which chemotherapy agent?
    A) Cisplatin
    B) Taxol
    C) Methotrexate
    D) Vincristine

141. Stage 1 lymphedema is:
    A) Pitting
    B) Nonpitting

C) Fibrotic
D) Not reduced with elevation

142. All of the following contributes to a cancer patient's fatigue **except**:
    A) Anemia
    B) Cytokine release (eg, tumor necrosis factor [TNF])
    C) Cachexia
    D) Release of testosterone

143. What type of cancer is usually associated with subacute motor neuropathy?
    A) Melanoma
    B) Lung cancer
    C) Lymphoma
    D) Colon cancer

144. Which medication is an effective antiemetic in cancer patients?
    A) Promethazine (Phenergan)
    B) Ondansetron (Zofran)
    C) Metoclopramide (Reglan)
    D) Diphenhydramine (Benadryl)

145. The most common cause of shoulder pain in breast cancer patients is:
    A) Rotator cuff tendinitis
    B) Posterior interosseous nerve injury
    C) C5/C6 radiculopathy
    D) Tight garments

146. Common side effects of bisphosphonates include:
    A) Hypocalcemia
    B) Renal toxicity
    C) Atypical femur fractures
    D) Gastrointestinal irritation

147. Treatment for chemotherapy-induced peripheral neuropathy (CIPN) includes:
    A) Neuropathic medications
    B) Bracing
    C) Education about skin care
    D) All of the above

148. Lymphedema is considered a:
    A) High-protein edema
    B) Low-protein edema
    C) Combination of low/high-protein edema
    D) Nonprotein edema

149. What is the most common symptom in cancer patients?
    A) Pain
    B) Fatigue
    C) Insomnia
    D) Nausea

150. Which of the following symptoms indicates delayed radiation myelopathy?
    A) Lower extremity paresthesias
    B) Deep vein thrombosis
    C) Decreased reflexes
    D) Macular rash

151. All of the following are manifestations of bone metastases in patients with multiple myeloma **except**:
    A) Fracture
    B) Dense lesions on x-ray
    C) Lytic lesions with sclerotic borders
    D) Bone pain

152. Postmastectomy pain syndrome can present with:
    A) Burning, stabbing pain in the chest wall
    B) Shoulder pain
    C) Hand weakness
    D) All of the above

153. Cancer pain is caused by:
    A) Tumor invasion
    B) Neuropathy
    C) Surgery
    D) All of the above

154. Radiation plexitis usually affects the:
    A) Ulnar nerve
    B) Upper trunk
    C) Middle trunk
    D) Radial nerve

155. A sign of impending pathologic fracture is:
    A) Pain with functional movement
    B) The size of lesion on x-ray
    C) Hypercalcemia
    D) Crepitus on palpation

156. Radiation therapy may cause peripheral nerve damage by all of the following **except**:
    A) Damaging the nerve itself
    B) Damaging the connective tissue of the nerve
    C) Damaging the anterior horn cell
    D) Damaging the vasa nervorum

157. What is the pathophysiology of radiation-induced transient myelopathy?
    A) Inflammation
    B) Transient demyelination
    C) Local edema
    D) Fibrosis

158. Which cancer is associated with blastic bone metastases?
    A) Lung
    B) Melanoma

    C) Prostate

    D) Colon

159. The nerve that is injured during a mastectomy, sometimes leading to postmastectomy pain syndrome, is:

    A) Intercostobrachial nerve

    B) Suprascapular nerve

    C) Musculocutaneous nerve

    D) Axillary nerve

160. Opioid analgesia dosing in the cancer patient should be limited only by:

    A) Side effects

    B) Fear of addiction

    C) Cost

    D) Opioids should not be used unless no other options exist

161. What is the usual presenting symptom of radiation plexitis?

    A) Pain

    B) Weakness

    C) Numbness/paresthesias

    D) Fasciculations

162. An unstable metastatic bony lesion is best treated by:

    A) Surgical fixation

    B) Radiation therapy

    C) Physical therapy

    D) Chemotherapy

163. The treatment for lymphedema includes:

    A) Antibiotics for cellulitis prophylaxis

    B) Oral steroids

    C) Manual lymphatic drainage

    D) Both (A) and (C)

164. Lymphedema is best treated with:

    A) Diuretics

    B) Manual lymphatic drainage (MLD)

    C) Antibiotics

    D) Dangling the limb to improve drainage

165. Complications of bone metastases include:

    A) Hypercalcemia

    B) Spinal cord compression

    C) Pathological fracture

    D) All of the above

166. The pain associated with post-thoracotomy pain syndrome is found in the:

    A) Intercostal nerve distribution

    B) External intercostals

    C) Internal intercostals

    D) Costochondral junction

167. A medication that reduces pain in bony metastases and reduces skeletal-related events (SREs) is:
    A) Bisphosphonates
    B) Opiates
    C) Nonsteroidal anti-inflammatory drugs
    D) Chemotherapy

168. Which cancer presents with lytic lesions?
    A) Multiple myeloma
    B) Non–small-lung cell cancer
    C) Renal cancer
    D) All of the above

169. The spine is considered unstable when there is tumor involvement of the:
    A) Middle column
    B) Two or more columns are involved
    C) Either (A) or (B)
    D) The anterior column

170. Myokymia on electromyography (EMG) is frequently seen in:
    A) Radiation plexopathy
    B) Radiculopathy
    C) Peripheral neuropathy
    D) Myopathy

171. What is the most common initial treatment for brain metastases?
    A) Corticosteroids
    B) Radiation
    C) Radiosurgery
    D) Chemotherapy

172. Multiple myeloma is caused by the proliferation of:
    A) Plasma cells
    B) Red blood cells
    C) White blood cells
    D) Platelets

173. Lymphedema is frequently seen in cancers of the:
    A) Breast
    B) Ovary
    C) Head and neck
    D) All of the above

174. Oncologists use this as a guide as to whether the patient should receive more chemotherapy:
    A) Functional status
    B) Patient's wishes
    C) Tumor response
    D) All of the above

175. Bone lesions that are **not** assessed by bone scan include:
    A) Prostate cancer
    B) Multiple myeloma

    C) Breast cancer
    D) Colon cancer

176. In a patient with bony metastases, the most common bone involved in the upper extremity is the:
    A) Humerus
    B) Radius
    C) Ulna
    D) Scaphoid

177. Brain tumors are best diagnosed by:
    A) Contrast MRI
    B) CT
    C) Bone scan
    D) Lumbar puncture

178. Which of the following is the most common rehabilitation issue for the patient with cancer?
    A) Pain
    B) Generalized weakness
    C) Activities of daily living (ADLs) deficits
    D) Ambulation

179. What primary cancer site is the most common cause of upper extremity lymphedema?
    A) Lung
    B) Breast
    C) Melanoma
    D) Osteosarcoma

180. Trismus, a condition that is common in patients with head and neck cancer who have had radiation therapy, is due to:
    A) Ectopic activity in the trigeminal nerve
    B) Ectopic activity in the facial nerve
    C) Ectopic activity in the mandibular nerve
    D) All of the above

181. The mechanism of action of ondansetron (Zofran), a common antiemetic given to cancer patients, is:
    A) Serotonin antagonist
    B) Antihistamine
    C) Anticholinergic
    D) None of the above

182. Bone scans can assess:
    A) Blastic activity
    B) Lytic activity
    C) Bone destruction
    D) Impending fracture site

183. The best screening test to assess for bony metastases is:
    A) X-ray
    B) Bone scan

C) CT

D) (A) and (B) together

184. The most common presenting symptom of a brain tumor is:
   A) Headache
   B) Weakness
   C) Paresthesias
   D) Bowel/bladder abnormality

185. Which diagnostic test is indicated when a cancer patient has silent aspiration?
   A) Chest x-ray
   B) Videofluoroscopic swallow study (VFSS)
   C) Esophagus manometry
   D) Barium swallow

186. In patients with radiation plexitis, which of the following can be seen on needle electromyography (EMG)?
   A) Myokymic discharges
   B) Fibrillation potentials
   C) Polyphasic motor unit action potentials
   D) Small motor unit action potentials

187. Trismus, a condition that is common in patients with head and neck cancer, results in:
   A) Difficulty with mouth opening
   B) Clenched jaw
   C) Difficulty chewing
   D) All of the above

188. Bony metastases are common in cancer of the:
   A) Breast
   B) Prostate
   C) Lung
   D) All of the above

189. The most common malignant bone tumor in children is:
   A) Osteosarcoma
   B) Ewing's sarcoma
   C) Neuroblastoma
   D) Osteochondromas

190. The most common site of spinal metastases is:
   A) Thoracic spine
   B) Cervical spine
   C) Lumbar spine
   D) All are equal

191. Swallowing disorders are often seen in:
   A) Central nervous system (CNS) tumors
   B) Lung tumors
   C) Breast cancers
   D) Spinal metastases

192. The earliest presentation of neoplastic spinal cord compromise is usually:
    A) Pain
    B) Weakness
    C) Sensory loss
    D) Bowel and bladder dysfunction

193. Which of the following cardiac disorders is a contraindication to intense exercise–related cardiac rehabilitation?
    A) Cardiac transplant
    B) Myocardial infarction
    C) Compensated heart failure
    D) Aortic dissection

194. In most cases of burn rehabilitation, immediate aggressive range of motion is indicated unless the burn affects:
    A) Tendons
    B) Face
    C) Hands and feet
    D) Genitalia

195. The most common etiology of cancer-related pain is:
    A) Antineoplastic therapy
    B) Direct tumor involvement
    C) Diagnostic procedures/evaluation
    D) Psychogenic pain

196. Which of the following treatments is most effective in improving dyspnea in chronic obstructive pulmonary disease (COPD) patients participating in pulmonary rehabilitation?
    A) Short-duration high-intensity training
    B) Long-duration mild-intensity training
    C) Inspiratory muscle training
    D) Chest physiotherapy

# Medical Rehabilitation (Cardiac, Pulmonary, Cancer, Burn, and Wound)

## ANSWERS

1. **B)** The TheraBite maintains the form of the mouth to prevent microstomia because of contractures of oral muscles in patients with facial burns.

2. **D)** A properly designed therapeutic exercise regimen will provide all of these benefits to the burn patient.

3. **D)** Firecrackers, matches, inflammable aerosols, and gasoline all contribute to flame burns in pediatric patients.

4. **D)** The goals of cardiac rehabilitation are not only to condition the heart to enhance exercise tolerance, but also to develop a long-term exercise plan that can be followed by the patient in the setting he or she will be in. Reversible risk factors, such as dyslipidemia, smoking, sedentary lifestyle, and compliance with medications, are some of the topics also addressed to reduce the risk of a future cardiac event.

5. **A)** Exercise therapy can significantly improve pain-free walking and the ability to carry out activities of daily living. A patient with intermittent claudication undergoing cardiac rehabilitation should be provided with sufficient rest in between periods of exercise until the therapy goals for cardiac rehabilitation are met.

6. **B)** COPD has a prevalence of roughly 10% among adults in the United States. It is estimated that 24 million adults in the United States have symptomatic COPD. It is more prevalent among men than women, in Whites than in African Americans, and among those of increased age. It is the fourth leading cause of mortality in the United States and is projected to become the third leading cause by 2020.

7. **C)** Emphysema is a pathological condition resulting in the destruction of the alveolar walls and enlargement of the distal airways. This causes hyperexpansion of the lungs and air trapping. Patients will often complain of shortness of breath and decreased exercise tolerance and may demonstrate characteristic "pursed-lip breathing."

8. **A)** The gold standard for diagnosing sleep apnea is an overnight polysomnography (PSG, or "sleep study"). Such studies are typically performed in the outpatient setting under the observation of a qualified technician. Indications for such a study include excessive daytime sleepiness, titration of continuous positive airway pressure (CPAP) therapy, unexplained pulmonary hypertension (HTN), or poorly controlled HTN, among others. PSG monitors sleep stages by monitoring an electroencephalograph, an electrooculography, respiratory flow/effort, oxyhemoglobin saturation, an electrocardiogram, and body position. PSG results will help to categorize central from obstructive sleep apnea.

9. **C)** Pursed-lip breathing is a technique where the patient inhales through the nose while keeping the mouth closed and then exhales slowly over the course of 4 to 6 seconds through pursed lips. The benefits of this technique include prevention of air trapping and promotion of better gas exchange in the distal airways. Overall, this technique also produces improved tidal volume and reduces dyspnea and the work of breathing. Controlled cough and huffing are techniques to maintain adequate airway secretion management.

10. **C)** Lung-volume reduction surgery may provide quality of life and survival benefits in very selected patients with severe emphysema. Targeted areas for resection include large peripheral focal areas with emphysematous tissue of one or both lungs. Studies have reported results of six randomized controlled studies that demonstrated reduced hyperinflation, improved pulmonary function tests, increased 6-minute walk testing, and improved quality of life.

11. **A)** In air shifting, the patient takes in a deep breath and holds it against a closed glottis for 5 seconds. During this breath hold, the air shifts to less-ventilated distal airspaces. Thereafter, the inhaled breath is exhaled through pursed lips, which helps to prolong the expiratory phase and keep distal airways patent.

12. **A)** The mechanism of action is not completely understood. Methylphenidate presumably activates the brain stem arousal system and the cortex to produce a stimulant effect. It blocks the reuptake of norepinephrine and dopamine into the presynaptic neuron and increases arousal.

13. **A)** Extramedullary (outside cord) compression accounts for more than 90% of spinal cord compression resulting from cancer. It includes epidural, intradural, and leptomeningeal disease. Intramedullary (inside the cord) spinal cord compression is seen in less than 5% of spinal cord tumors and includes gliomas, ependymomas, and astrocytomas.

14. **D)** The elbow is the most common joint to develop heterotopic ossification in burn patients. Posterior elbow burns that are open for prolonged periods are at highest risk.

15. **A)** Active range of motion is preferable to passive because it involves the patient's muscles. Working against the contractile force of the healing scar tissue will help keep the tissue loose. Ranging toward the force of a contracting scar would not help counteract the contractile force.

16. **C)** The systemic response to burn includes fluid extravasation. This can be so severe that it leads to hypovolemic shock (especially in large body surface area burns).

17. **A)** Patients with heart transplant lack vagal innervation to the heart, resulting in a higher baseline heart rate and slow return to baseline after exercise. Another cause of a higher baseline heart rate posttransplant is antirejection medication. Rate control is mediated mostly by hemodynamic changes and catecholamines.

18. **B)** The goal of therapy for a patient with frequent stable arrhythmias is to condition the body to increase efficiency while maintaining the pulse under the heart rate when arrhythmias frequently occur. Closer cardiac monitoring and gradual cooldown phase are also required to reduce episodes of arrhythmia.

19. **D)** MET is an important ratio of work to resting metabolic rate used as a guideline for physical activity. Activities are assigned a MET value that is used as a reference to guide therapy and evaluate the patient for return to employment. Although the decision to return to employment is based on the type of work, patients with METs higher than 7 can return to work on most jobs and those with METs lower than 4 should not return to employment because of a decreased level of function.

20. **A)** PFT involves a series of tests that measure how well the lungs move volumes of air and exchange oxygen. PFTs can include simple screening spirometry, formal lung volume measurement, diffusing capacity for carbon monoxide, and arterial blood gases. PFTs, especially the spirometry component, are the main method of diagnosing chronic obstructive pulmonary disease (COPD).

21. **B)** Mechanical insufflator-exsufflator is indicated for secretion management in conditions such as neuromuscular disease, high cervical spinal cord injuries, traumatic brain injuries, and cerebral palsy where patients may have less than 5 L/sec peak cough flows (PCFs). Such cough-assist devices are contraindicated in bullous emphysema, pneumothorax, pneumomediastinum, barotrauma, or impaired consciousness.

22. **A)** In C5 tetraplegic patients, some innervation to the diaphragm remains intact. However, the abdominal contents may tend to sag secondary to weakened abdominal muscles. When tetraplegic patients go from a supine to sitting posture, the diaphragmatic excursion decreases as it becomes pulled down by the sagging abdominal contents and the vital capacity reduces. It has been found that using an abdominal binder while sitting may reduce this drop in vital capacity.

23. **B)** The literary misnomer known as *Ondine's curse* refers to a rare hereditary disorder characterized by congenital central hypoventilation. Recent research suggests that this disorder is more consistent with a generalized dysfunction of the regulation of the body's autonomic nervous system. Patients usually present in infancy with respiratory distress soon after birth requiring mechanical assistance. They may also develop more normal patterns of breathing during wakefulness with episodes of apnea during sleep.

24. **C)** By far, smoking cessation is the most cost effective and clinically effective way to prevent COPD.

25. **A)** Several benefits of supplemental home oxygen use for COPD patients have been identified. Home oxygen use has been found to reduce polycythemia, improve pulmonary hypertension, reduce subjective effort during activity, prolong survival, improve cognitive function, and reduce rehospitalization. Of course, smoking cessation should be emphasized.

26. **B)** Neoplastic-related spinal cord compression comprises up to 14% of new onset SCI. The vast majority is metastatic (up to 85% of the cases). Spinal metastasis is seen in 15% to 40% of all systemic cancers. The primary cancer site for spinal metastasis is most commonly breast, lung, and prostate.

27. **A)** Viable tissue must be available for healing to occur. Debridement uncovers that viable tissue. Burn wounds are unsightly, even if they are grafted. Debridement has real physiologic benefit for wound healing, not just placebo. The depth of a burn wound can be determined, even in the presence of an eschar.

28. **C)** Scar tissue forms 24 hours a day in a healing burn, so pressure needs to be maintained to minimize scarring. The pressure garment may be removed for a short period of time for hygiene.

29. **C)** Blood flow can be compromised to involved tissues in both heat and cold injuries.

30. **B)** The Borg scale is a widely used scale that quantifies exertion by the patient and helps tailor rehabilitation for the patient. The original Borg scale was a 15-point scale, whereas the modified Borg scale consists of 10 points (from no exertion to maximal exertion). Patients should be maintained on moderate exertion during the first two phases of cardiac rehabilitation.

31. **C)** Patients undergoing cardiac rehabilitation are at a higher risk for postexercise hypotension or even syncope if a slow cooldown phase is not incorporated into the exercise regimen. The heart continues to generate a higher cardiac output based on the increased demand during the conditioning phase and an abrupt stop in exercise may result in a drop in blood pressure causing hypotension.

32. **D)** Although a patient with congestive heart failure will be unable to tolerate prolonged exercise programs initially, exercise duration and efficiency can increase up to 18% to 34% with continued cardiac rehabilitation. With impaired contractility, an increase in heart rate would result in decreased ejection fraction, lower stroke volume, and hypotension that may even result in a syncopal episode. Rehabilitation should be tailored to the patient's cardiac function to provide maximum benefit.

33. **D)** The diaphragm is supplied by the phrenic nerve (C3–5 nerve roots). The long thoracic nerve (C5–7) supplies serratus anterior. The thoracodorsal nerve (C7–8) supplies latissimus dorsi, and the lateral pectoral nerve (C5–7) supplies the pectoralis major muscle.

34. **A)** A mechanical insufflator-exsufflator (eg, cough assist) is a device that aids in the clearance of bronchopulmonary secretions in patients who have conditions such as neuromuscular disease, traumatic brain injury, cerebral palsy, and tetraplegia. This machine delivers deep inspiration through a face mask or adapter connecting to the patient's tracheostomy tube, followed immediately by a suction pressure (negative pressure). This device can be adjusted so that at least 2 to 4 seconds are allotted to allow for maximal chest expansion before rapid lung emptying.

35. **B)** Normal respiratory function decline, represented by $FEV_1$, decreases by 30 mL/year in non-smokers starting at about 25 years of age. In smokers, this rate of decline significantly increases to as high as 60 mL/year or more.

36. **C)** The American College of Sports Medicine defines aerobic exercise as "any activity that uses large muscle groups, can be maintained continuously, and is rhythmic in nature" with the goals of producing physiological adjustments to the cardiovascular system in response to the exercise. Examples of aerobic activity include walking, jogging/running, aerobics, upper extremity ergometer use, or stationary bike.

37. **D)** Central chemoreceptors in the medulla are sensitive to, both, changes in pH and rising $CO_2$ levels within the cerebrospinal fluid of the fourth ventricle. There are peripheral chemoreceptors as well, which are sensitive to pH, $pCO_2$, and $pO_2$ levels. Such receptors are located in the aortic arch as well as the carotid bodies.

38. **B)** A flutter valve (acapella) is a portable and relatively inexpensive device that is used to clear airway secretions by vibrating the airways to dislodge mucous, facilitating positive airway pressure in the airways to promote their patency, and ultimately allowing for the secretions to be coughed up for expectoration. This device can be used in combination with other manual modalities and is easy to use. It may achieve mucous clearance in patients who acutely produce a lot of airway secretions, or for patients at the subacute level who have cystic fibrosis or chronic obstructive pulmonary disease (COPD).

39. **A)** Meningiomas arise from the arachnoid "cap" cells of the arachnoid villi. They are usually benign and are cured by surgical resection. They may present with focal seizures, weakness, aphasia, or increased intracranial pressure.

40. **B)** Children, especially infants and toddlers, who have burns in a stocking distribution, especially on both feet, should be suspected of having been abused. Complex regional pain syndrome can cause skin changes in a limb, but would be unusual in a child and is usually unilateral. Food allergy would cause systemic symptoms, possibly including skin manifestations, but would not resemble a burn in a stocking distribution. Malnourishment has no pathophysiologic relation to foot burns.

41. **B)** Part of the healing process in the first few days after grafting is thought to be facilitated by a semipermeable membrane effect between the surface of the graft and the underlying surface of the recipient wound site. Blood and pus interrupt this effect and impede the diffusion of nutrients and gases prior to the formation of new capillaries in the graft. Also, pus is usually a sign of infection and should never be treated as an incidental finding or as a sign of graft taking.

42. **D)** Burns of the eyes, ears, face, perineum, and genitalia are always considered to be major burns. Burns in other parts of the body, including the hands, are considered mild, moderate, or severe depending on the percentage of total body surface area involved.

43. **A)** Phase 1 is the first acute inpatient rehabilitation phase that can last from 1 to 14 days. The focus of this phase is to closely monitor the patient while increasing metabolic equivalents (MET) by 1 to 2 each day until a MET of 4 is reached. This should start on the acute care floor, usually in the critical care unit (CCU), and continue in acute rehabilitation. Cardiac patients should not wait to start therapy until they are on the rehabilitation floor. Phases are tailored to the individual. It is possible to skip phase 1 in some patients and go directly to phase 2 (intermediate outpatient phase after a noninvasive procedure).

44. **C)** Stroke volume increases at rest and during exercise, whereas heart rate decreases in response to exercise therapy. Recall that cardiac output is the product of stroke volume and heart rate, so an increase in stroke volume will require a reduction of heart rate. Myocardial oxygen capacity does not change, and peripheral resistance decreases in response to exercise therapy.

45. **D)** When exercise tolerance testing or exercise echocardiography cannot be used to evaluate cardiac function, pharmacologic stress testing can be performed using dobutamine, dipyridamole, or adenosine. A stress test is used in cardiac rehabilitation to evaluate cardiac function and guide therapy rather than for diagnostic benefits of the tests.

46. **C)** Cystic fibrosis is an autosomal recessive disease with a gene mutation resulting in the formation of inactive cystic fibrosis transmembrane receptor (CFTR) protein or the complete absence of it. Consequently, abnormalities of the chloride ion channels of exocrine glands fail to adequately remove secretions in the respiratory tract. This is a multisystem disease that also affects the gastrointestinal tract and genitourinary system.

47. **C)** The MIC is the largest volume of air that can be held by a patient against a closed glottis. The MIC is achieved by "air stacking" consecutively delivered volumes of air that are delivered by an external resuscitator or volume ventilator with a nasal piece or mouthpiece interface. Determining the MIC has been used in tracking therapies for patients with neuromuscular disease who have compromised inspiratory and expiratory muscle strength. Owing to their impaired ability to fully expand the lungs secondary to weakness, there is a decline in lung compliance. If a patient can maintain an MIC greater than his or her VC through air stacking techniques, he or she may be able to forgo the need for a tracheostomy and be maintained on noninvasive ventilatory support alone, assuming that there is no bulbar weakness.

48. **C)** Sarcoidosis is a systemic disease characterized by noncaseating epithelioid granulomas containing giant cells. It is systemic, but commonly affects the lungs and lymph tissue. The most common presenting symptoms are cough and dyspnea. This condition occurs most commonly among adults aged 20 to 40 years and is slightly higher among women than men.

49. **D)** The GOLD criteria is the result of a collaborative effort by the National Institute of Health and the World Health Organization to devise a staging system for COPD. The GOLD criteria stages patients from 0 to 4 depending on the degree of airflow limitation (decline in $FEV_1$) measured during pulmonary function testing. Stage 0 (at risk) includes those at risk who have normal spirometry results; stage 1 (mild COPD) is $FEV_1/FVC$ ratio of lower than 70% predicted with $FEV_1$ of 80% predicted or higher; stage 2 (moderate COPD) is $FEV_1/FVC$ lower than 70% predicted and $FEV_1$ 50% to 79% predicted; stage 3 (severe COPD) is $FEV_1/FVC$ lower than 70% and $FEV_1$ 30% to 49% predicted; stage 4 (very severe COPD) is $FEV_1/FVC$ lower than 70% predicted and $FEV_1$ lower than 30% predicted.

50. **D)** Central respiratory centers are located in the medulla (specifically in the dorsal respiratory group), and they initiate the rhythm of breathing. Other respiratory centers are located in other parts of the medulla as well as the pons.

51. **B)** Diaphragm rest can be provided by using intermittent positive pressure ventilation through a mouthpiece or nasal piece, usually at bedtime. Benefits of respiratory muscle rest have been shown to decrease oxygen consumption, thereby improving daytime arterial blood gas values, vital capacity, dyspnea symptoms, 12-minute walk test distances, and overall quality of life. There is a risk of air trapping; however, this does not outweigh the potential benefits.

52. **A)** Cerebellar astrocytoma is the most common posterior fossa tumor in children and carries a favorable prognosis. Medulloblastoma and brain stem gliomas are the second and third most frequent posterior fossa tumors in children. Depending on the grade of the tumor, cerebellar astrocytomas are typically treated by observation, surgery, and/or radiation. With complete surgical removal, these tumors rarely return and the long-term outcome is usually very good.

53. **C)** Scald burns represent 40% to 50% of the burns in the pediatric population.

54. **A)** Bacteria can contaminate the Hubbard tank and theoretically cause severe bacterial infections of wounds.

55. **B)** Burns of the epidermis with no dermal involvement should heal in less than a week and require only acetaminophen or over-the-counter doses of nonsteroidal anti-inflammatory drugs (NSAIDs).

56. **A)** Although cardiac rehabilitation increases maximum cardiac output, it does not increase resting cardiac output. Cardiac rehabilitation has been shown to reduce the rate of recurrent MI by 17%, decrease mortality secondary to MI by 15% to 20%, and increase LV ejection fraction after MI.

57. **B)** The target heart rate is usually 60% to 80% of maximum heart rate, but in patients taking a beta-blocker, the heart rate may not reflect the exercise demand on the heart as any negative inotropic agents tend to slow the heart rate.

58. **B)** The coronary arteries begin at the aortic root and provide oxygen-rich blood to the myocardium during diastole. Although coronary arteries do not completely collapse during systole, the majority of the myocardial perfusion takes place during the diastolic phase. As the heart rate increases, the heart spends less time in diastole and can lead to an ischemic event if not monitored closely during cardiac rehabilitation.

59. **C)** Tidal volume is the volume of air moved in and out of the lungs during normal respiration. VC represents the volume of air that can be exhaled following maximal inspiration. TLC is achieved following maximal effort of the muscles of inspiration to expand the lungs. The FVC is the total volume of air expired after a full inspiration.

60. **D)** Pulmonary dysfunction is usually categorized into obstructive disease and restrictive disease. Obstructive lung disease usually involves the impaired movement of exhaled air due to airway narrowing, whereas restrictive disease impairs the ability to fully expand the lungs. Examples of obstructive disease include chronic obstructive pulmonary disease (COPD), asthma, and bronchitis. Restrictive diseases usually are conditions that affect the lung tissue itself (eg, interstitial lung diseases) or the chest wall (eg, paralysis and Guillain-Barré syndrome).

61. **C)** In the three-zone model of pulmonary blood flow, the interrelationship among alveolar pressure ($P_A$), pulmonary arterial pressure ($P_a$), and pulmonary venous pressure ($P_V$) is described. In zone 1, $P_A$ exceeds $P_a$, and therefore ventilation occurs in excess of perfusion. In zone 2, the following relationship occurs where $P_a$ is greater than $P_A$, which is in turn greater than $P_V$, so ventilation and perfusion are fairly equal. Finally, in zone 3, $P_a$ is greater than $P_V$, which is in turn greater than $P_A$, so flow is dependent on the arterial and venous pressure difference and has the highest rate of perfusion relative to the other two zones. Of course, perfusion of the lung is dependent on posture, and the above is assuming an upright posture.

62. **C)** Postural drainage uses gravity-assisted positioning to clear the airways. Common positions include Trendelenburg with the patient side-lying, supine, or prone depending on which lobe is being drained. Such techniques should be avoided in patients with significant pulmonary edema, congestive heart failure, acute dyspnea, or aspiration problems.

63. **A)** Electrodiagnostic studies of the phrenic nerve are necessary to determine whether a patient is a candidate for phrenic nerve pacing. Phrenic pacing is an increasingly used method to provide ventilation to high-level spinal cord injury (SCI) patients (C1–C2) besides chronic ventilator use. Ideal candidates for pacing have an intact diaphragm and phrenic nerve, but impaired respiratory function because of a higher lesion (as in central hypoventilation syndrome, brain stem injury, or high [C1–C2] cervical lesions).

64. **C)** Emphysema is an abnormal permanent enlargement of the airspaces distal to the terminal bronchioles. Airflow limitation is the result of the loss of elastic recoil and decreased airway tethering. Airflow limitations are due to narrowed airway caliber and increased airway resistance.

65. **C)** Brain metastasis occurs in 25% of patients with cancer, making it the most common type of brain cancer. Rehabilitation of such tumors is heavily dependent on the site of the lesion, similar to primary brain tumors.

66. **A)** The rule of nines refers to the percentage of the body comprised by the major surface body parts. It is modified in children. There is no preset clinical limit to the number of therapy sessions in a burn rehab regimen—the number of sessions is determined in each clinical case. Family members are encouraged to visit, unless they are ill. Certain isolation precautions may apply. The amount of time required for a burn to develop depends on the temperature of the agent causing the burn.

67. **B)** The raised epidermis and blister fluid act as a natural and already sterile dressing. Eventually, the epidermis will break on its own because of the effect of the fluid.

68. **A)** Fat cells in the nonburned regions of the body still function in the normal way. Burn patients still can develop obesity and may have significant disfigurement if large areas of fat cells have been burned away and subsequently cannot regenerate.

69. **D)** MET is an important ratio of work to resting metabolic rate used as a guideline for physical activity. Activities are assigned a MET value that is used as a reference during different stages of cardiac rehabilitation. Examples of low MET values corresponding to light activities are eating, sleeping, and writing (MET values below 2.0). Interestingly, using a bedside commode is about 3.6 METS, whereas using a bedpan is about 4.7 METS. A brisk walk is about 5 METS, whereas shoveling snow is about 7 METS.

70. **D)** Cardiac rehabilitation will not change the heart rate at which the angina will occur, nor will it change the myocardial oxygen consumption. However, conditioning and increased efficiency below the angina threshold will help patients cope with the limitations caused by the chest pain.

71. **A)** Hypertrophic cardiomyopathy is not an absolute contraindication for cardiac rehabilitation, but requires hemodynamic studies and closer monitoring during exercises. The goal of therapy in patients with hypertrophic cardiomyopathy is to optimize conditioning if the patient is not a candidate for pacemaker placement. The other answer choices are absolute contraindications for exercise testing.

72. **A)** The FRC is the volume of air remaining at the end of a normal exhalation. VC represents the volume of air that can be exhaled after maximal inspiration. The RV is the volume remaining in the lungs after maximal exhalation. The ERV is the amount of air that can be exhaled after a normal expiration.

73. **B)** A non-rebreathing mask has a reservoir bag and a one-way valve that prevents exhaled gases from entering the reservoir, thereby maximizing the $FiO_2$ to approximately 80% to 90%. A Venturi mask allows for a more precise administration of oxygen than nasal cannula. Blow-by oxygen is administered by holding oxygen close to a patient's face. This is not an efficient delivery system for adults, but may be used in infants or small children who may not tolerate a mask.

74. **A)** Persons with SCI typically have a restrictive form of pulmonary disease where all lung volumes are reduced except for the residual volume (RV), which increases.

75. **A)** During normal respiration, the vocal cords partially abduct (open) during inspiration and partially adduct (close) during end-exhalation. In vocal cord dysfunction (paradoxical vocal cord motion), the vocal cords adduct during inhalation, resulting in airflow obstruction at the level of the larynx. This diagnosis can be confirmed by visualization with a laryngoscope.

76. **D)** Pneumonia is the leading cause of mortality among SCI patients, particularly those who have tetraplegia. Heart disease is the second most common cause, whereas septicemia (from pressure injuries, urinary tract infections, or respiratory infections) is third.

77. **D)** PCF can be measured using a peak flow meter, and it is measured in liters per minute or liters per second (liters per minute divided by 60 seconds). Measuring the PCF is an acceptable way to measure expiratory muscle force, particularly in patients who have muscle weakness (as in Duchenne muscular dystrophy or amyotrophic lateral sclerosis). This value correlates with what is called the *maximal expiratory pressure* (MEP), another indicator of expiratory muscle force, which is harder to measure in patients with facial muscle weakness. Measuring and tracking the PCF and MEP in patients with neuromuscular weakness is important in assessing such patients' ability to produce efficient and productive coughs for the clearance of airway irritants and/or secretions. Weakness or inability to produce this physiologic mechanism can result in respiratory infection and ultimate failure.

78. **B)** Steroid myopathy is usually an insidious disease process that causes weakness mainly to the proximal muscles of the upper and lower limbs and to the neck flexors. Patients typically complain of a progressive inability to rise from chairs, climb stairs, and perform overhead activities. This condition can develop after prolonged administration of prednisone at a dose of 40 to 60 mg. Although there is no clear length of time, the onset of weakness has been found to occur within weeks to years following the initiation of corticosteroid administration. Steroid myopathy affects type II muscle fibers. Therefore, electromyographic (EMG) needle testing is usually normal.

79. **C)** Electrical exposure sufficient to cause a burn can interfere with the intrinsic electrical activity of the heart, causing arrhythmias. Cardiac monitoring is indicated.

80. **D)** Pain relief and prevention of further injury while epithelialization occurs are the goals of treating first- and second-degree burns. First- and second-degree burns are inexpensive to treat and are not sufficient cause for a person to be certified as disabled. These burns rarely have any lasting cosmetic effects or implications for a patient's self-esteem.

81. **C)** Burns represent a significant trauma that can lead to posttraumatic stress disorder. Depression has also been shown to develop in about half of patients with burn injuries.

82. **A)** Cardiac output is defined as the product of the heart rate and stroke volume. The resting cardiac output does not change with cardiac rehabilitation, but studies show that rehabilitation increases the maximum cardiac output over time.

83. **A)** Prosthetic ambulation consumes more energy than normal ambulation. Ambulation with the use of crutches can increase the energy expenditure by 15%, whereas patients with prosthetic limbs consume 10% to 280% more energy depending on the type of prosthetic. For example, a unilateral below knee prosthesis can increase energy cost by 9% to 28%, whereas a bilateral above knee prosthesis can increase energy cost by 280%. Most patients slow their gait to decrease energy expenditure. Any functional or structural change in demand should be understood in patients undergoing cardiac rehabilitation.

84. **B)** Near-maximum stroke volume is obtained in supine position at rest, whereas exercising in this position decreases stroke volume in a linear fashion. While standing, the stroke volume increases in a curvilinear fashion until it reaches maximum. As stroke volume changes minimally during exercises in supine position, this position can be utilized for patients with impaired compensatory stroke volume changes.

85. **D)** TLC is achieved after maximal effort of the muscles of inspiration to expand the lungs. The FRC is the volume of air remaining at the end of a normal exhalation. The RV is the volume remaining in the lungs after maximal exhalation. VC represents the volume of air that can be exhaled after maximal inspiration.

86. **A)** For an adult patient who has a minimal supplemental oxygen requirement, nasal cannula would be the best interface for oxygen delivery. One liter per minute via nasal cannula is roughly equal to an $FiO_2$ of 24%, with each additional liter increasing the $FiO_2$ by 4%.

87. **D)** Nasal CPAP (n-CPAP) is the most effective treatment for obstructive sleep apnea syndrome. Polysomnography studies will help in the quantification of the severity of OSA in the form of a respiratory disturbance index (RDI). CPAP is generally prescribed for patients with an RDI higher than 20 or those with lower RDIs with additional symptoms such as daytime somnolence. Overall n-CPAP has been found to ameliorate daytime sleepiness, depressive symptoms, and elevated diastolic blood pressure.

88. **C)** Deficiency of A1AT protein is the only genetic abnormality linked to COPD. Symptoms of COPD related to A1AT typically manifest in the fourth decade of life and include exertional dyspnea, cough, and wheeze. Forced expiratory volume at 1 second ($FEV_1$) is usually at or below 50% predicted normal and declines at a rate of 50 to 80 mL/year for ex-smokers or nonsmokers and 100 to 130 mL/year for smokers. Smoking cessation is the cornerstone of treatment in this population. In some limited cases, A1AT replacement has been used as a treatment strategy as well.

89. **C)** PEEP is pressure above atmospheric pressure mechanically exerted on the airways to keep them patent. The overall effect of PEEP, if applied during mechanical ventilation, is to increase lung compliance and oxygenation while decreasing shunt fraction and the work of breathing.

90. **A)** $VO_{2max}$ (maximum aerobic capacity or maximal oxygen consumption) represents the maximum ability of an individual to take in, consume, and utilize oxygen. This value defines an individual's level of physical fitness. This value is defined by the Fick equation: $VO_2 = HR \times SV \times$ a-$VO_{2diff}$. $VO_{2max}$ is considered the single best measure of cardiopulmonary fitness.

91. **D)** Even at physiologic doses of glucocorticoids, bone loss can occur. Any patient receiving the equivalent of prednisone 5 mg for more than 3 months is at risk for bone loss. ACR guidelines recommend the above for prevention of bone loss and fractures.

92. **B)** Superficial burns involve only the epidermis, whereas full thickness burns include the whole depth of the dermis and would include any burn with an eschar. Partial thickness burns affect part of the dermis. Unstageable is not used in classifying burns, rather it refers to decubitus ulcers with an eschar making their true depth indeterminate.

93. **A)** Older adults die from their burns more frequently than do younger adults. Men are burned more frequently than women.

94. **C)** Burns cause significant pain. Opioid analgesics are appropriate to use. Scheduling the medication prior to wound care ensures that there is sufficient opioid in the patient's system to be effective, whereas an "as-needed" regimen might cause pain and anxiety. The environment in which wound care occurs can put the patient at psychological ease, which can increase trust and minimize pain.

95. **C)** Oxygen extraction can be assessed by the ratio of oxygen delivery and oxygen consumption in any organ system of the body. The heart has the highest percentage of oxygen extraction.

96. **D)** Isometric exercises can raise the heart rate and demand on the heart. Although isometric exercises are initially held during cardiac rehabilitation, they are introduced later in short durations to condition the heart to handle increased demand. Valsalva maneuvers can cause arrhythmias and should be avoided in the acute phase of cardiac rehabilitation. Raising the legs above the heart can increase preload.

97. **C)** After the closely monitored outpatient–phase 2 cardiac rehabilitation and determination of hemodynamic ability of the heart with exercise-tolerance testing, phase 3 begins. This phase sets a higher target heart rate for the patient and sets a goal to maximize the therapeutic benefit of cardiac rehabilitation before the maintenance phase begins.

98. **A)** During quiet respiration, the primary muscle of respiration is the diaphragm. During exercise, additional muscles become involved (such as the external intercostals during inspiration, the abdominal muscles, and the scalenus).

99. **D)** Stridor is a high-pitched sound that is usually caused by a partial obstruction in the upper airways. Stridor is a symptom that may occur at various phases in respiration (inspiration, expiration, or biphasic). When stridor occurs during inspiration, it usually signifies laryngeal obstruction, whereas expiratory stridor implies tracheobronchial obstruction.

100. **C)** According to the Consensus Conference Report on Cystic Fibrosis (2004), the best predictor of survival in CF is the $FEV_1$. Patients with an $FEV_1$ of under 30% predicted value will have a 50% incidence of 2-year mortality.

101. **B)** Significant weight loss and hypermetabolism are common in moderate to severe cases of COPD. This is due in part to increased work of breathing and catabolic state as well as decreased oral intake related to the interference of dyspnea and limitations of energy. A comprehensive pulmonary rehabilitation program should include nutritional counseling and supplementation.

102. **D)** SIMV allows the ventilator to become sensitized to the patient's respiratory pattern and deliver ventilator-assisted breaths in synchrony with the patient. ACV is usually the initial mode of ventilation for patients intubated for respiratory failure. The ventilator is set at a selected backup rate and is able to deliver breaths for every patient-initiated effort as well as when the patient's respiratory rate falls below the preset backup rate. PSV provides augmentation of patient's spontaneous respiratory effort and can be used during weaning trials.

103. **C)** The most widely accepted guideline for the prescription of supplemental oxygen therapy during exercise is when the $SpO_2$ falls below 90% during exercise. It is recommended, however, that individual patients also be monitored for response in dyspnea and endurance with and without supplemental oxygen to see whether there is an objective benefit.

104. **D)** Patients with brain tumors are frequently given seizure prophylaxis. Diffuse, macular rash can be seen as a result of phenytoin allergy. Other side effects include cognitive dysfunction, fatigue, and drowsiness. Phenytoin and phenobarbital are used less frequently because of an increased rate of cognitive dysfunction.

105. **D)** Fibroblasts lay down new collagen. If the patient is positioned such that there is no stretch on the wound, the new collagen will not stretch enough to allow full premorbid range of motion.

106. **C)** Medical and surgical advancements have decreased the mortality rate and allowed patients with larger wounds to survive.

107. **D)** All of these complications can occur in burns of the lower extremities, depending on which structures are involved in the burn.

108. **B)** Irreversible risk factors for coronary artery disease include age, male gender, family history of coronary artery disease (CAD), past history of CAD, peripheral vascular disease (PVD), or stroke. Reversible risk factors include hypertension, cigarette smoking, hyperlipidemia, diabetes, obesity, sedentary lifestyle, or hyperinsulinemia.

109. **B)** Phase 2 is a supervised ambulatory outpatient program lasting 3 to 6 months. An exercise-tolerance test is usually performed at this phase to guide further rehabilitation. This is the immediate outpatient phase that requires a higher level of monitoring.

110. **D)** Although all modifiable risk factors are important and should be addressed in a cardiac rehab patient, smoking cessation is associated with a 30% decrease in 10-year mortality and is the single greatest modifiable risk factor for cardiac disease.

111. **C)** Supplemental oxygen therapy is a major component to the management of moderate to severe COPD. Oxygen ($O_2$) is generally prescribed to those patients who have a $PO_2$ of less than 55 mmHg or an $O_2$ saturation of less than 88% regardless of whether hypercapnia is present. The use of long-term oxygen therapy in chronic respiratory illness has been shown to improve survival, exercise capacity, and mental status, and has beneficial effects on hemodynamics. Although pulmonary rehabilitation has not been shown to decrease mortality, it has been shown to improve quality of life.

112. **D)** The FVC is the volume of air that can be maximally and forcibly exhaled from the lungs after having taken in the deepest breath possible. $FEV_1$ represents the volume of air forcibly exhaled in the first second of forced exhalation. The $FEV_1/FVC$ expresses the volume of FVC expelled in the first second as a ratio of the total FVC.

113. **B)** Exercise is a common precipitant of acute asthma exacerbations in asthmatic patients. In some asthmatic patients, exercise is the only precipitant of symptoms. Those with EIA tend to be more sensitive to humidity and temperature changes. During exercise, the air that is inhaled through the mouth tends to be cooler and drier, precipitating symptoms of cough, chest tightness, and/or wheezing. Symptoms may appear 5 to 20 minutes after the initiation of exercise. Prophylactic use of short-acting bronchodilators, beta-2 agonists, or mast cell stabilizers, such as cromolyn sodium, can be used 15 to 30 minutes before starting exercise to decrease symptoms.

114. **D)** Tracheostomy tubes have various features depending on what is needed for the patient. Cuffed tubes allow for good air seals and protection from aspiration, but do not allow the patient to speak. Uncuffed tubes provide a looser fit and poorer air seal, but allow for the patient to verbally communicate when needed. Fenestrated tubes are appropriate for patients able to speak and who intermittently require ventilator support. Nonfenestrated tubes are for patients requiring continuous mechanical ventilation or who cannot protect the airway from aspiration. Passy-Muir valve is a brand of talking tube that has a one-way valve to facilitate speech with a tracheostomy.

115. **C)** Incentive spirometry, also known as sustained maximal inspiration (SMI), is a device used to encourage patients to take maximal inspirations to improve inspiratory lung volumes and inspiratory muscle performance. This is particularly useful in the postoperative period after general anesthesia as a way to reverse lung atelectasis and maintain airway patency.

116. **D)** IAPV is a body ventilator that consists of an elastic air sac, which is worn underneath the clothing by patients who have respiratory muscle weakness. When the elastic bladder inflates with air by an external positive pressure ventilator, it causes the diaphragm to move upward. Once it deflates, the abdominal contents sag and pull the diaphragm down, allowing inspiration to occur passively. This technique can augment tidal volume by at least 300 mL or even higher if the patient has any degree of inspiratory capacity.

117. **C)** There is a high rate of dysphagia and subsequent aspiration in patients with brain tumors. This can be as a result of weakness or cognitive abnormalities from the tumor itself, or as a complication of radiation therapy. Dysphagia can be evaluated with a modified barium swallow. Patients with brain tumors respond to swallowing therapy comparably to stroke patients.

118. **A)** Burns cause tissue destruction, which puts the body into a catabolic state, sometimes requiring 5,000 to 10,000 calories/day. This can be treated with increased caloric intake and/or an anabolic steroid, usually oxandrolone.

119. **A)** The presence of dermal appendages in split thickness skin grafts provides centers for growth.

120. **D)** Prolonged bed rest, especially when combined with the potential of burn wounds to contract, can cause scoliosis and hip contractures. Bed rest for any reason causes a decline in cardiovascular conditioning, which can be particularly pronounced if the bed rest lasts for several weeks (as it can in severe body surface area burns).

121. **B)** Melanocytes produce skin pigmentation, and if they are destroyed, the skin pigmentation will be decreased.

122. **C)** The Frank-Starling law is an important concept to understand in patients undergoing cardiac rehabilitation. The law states that when venous return and the end-diastolic volume increase, the force generated by the myocardium increases resulting in a higher stroke volume. This law is particularly important in heart transplant patients, where the heart compensates to change in demand primarily due to hemodynamic changes and catecholamines rather than autonomic innervation. In the case of increased afterload, the heart reduces stroke volume to compensate. Recall here that cardiac output is the product of stroke volume and heart rate.

123. **D)** The maintenance phase, also known as phase 4 of cardiac rehabilitation, focuses on maintaining the goals met during the initial phases of rehabilitation by incorporating a home exercise program and continuing risk factor management. Initial gains made during the first three rehabilitation phases may decrease with time if the patient does not continue with exercises to maintain conditioning.

124. **C)** Smoking is by far the most common risk factor for COPD. It results in the greatest annual rate of decline in forced expiratory volume in the first second ($FEV_1$) from normal rates. Smoking cessation is an important prerequisite for a pulmonary rehabilitation program.

125. **C)** The phrenic nerve originates from the C3, C4, and C5 nerve roots.

126. **C)** According to the American Thoracic Society, pulmonary rehabilitation is a multidisciplinary program of care for patients with chronic respiratory impairment that is individually tailored and designed for patients to maximize their functional independence and functioning in the community. Potential benefits of pulmonary rehabilitation are improved exercise tolerance, improved symptoms of dyspnea, and quality of life. Also cited are less frequent hospitalizations for exacerbations.

127. **B)** Chest percussion involves the use of a cupped hand, or mechanical percussor, and providing rhythmic strikes to the chest wall and rib cage to loosen mucous. Contraindications for such therapy include increased intracranial pressure, increased intraocular pressure, cardiovascular collapse or instability, aortic aneurysm, and gross tumor. Precautionary measures should be taken for conditions where patients are on anticoagulation therapy, or have thrombocytopenia, rib fractures, or severe osteoporosis; however, these are not contraindications.

128. **B)** The American Thoracic Society has issued guidelines on the administration of the 6-minute walk test. This test is safe to administer relative to other walk tests, is better tolerated, and better reflective of activities of daily living (ADL) performance. The primary measurement during this test is 6-minute walk distance. Other parameters are also measured, such as patient's blood oxygen saturation and symptoms. This walk test can be used before, during, and after pulmonary rehabilitation to track the patient's progress and response.

129. **C)** Patients who have severely limited vital capacity and inspiratory muscle weakness can be trained in the technique of GPB. This strategy involves the patient being able to take in several successive "gulps" of air and closing the glottis after each one. With proper coordination, patients can manage to take in several hundred milliliters of air and thereby maintain alveolar ventilation while off of the ventilator. This technique cannot be used by patients with a tracheostomy or even a capped tracheostomy because of air leakage around the stoma.

130. **D)** Cognitive dysfunction, nausea, and fatigue are all side effects of radiation therapy. Fatigue can persist for several months. In the long term, a decline in cognitive dysfunction is the most prominent side effect of radiation treatment in brain tumors.

131. **A)** MRI remains the best diagnostic tool for detecting spinal metastases. It has a sensitivity of 83% to 93% with a specificity of 90% to 97%. The use of diffusion-weighted and contrast enhancement allows for differentiation between benign and malignant tissue.

132. **A)** It is prudent to not use resistive exercises on a limb that has a metastatic lesion to prevent causing a pathologic fracture.

133. **A)** Pain is the most common presenting symptom of metastatic bone disease as the tumor invades the bone. As the tumor grows and the bone remodels, pain can significantly affect the patient's functional status. The pathophysiology of bone pain is complex and includes both mechanical and chemical factors. Metastatic bone disease frequently presents with pain that is nonmechanical in nature. Nighttime pain is common. Pain is usually dull and constant and increases in severity. Breakthrough pain (episodes of extreme pain throughout the day) is common.

134. **A)** Secondary lymphedema, or acquired lymphedema, can be caused by lymph node surgery. Radiation therapy can cause scar tissue to form within the lymphatic system, leading to lymphedema. Primary lymphedema is not directly attributed to another medical cause.

135. **B)** Prostaglandin release is one of the mechanisms of bone pain in patients with bone metastases. NSAIDs inhibit prostaglandin synthesis and are effective first-line therapy for bone pain due to metastases.

136. **A)** The axial skeleton is the most common site of bone metastases followed by the femur and the humerus.

137. **B)** Participation in cardiac rehabilitation has shown a 20% to 30% decrease in mortality following myocardial infarction. Utilization of regular physical activity and secondary prevention (tobacco cessation, nutritional counseling, weight management, and blood pressure control) reduces morbidity and mortality after myocardial infarction.

138. **A)** The most common site of vertebral metastases is the vertebral body, most commonly in the thoracic spine.

139. **A)** Bisphosphonates inhibit osteoclastic bone resorption.

140. **A)** Platinum-based chemotherapy agents are associated with cochleotoxicity, presenting with high-frequency hearing loss. Tinnitus can also occur with these agents.

141. **A)** Stage 1 (pitting edema) is edema that gets worse throughout the day but is almost normal in size by the morning; it is partly, if not entirely, reversed with elevation of the affected limb. Stage 2 (nonpitting edema) is characterized by fibrosis. This marks the beginning of hardening of the skin and an increase in size. In stage 3, the swelling is irreversible and the affected area is very large. The tissue is fibrotic and unresponsive.

142. **D)** Fatigue in a cancer patient is multifactorial. The main reasons for a cancer patient's fatigue include anemia, cytokine release (eg, TNF), cachexia, deconditioning, and pain. Testosterone may be used to decrease weight loss and improve strength in cancer patients.

143. **C)** Subacute motor neuropathy can be seen with lymphoma.

144. **B)** Ondansetron (Zofran) is a 5-HT receptor blocker and is an effective antiemetic medication for cancer patients.

145. **A)** Rotator cuff tendonitis is among the most common causes of shoulder pain in patients who have breast cancer. The pathophysiology is impingement of the rotator cuff tendon between the coracoacromial arch and the humeral head. Weakness of the rotator cuff muscles contributes to this and can be multifactorial—from disuse following surgery due to pain, C5/C6 root damage from radiation and chemotherapy, or brachial plexopathy.

146. **D)** Bisphosphonates can cause inflammation of the esophagus and lead to erosions of the surface of the esophagus. Renal toxicity rarely occurs and is usually seen in patients who already have significant renal impairment. Atypical femur fractures are very rare fractures in patients taking bisphosphonate therapy for prolonged periods (more than 5 years). Although studies vary, some show that bisphosphonate use was associated with a 47% lower risk for classic fracture in patients with osteoporosis.

147. **D)** Treatment of CIPN is multifactorial. It can include medications (gabapentin, pregabalin, duloxetine, lidoderm patch, capsaicin cream). For patients who have more motor involvement, bracing may be needed, for example, an ankle-foot orthosis for a foot drop. Patients with numbness and insensate skin need education on proper skin hygiene, including washing with soap, daily moisturizing, and daily skin checks. In addition, patients should be instructed not to walk barefoot.

148. **A)** Lymphedema is a debilitating condition where there is a buildup of interstitial fluid containing high–molecular weight proteins. The rate of production of interstitial fluid is greater than lymphatic return because of an impairment of the lymphatic system. This leads to accumulation of proteins. The higher oncotic pressure draws more water into the interstitium. In the interstitium, protein and fluid accumulation sets off an inflammatory response, which leads to collagen deposition. In the United States, lymphedema is seen most commonly after breast cancer surgery, especially after undergoing an axillary lymphadenectomy. It can also be seen after head and neck surgery as well as pelvic surgery.

149. **B)** Although all of these symptoms are common in cancer or its treatment, the most common symptom among patients with cancer is fatigue.

150. **A)** The symptoms of delayed radiation myelopathy include lower extremity paresthesias, weakness, and pain.

151. **B)** Patients with multiple myeloma and bone metastasis may suffer from bone fracture, osteoporosis, bone pain, hypercalcemia, and/or lytic lesions with sclerotic borders.

152. **A)** Postmastectomy pain syndrome is a disorder characterized by burning, stabbing pain in the axilla, anterior chest wall, medial arm, and incision site. It is associated with paresthesias and allodynia. Injury to the intercostobrachial cutaneous nerve contributes to this disorder.

153. **D)** Acute cancer pain is usually caused by treatment, which can include pain from surgical intervention, chemotherapy-induced neuropathy, or radiation therapy. These can sometimes produce significant pain persisting long after the disease has been cured. Tumors can cause pain by activating nociceptors or by irritating or damaging somatosensory nerves.

154. **B)** Radiation plexopathy can occur when radiation is directed at the chest, axillary region, thoracic outlet, or neck. Damage occurs from fibrosis and ischemia of neural structures. Radiation plexopathy usually affects the upper trunk and is usually painless.

155. **A)** Pain with function of the involved extremity is considered a sign that a patient needs a prophylactic fixation. In a study that examined different bone lesions that went on to fracture, none of the other factors (weight-bearing versus non–weight-bearing bone, lytic versus blastic) had as much predictive value as functional pain.

156. **C)** Radiation therapy may damage the vasa nervorum. In addition, the secondary coagulation response leads to the accumulation of fibrin and the formation of fibrotic tissue. This leads to damage of the nerve, vascular, and connective tissues.

157. **B)** The main mechanism of radiation-induced myelopathy is transient demyelination.

158. **C)** Prostate cancer is associated with blastic bone metastases.

159. **A)** The intercostobrachial nerve is the lateral cutaneous nerve of the second thoracic nerve root. It provides sensation to the medial, posterior portion of the arm and axilla and the lateral portion of the chest wall. It is affected by axillary lymph node dissection and presents with absent or abnormal sensation and neuropathic pain.

160. **A)** Common side effects of opiate therapy include nausea/vomiting, constipation, drowsiness, dizziness, and tolerance. Opioids should be prescribed at the lowest possible dose to provide analgesia and to improve the patient's function. Tolerance, or loss of analgesic potency, is one of the most common complications of opioid therapy leading to decreased effectiveness over time. Constipation is a common problem occurring in almost all patients using opiates. Severe constipation may force the patient to stop opioid use. A comprehensive bowel program must be part of opioid prescription in the cancer setting.

161. **C)** Plexopathy resulting from radiation can take months or years to develop. It usually presents with numbness and paresthesias. It must be differentiated from tumor recurrence, which can cause brachial plexopathy. An MRI of the brachial plexus with contrast can rule out axillary recurrence of breast cancer. Electrodiagnostic testing can help differentiate brachial plexopathy from other neurologic conditions. Typical findings include myokymia on needle electromyography.

162. **A)** An unstable metastatic lesion is best treated with fixation. Much has been done to try to develop a way to tell which lesions are unstable. Lytic lesions that measure more than 2/3 of the cortex and those that present with functional pain are at greater chance for pathologic fracture.

163. **C)** Antibiotics have not shown to be effective in lymphedema treatment. Patients who have lymphedema are predisposed to cellulitis, for which antibiotic treatment is needed. The treatment of lymphedema is with manual lymphatic drainage, compression garments, and patient education.

164. **B)** MLD is a gentle massage that increases the natural drainage of the lymph from the body. It simulates the rhythmic contractions of smooth muscle cells in the walls of lymph vessels. MLD uses a specific amount of pressure and rhythmic circular movements to stimulate lymph flow. Compression garments are worn both as therapeutic and maintenance modalities.

165. **D)** Pathologic fractures can be a complication of or the initial presentation of bone metastases. They usually occur as a result of the progression of bony disease. Hypercalcemia in patients with cancer is primarily due to increased bone resorption and the release of calcium from bone. Epidural metastasis is the most ominous complication of bone metastasis to the vertebral spine and is a medical emergency. The tumor enters the epidural space by contiguous spread from adjacent vertebral metastasis. Failure to properly diagnose this condition can lead to spinal cord injury and permanent neurological damage. Signs of spinal cord compression include motor, sensory, and autonomic (bladder and bowel) dysfunction.

166. **A)** Post-thoracotomy pain syndrome presents as pain lasting more than 2 months at the incision site/distribution of the intercostal nerve. It can result from dissection of latissimus dorsi, serratus, and separation of the ribs. Clinically, it presents with lancinating pain in the distribution of the nerve, allodynia, and dysesthesias.

167. **A)** There is increasing evidence that bisphosphonates can prevent bony complications in metastatic malignant diseases and may even improve survival in patients with multiple myeloma with lytic bone lesions. Bisphosphonates inhibit osteoclastic bone resorption. They have been proven to reduce pain and SREs, including fractures, need for radiation or surgery, and hypercalcemia.

168. **D)** Lytic lesions predominate in the cancers listed as well as cancers of melanoma, thyroid, and non-Hodgkin's lymphoma.

169. **C)** When assessing spine stability, the spine can be divided into three columns. The anterior column consists of anterior longitudinal ligament, anterior annulus, and anterior 2/3 of vertebral body. The middle column consists of the posterior 1/3 of the vertebral body, posterior annulus, and posterior longitudinal ligament. The posterior column consists of the pedicles, facets, lamina, spinous process, and posterior ligaments. The spine is considered stable if only one column is affected, unless it is the middle column. It is considered unstable if two or more columns are involved. It is also considered unstable if there is a 20° or greater angulation. The spine stability system was developed for the traumatic spine. However, the issues are more complex in cancer. Metastatic bone disease is a dynamic disease, with both mechanical and chemical forces acting on the bone.

170. **A)** Myokymic discharges are groups of motor unit action potentials that fire synchronously. On needle EMG, it is classically noted in radiation plexopathy. The sound of the discharge has been described as "marching soldiers."

171. **A)** Corticosteroids are usually considered the initial therapy for brain lesions in cancer patients. Corticosteroids can reduce peritumoral edema and local brain compression.

172. **A)** In multiple myeloma, collections of abnormal plasma cells accumulate in the bone marrow, where they produce a paraprotein, which can cause kidney disease, bone lesions (lytic), and hypercalcemia.

173. **D)** Lymphedema is a high-protein edema, which is caused by a blockage in the lymphatic system. It is seen most commonly in breast cancer surgery with lymph node removal and also in pelvic surgery as well as head and neck surgery. It is graded from 1 to 3. Grade 1 is pitting edema, which is partially reversible with elevation, grade 2 is nonpitting edema, which is not reduced by elevation. Grade 3—such as in elephantiasis—is enormous swelling of the involved area.

174. **D)** Oncologists use tumor response, patient wishes, and patient's functional status to decide whether a patient should have more chemotherapy. The Karnofsky performance scale index allows patients to be classified as to their functional impairment. The scoring is from 0 to 100, with a 100 being normal. It can be used to compare the effectiveness of different therapies and to assess the prognosis in individual patients. The lower the Karnofsky score, the worse the chances of survival for most serious illnesses.

175. **B)** Bone scan will be negative in lytic lesions, as seen in multiple myeloma. Bone scans should be ordered along with x-ray.

176. **A)** The most common upper extremity bone involved in bony metastases is the humerus (20%). Although the humerus is not normally a weight-bearing bone, in patients who have functional impairments, there may be a greater dependence on upper extremity for weight bearing during transfers as well as using an assistive device. Special walkers to offload the involved extremity may be needed.

177. **A)** Contrast MRI is the best radiologic tool to diagnose brain tumors.

178. **B)** Generalized weakness is considered the most common rehabilitation problem for patients with cancer.

179. **B)** Breast cancer (and its treatment) is the most common cause of upper extremity lymphedema.

180. **A)** Radiation-induced ectopic activity in the trigeminal nerve leads to neuropathic pain, weakness, and spasm of the masseter muscle.

181. **A)** Ondansetron is a selective serotonin 5-$HT_3$ receptor antagonist. It is thought that chemotherapeutic agents produce nausea and vomiting by releasing serotonin from the enterochromaffin cells of the small intestines. The released serotonin then activates 5-$HT_3$ receptors located on vagal efferents to initiate the vomiting reflex. Ondansetron works by blocking the reception of serotonin at these 5-$HT_3$ receptors.

182. **A)** Tracer accumulates in new bone that is formed in response to a new lesion and can occur at any site with bone turnover. It is extremely nonspecific; only 50% of foci represent cancer. Positive scans require further radiologic confirmation.

183. **D)** X-rays have poor sensitivity for bony lesions. Fifty percent of bone mass must be destroyed before a bony lesion is seen on a radiograph. Bone scans have good sensitivity, but very poor specificity. The test will be positive at any site where there is bone turnover. Together, the two

are good first-screening tests. In a patient with a high suspicion of metastatic disease, often PET scan, CT, or MRI will be used.

184. **A)** The most common initial clinical presentation of brain tumors is headache. The pain is usually intermittent, moderate to severe in intensity, and progressive. Other symptoms include nausea/vomiting, ataxia, weakness, speech deficits, and sensory abnormalities. Symptoms will depend on the size, location, and type of tumor. A complete neurologic examination is essential.

185. **B)** One indication for VFSS is silent aspiration among cancer patients.

186. **A)** EMG can reveal myokymic discharges in patients with radiation plexitis. Fibrillation potentials are seen with denervation; polyphasic potentials suggest a chronic process of denervation and reinnervation. Small-amplitude motor units are typically seen in myopathy.

187. **D)** Trismus, a condition seen as a sequela of radiation therapy in head and neck cancer, is the inability to open the mouth fully as a result of spasm in the masseter and lateral pterygoid muscles. In addition, radiation therapy can affect the surrounding local connective tissue, which contributes to the spasm.

188. **D)** Breast, prostate, and lung are the most common cancers to metastasize to bone.

189. **A)** Osteogenic sarcoma is the sixth most common cancer in children below age 15 years. A second peak in incidence occurs in the elderly, usually associated with an underlying bone pathology, such as Paget's disease or a prior history of radiation. Osteochondromas are benign.

190. **A)** The most common site of metastases is the vertebral bodies of the thoracic spine (70%).

191. **A)** Swallowing disorders are very commonly seen in CNS tumors and may be due to the tumor itself, surgery, chemotherapy, or radiation therapy. Patients with head and neck tumors present with swallowing dysfunction due to their tumor and/or as a result of radiation therapy. Radiation therapy leads to fibrosis of the pharyngeal muscles. Cognitive impairment is also associated with swallowing dysfunction.

192. **A)** Pain is usually the classic presenting symptom, preceding the others. An acute onset of back pain in a patient with cancer is metastasis until proven otherwise. Pain is usually progressive, not relieved with rest, and worse at night. Weakness and bowel/bladder dysfunction in a cancer patient is suspicious for spinal cord compression.

193. **D)** Contraindications to cardiac rehabilitation are related to the risk of intense physical activity. The most common disorders in which exercise is contraindicated include aortic dissection, aortic aneurysm, unstable angina, recent pulmonary embolism, and severe aortic stenosis. Although strenuous exercise is prohibited, other components of cardiac rehabilitation, such as heart-healthy nutrition education, minimizing risk factors, and optimizing mental health should be implemented.

194. **A)** Intense active and passive range-of-motion exercises are critical in burn patients for prevention of contractures. However, immobilization is indicated in patients with bone and tendon injury, recent skin grafts, and open wounds. Stretching of damaged tendons due to burn may lead to rupture. Immediate range of motion for burns to the face, hands/feet, and genitalia is critical. Facial burns are known to cause contractures to the eyelids and commissures of the mouth. Hands and feet are prone to contractures of the webbing between fingers and toes. Finally, burn wounds around genitalia may lead to complications in voiding.

195. **B)** Up to 60% of chronic cancer patients will experience pain. The most common cause of pain in cancer patients is compression of the tumor onto bones, nerves, spinal cord, and other internal organs.

196. **B)** The ultimate goal for COPD patients participating in pulmonary rehabilitation is to decrease dyspnea by increasing endurance. Long-duration, as opposed to short-duration, exercises have been found to optimize function and reduce dyspnea over time. Inspiratory muscle training and chest physiotherapy are less effective and thus adjuncts in treatment of COPD patients in pulmonary rehabilitation.

# Prosthetics, Orthotics, Assistive Devices, and Gait

## QUESTIONS

1. Which is **not** a pressure-sensitive area in regard to lower extremity prosthetics?
   A) Pretibial muscles
   B) Hamstring tendons
   C) Patella
   D) Distal tibia

2. When compared with normal walking without a prosthesis or assistive device, which condition requires the greatest increase in energy expenditure?
   A) Transtibial amputation
   B) Transfemoral amputation
   C) Bilateral transtibial
   D) Wheelchair use

3. What is the most common congenital upper extremity limb deficiency?
   A) Transradial
   B) Transhumeral
   C) Absence of ulna
   D) Absence of carpal, metacarpals, and phalanges

4. How is myodesis different from myoplasty?
   A) Myodesis refers to suturing agonist-antagonist muscles to each other
   B) Myoplasty refers to suturing agonist muscles to each other
   C) Myodesis refers to directly suturing residual muscle or tendon to bone/periosteum
   D) Myodesis refers to suturing tendons together

5. Which of the following is a common dermatological problem in patients with prosthetic devices?
   A) Hyperhidrosis
   B) Acne
   C) Melanoma
   D) Erysipelas

6. What is the "safe" position of the hand (to prevent claw deformity)?
   A) Wrist extended, metacarpophalangeal (MCP) joint flexed, proximal interphalangeal (PIP) joint extended, distal interphalangeal (DIP) joint extended
   B) Wrist flexed, MCP flexed, PIP flexed, DIP flexed
   C) Wrist extended, MCP extended, PIP extended, DIP extended
   D) Wrist flexed, MCP extended, PIP flexed, DIP flexed

ANSWERS TO THIS SECTION CAN BE FOUND ON PAGE 289

7. This device is used for cubital tunnel syndrome:
   A) Long arm splint
   B) Flail arm splint
   C) Elbow flexion splint
   D) Wrist flexion splint

8. Which of these devices assists with plantar flexion?
   A) Anterior stop
   B) Posterior stop
   C) Anterior spring
   D) Posterior spring

9. Which orthosis is useful for anterior cruciate ligament (ACL) tears or postop repair?
   A) Cho-Pat strap
   B) Swedish knee cage
   C) Craig-Scott orthosis
   D) Lenox Hill derotation orthosis

10. Where does most of cervical rotation occur?
    A) C1 to C2
    B) C3 to C4
    C) C4 to C5
    D) C6 to C7

11. Which of these thoracolumbosacral orthoses (TLSO) cannot be used on an unstable thoracolumbar spine fracture?
    A) Jewett brace
    B) Cruciform anterior spinal hyperextension (CASH) brace
    C) Molded plastic TLSO
    D) Taylor's brace

*Changing Q be word says these are all CI in unstable except for one. One of these is least stable. Two are intermed stable. One is most stable for unstable fx*

12. When using standard crutches, how many inches should the patient be able to raise the body with complete elbow extension?
    A) 0 to 1 in.
    B) 1 to 2 in.
    C) 2 to 3 in.
    D) 3 to 4 in.

13. A rocker knife and bottle stabilizer are beneficial in an individual with which of the following conditions?
    A) Hemiplegia
    B) Paraplegia
    C) Shoulder pain
    D) Spasticity

14. All of the following are pressure-tolerant areas for a below-knee amputation prosthetic except:
    A) Patellar tendon
    B) Medial tibial flare
    C) Fibular head
    D) Popliteal fossa—gastroc-soleus muscles

15. All of the following are reasonable pharmacologic interventions for the treatment of phantom pain **except**:
    A) Tricyclic antidepressants
    B) Serotonin reuptake inhibitors
    C) Narcotics
    D) Anticonvulsants

16. Which amputation allows a patient to stand easily and walk on the end of the residual limb without wearing a prosthesis for short household distances?
    A) Long transtibial
    B) Syme's
    C) Short transtibial
    D) Hemicorporectomy

17. What does the term *prehensile* mean?
    A) Balance
    B) Grasp by wrapping around
    C) Weakness in the arm
    D) Apprehension

18. How often does a prosthesis need to be replaced in a child age 0 to 5 years?
    A) Every 6 months
    B) Every 12 months
    C) Every 18 months
    D) Every 24 months

19. What is the natural position caused by the resting muscle tension of the hand?
    A) Wrist flexed, metacarpophalangeal (MCP) joint flexed, proximal interphalangeal (PIP) joint flexed, distal interphalangeal (DIP) joint flexed
    B) Wrist extended, MCP extended, PIP flexed, DIP flexed
    C) Wrist flexed, MCP extended, PIP flexed, DIP flexed
    D) Wrist extended, MCP extended, PIP extended, DIP extended

20. A patient with a C6-level spinal cord injury would find this splint useful to help pick up small objects using a three-jaw chuck pinch:
    A) Kleinert splint
    B) Adaptive usage device splint
    C) Dynamic splint
    D) Rehabilitation Institute of Chicago tenodesis splint

21. Which of these are considerations for an orthosis to prevent diabetic foot ulcers?
    A) Increase friction to reduce slippage
    B) Cosmesis
    C) Reduce shear forces
    D) Allow for wound healing

22. What would you **not** tell a paraplegic patient who is inquiring about using a knee-ankle-foot orthosis (KAFO)?
    A) Using a KAFO requires a lot of energy
    B) Your KAFO can replace your wheelchair as your primary means of locomotion in time

C) You should use forearm crutches while walking with a KAFO

D) Ambulation with a KAFO uses a swing-through gait

23. Which spinal segment has the greatest range of motion?
   A) Cervical
   B) Thoracic
   C) Lumbar
   D) Sacral

24. What is the highest thoracic spine level for which a clamshell brace is effective in immobilizing the lower trunk?
   A) T1
   B) T5
   C) T8
   D) T11

25. When the patient is standing upright, the top of a walker should reach which anatomic location?
   A) Xiphoid process
   B) Greater trochanter
   C) Pubic symphysis
   D) Iliac crest

26. All of the following are components of a transtibial prosthesis **except**:
   A) Socket
   B) Rotor
   C) Shank
   D) Suspension

27. Which of the following describes an awareness of a nonpainful sensation in the amputated part?
   A) Allodynia
   B) Phantom pain
   C) Hyperalgesia
   D) Phantom sensation

28. The surgical removal of the entire lower limb plus all or a major portion of the ileum is known as what type of amputation?
   A) Hemipelvectomy
   B) Hip disarticulation
   C) Boyd's amputation
   D) Pirogoff's amputation

29. What is a forequarter amputation?
   A) Involves removal of part of the humerus
   B) Involves removal of part of the radius and ulna
   C) Involves removal of the entire humerus, radius, ulna, carpals, metacarpals, and phalanges
   D) Involves removal of the scapula, part or all of the clavicle, entire humerus, radius, ulna, carpals, metacarpals, and phalanges

30. What is the preferred term for the remaining portion of the limb after amputation?
   A) Residual limb
   B) Stump

C) Stub
D) Postsurgical limb

31. What often occurs in a child with a congenital limb deficiency?
    A) The prosthesis is perceived as an aid rather than a replacement
    B) The child usually experiences a sense of loss as the limb was absent from birth
    C) The child puts limitations on himself or herself
    D) Phantom pain is common

32. What type of splint would you use on a boxer's fracture?
    A) Stax splint
    B) Resting hand splint
    C) Ulnar gutter splint
    D) Wrist splint

33. A patient has weakened peroneus longus muscles. What kind of foot orthotic should be placed in his or her shoe to prevent the ankle from rolling?
    A) Medial wedge
    B) Lateral wedge
    C) Heel cushion
    D) Rocker bar

34. What type of T-strap is used for someone with a valgus ankle deformity?
    A) Medial T-strap
    B) Lateral T-strap
    C) Superior T-strap
    D) Posterior T-strap

35. Which can occur when using a spinal orthoses?
    A) Strengthening of upper extremity muscles
    B) Weakening of axial muscles
    C) Weakening of lower extremity muscles
    D) Weakening of upper extremity muscles

36. Which orthosis is used for low-back pain during pregnancy?
    A) Lumbosacral orthosis (LSO) with a rigid frame
    B) Corset
    C) Wide belt
    D) Rainey orthosis

37. A patient with which nerve palsy would most benefit from the activities of daily living (ADL) splint seen here?
    A) Median
    B) Ulnar
    C) Radial
    D) Musculocutaneous

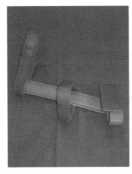
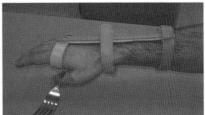

38. Which of the following would be acceptable in contracture prevention for the patient with a transtibial amputation?
    A) Sitting with the knee extended on a towel-wrapped board under the wheelchair cushion
    B) Sitting with the residual limb hanging over the edge of the bed
    C) Sitting with a pillow placed under the knee
    D) Sitting with a pillow placed between the legs

39. Which dermatologic complication results from inadequate socket-wall contact with subsequent edema formation causing wart-like skin overgrowth?
    A) Tinea corporis
    B) Verrucous hyperplasia
    C) Hyperhidrosis
    D) Folliculitis

40. Which of the following is **not** a cause for a circumducted gait in a transfemoral amputee patient with a prosthesis?
    A) Prosthesis is too long
    B) Inadequate suspension
    C) Abduction contracture of the residual limb
    D) Too much adduction built into the prosthesis

41. Which of the following acquired upper-extremity amputations is the most common in the United States?
    A) Above the elbow/transhumeral
    B) Below the elbow/transradial
    C) Wrist disarticulation
    D) Shoulder disarticulation

42. What is the name for the amputation that removes the entire radius, ulna, carpals, metacarpals, and phalanges?
    A) Below the elbow
    B) Above the elbow
    C) Mid-elbow
    D) Elbow disarticulation

43. Which of the following body actions will **not** activate the terminal device on an upper-extremity prosthetic?
    A) Scapular abduction
    B) Shoulder extension
    C) Chest expansion
    D) Humeral flexion

44. With finger sprains, what is the best position for the digits?
    A) Proximal interphalangeal joint (PIP) flexed, allowed distal interphalangeal joint (DIP) flexion
    B) PIP extended, allowed DIP flexion
    C) PIP flexed, DIP fixed extended
    D) PIP extended, DIP fixed extended

45. A patient with a leg length discrepancy needs a 1-in. heel lift. How high should the outer sole be?
    A) 1/4 in.
    B) 1/2 in.

C) 3/4 in.
D) 1 in.

46. What can be placed on a double metal upright type ankle-foot orthotic (AFO) for someone with mediolateral ankle instability?
   A) Figure 8 strap
   B) T-strap
   C) Posterior stop
   D) Anterior stop

47. What adjustments to the shoe would be good for a patient with pes planus?
   A) Lateral sole flare
   B) Thomas' heel
   C) Reverse Thomas' heel
   D) Rocker bottom sole

48. Which truncal orthosis uses a three-point pressure system to allow for extension but limit flexion?
   A) Jewett brace
   B) Williams' brace
   C) Taylor's brace
   D) Clamshell brace

49. Which of the following assistive devices would be **most** appropriate for a patient with Parkinson's disease?

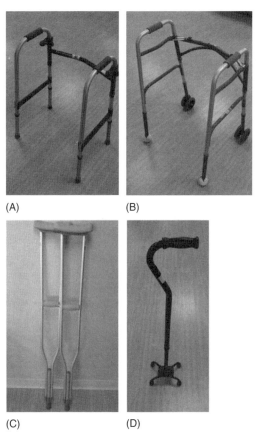

(A)          (B)

(C)          (D)

50. In the postoperative management of the residual limb, a "shrinker" should be worn for how many hours out of the day?
    A) 24
    B) 12
    C) 8
    D) Shrinkers are not used after amputation

51. Brawny edema, induration, and discoloration of the skin of the distal stump in a circular shape may indicate which dermatologic complication in an amputee patient?
    A) Allergic dermatitis
    B) Epidermoid cyst
    C) Folliculitis
    D) Choked stump syndrome

52. When assessing gait for the transtibial amputee patient, which is the cause of high pressure against the patella throughout most of the stance phase, as well as the heel being off the floor when standing?
    A) Foot too far posterior
    B) Foot too dorsiflexed
    C) Foot too plantar-flexed
    D) Foot too far anterior

53. What is a congenital terminal limb deficiency?
    A) A deficiency in the long axis
    B) A deficiency in the short or transverse axis
    C) A deficiency of both long and short axes
    D) An absence of a joint

54. Which of the following is important in the acute postop period for the new amputee patient?
    A) Immediate fitting of the prosthesis
    B) Skin desensitization
    C) Maintaining bed rest to ensure adequate healing
    D) Keeping the extremity dependent to encourage drainage

55. Which of the following is **not** a key function of the prosthetic socket?
    A) Adequate cosmesis
    B) Secure suspension of prosthesis
    C) Efficient energy transference to the prosthesis
    D) Grasp objects

56. What type of injury is lateral epicondylitis?
    A) Tendonitis
    B) Tenosynovitis
    C) Enthesopathy
    D) Sprain

57. What is the longest leg-length discrepancy that would **not** need correction?
    A) 1/4 in.
    B) 1/2 in.
    C) 1 in.
    D) 2 in.

**58.** How is the hip placed in an orthosis for someone with Legg-Calvè-Perthes (LCP) disease?
A) Abduction and external rotation
B) Adduction and internal rotation
C) Abduction and internal rotation
D) Adduction and external rotation

**59.** Which of the following does **not** promote knee flexion?
A) Cushioned heel
B) Posterior stop
C) Posterior ground reactive force
D) Ankle dorsiflexion

**60.** Which of these back braces is primarily used for stable vertebral anterior compression fractures?
A) Williams' brace
B) Chairback brace
C) Taylor's brace
D) Knight brace

**61.** This cervical orthosis is useful for bedridden patients with a C1 fracture as it does **not** have posterior uprights:
A) Minerva brace
B) Miami collar
C) Sterno-occipital-mandibular immobilizer (SOMI)
D) Halo Vest

**62.** What is the ideal shape for a transtibial residual limb?
A) Rectangular
B) Conical
C) Pyramidal
D) Cylindrical

**63.** Which of the following knee units **cannot** be used with a bilateral transfemoral amputee patient?
A) Polycentric/four-bar knee
B) Manual locking knee
C) Stance-control knee
D) Fluid-controlled knee unit

**64.** In describing prosthetic feet, what does SACH stand for?
A) Solid action cushioned heel
B) Single-axis ankle cooperative heel
C) Single assembly coordinated heel
D) Solid ankle cushioned heel

**65.** Why is a disarticulation (separation at the joint level) of upper extremity amputation preferred in children?
A) More cosmetic
B) Preserves epiphyses
C) Easier to fit with a prosthesis
D) Easier to perform activities of daily living (ADLs)

66. Which of the following is true about amputee patients?
    A) It is okay to delay a visit to the rehabilitation physician and prosthetic team until 6 months postamputation
    B) It is best for the patient to be seen by the rehabilitation physician and prosthetic team prior to surgery
    C) It is best for the patient to be seen by the rehabilitation physician and prosthetic team 2 to 4 weeks after surgery
    D) It is best for the patient to be seen by the rehabilitation physician and prosthetic team only after the residual limb has healed

67. What is a benefit of an immediate postop rigid dressing (IPORD)?
    A) Desensitization of the residual limb
    B) Prevent falls
    C) Improve gait training
    D) Decrease cost

68. A patient presents with wrist pain. He has pain when gripping a cup handle. You notice a positive Finkelstein's test. What brace would you recommend for this patient?
    A) Volar wrist splint
    B) Radial nerve palsy splint
    C) Resting hand splint
    D) Thumb spica splint

69. Which hand orthosis employs wrist extension for closing the hand?
    A) Wrist-hand orthosis
    B) Wrist orthosis
    C) Tenodesis orthosis
    D) Kleinert orthosis

70. A patient wearing a new ankle-foot orthotic (AFO) starts complaining of numbness in his foot. He says that it feels a little tight on the upper part of the orthosis. You notice that the top of the AFO is at the level of the fibular head. What can you suggest to this patient?
    A) Widen the upper brim of the orthosis
    B) Add some padding to the upper brim
    C) Find another orthotist
    D) Adjust the AFO by taking away 1 in. from the upper brim

71. A patient has weak plantar flexors. What adjustments to his shoes can you make to assist him?
    A) A rocker bar at the sole of the shoe
    B) Thomas' orthopedic heel
    C) Medial sole and heel wedging
    D) Reverse Thomas' heel

72. A patient has a stable C4 fracture. Which cervical orthosis would be appropriate?
    A) Soft collar
    B) Philadelphia collar
    C) Halo Vest
    D) Minerva

73. This lumbosacral brace has two posterior uprights that prevent extension, and an anterior apron with two anterior straps: one at the thorax and one at the pelvis that limit flexion:
    A) Rainey jacket
    B) Clamshell brace
    C) Milwaukee brace
    D) Chairback brace

74. A weighted utensil as shown here would be most beneficial for an individual with which of the following conditions?
    A) Parkinson's disease
    B) Hemiplegia
    C) Paraplegia
    D) Osteoarthritis

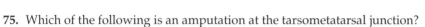

75. Which of the following is an amputation at the tarsometatarsal junction?
    A) Transmetatarsal
    B) Syme's
    C) Lisfranc
    D) Chopart's

76. The Silesian belt, total elastic suspension belt, and pelvic band are all types of suspension for which type of prosthesis?
    A) Below-knee amputation (transtibial)
    B) Above-knee amputation (transfemoral)
    C) Hip disarticulation
    D) Syme's amputation

77. Which level patient, in following Medicare regulations, is **not** a candidate for a prosthesis?
    A) Level 0
    B) Level 1
    C) Level 2
    D) Level 3

78. What is the most commonly used suspension for a transradial amputee patient?
    A) Suction
    B) Figure 8 (O ring) harness
    C) Figure 9 harness
    D) Chest strap with shoulder saddle

79. What is the best type of medication for the treatment of phantom pain?
    A) Opioid
    B) Selective serotonin reuptake inhibitor (SSRI)
    C) Tricyclic antidepressant (TCA)
    D) Acetaminophen

80. What is true about edema as a complication following upper amputation surgery?
    A) It is an uncommon complication
    B) A figure 8 dressing should not be used
    C) The ideal shape of the residual limb is cylindrical
    D) It is okay to rewrap the residual limb every 24 hours to provide optimum edema control

81. What type of splint is a swan-neck splint?
    A) Static motion blocking
    B) Static progressive
    C) Serial static
    D) Nonarticular

82. This device holds the arm in abduction to help prevent contractures after an axillary burn or to ensure healing after a shoulder fusion:
    A) Airplane splint
    B) Shoulder sling
    C) Jewett brace
    D) Balanced forearm orthosis

83. Which ankle-foot orthosis (AFO) can be used for someone with a foot drop and weak quadriceps?
    A) AFO with posterior foot stop
    B) Solid AFO
    C) AFO with posterior stop with a Klenzak joint
    D) Solid AFO with anterior and posterior stops

84. You notice that your patient has a valgus deformity at the ankle when he walks. What adjustments to his shoe can you suggest so that his gait is more stable?
    A) Cushioned heel
    B) Medial heel flare
    C) Lateral heel flare
    D) Heel lift

85. A patient with a C2 fracture is placed on a Halo Vest. How long does he have to wear the vest?
    A) 6 weeks
    B) 9 weeks
    C) 12 weeks
    D) 18 weeks

86. This brace is used in patients with spondylolisthesis. It restricts extension, but allows flexion, as the front is made up of an elastic band. It also has side uprights that prevent lateral bending:
    A) Williams' brace
    B) Chairback brace
    C) Rainey jacket
    D) Taylor's brace

87. A scoop dish or plate guard, as depicted here, would be most beneficial in an individual with which of the following conditions?
    A) Parkinson's disease
    B) Hemiplegia
    C) Paraplegia
    D) Osteoarthritis

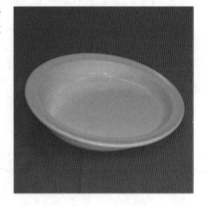

88. In a standard transtibial amputation, the amputation is approximately what percentage of the tibial length?
    A) Less than 20
    B) 20 to 50
    C) Greater than 50
    D) Greater than 75

89. Tenderness on the anterior distal femur, lateral lurch when walking, and increased skin irritation at the ischium and pubis are all disadvantages of which above-knee amputation socket?
    A) Narrow mediolateral
    B) Ischial containment
    C) Contoured adductor trochanteric-controlled alignment method (CAT-CAM)
    D) Quadrilateral transfemoral

90. According to Medicare regulations, what is the reimbursement level (K-level) for unilateral transtibial or transfemoral prosthesis where the patient has the ability or potential to ambulate with variable cadence and traverse environmental barriers?
    A) Level 1
    B) Level 2
    C) Level 3
    D) Level 4

91. What is the most commonly used type of terminal device in the upper extremity?
    A) Passive
    B) Voluntary closing
    C) Voluntary opening
    D) Myoelectric

92. What is the difference between phantom sensation and phantom pain?
    A) Phantom pain is pain perceived in the intact part of the limb
    B) Phantom pain is the same as phantom sensation
    C) Phantom sensation is nonpainful perception of the missing part of the limb
    D) Phantom sensation is painful perception of the missing part of the limb

93. What is a benefit of elbow disarticulation surgery as opposed to transradial or transhumeral?
    A) Less blood loss
    B) Better functional outcomes
    C) Better prosthetic fit
    D) Better cosmesis

94. What type of splint is a gel shell splint?
    A) Static
    B) Dynamic
    C) Nonarticular
    D) Adaptive

95. Which one of these hand functions would a monkey be able to perform?
    A) Give an "okay" sign
    B) Hold onto a handrail
    C) Turn a key in a lock
    D) Hold onto a baseball and throw it with one hand

96. Which of the following is an ankle-foot orthosis (AFO) with the footplate set in slight plantar flexion to help with stability at the knee during full extension for patients with weak quadriceps?
    A) Posterior assist AFO
    B) Posterior stop AFO
    C) Anterior stop AFO
    D) Floor reaction AFO

97. Which one of these does **not** promote knee extension?
    A) Cushioned heel
    B) Ankle plantar flexion
    C) Anterior ground reactive force
    D) Posterior stop

98. Which of the following cervical orthoses does **not** limit rotation?
    A) Halo Vest
    B) Minerva brace
    C) Aspen collar
    D) Sterno-occipital-mandibular immobilizer (SOMI)

99. This cervical orthosis consists of one anterior poster supporting the chin and one posterior poster supporting the occiput that attaches to a thoracic jacket:
    A) Rainey orthosis
    B) Sterno-occipital-mandibular immobilizer (SOMI)
    C) Minerva brace
    D) Aspen collar

100. This assistive device is helpful when putting on which garment?
    A) Gloves
    B) Socks
    C) Pants
    D) Shoes

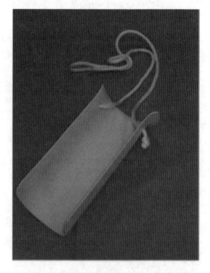

101. In general, what is the most common type of amputation seen among new amputee patients?
    A) Transfemoral
    B) Syme's
    C) Transtibial
    D) Hip disarticulation

102. Which of the following prosthetic options would allow for participation in the most vigorous of sports?
    A) Flex-foot
    B) Single-axis foot
    C) Rigid keel
    D) Multi-axis foot

103. What will be the result of a heel cushion that is too soft, or a prosthetic foot in excessive plantarflexion?
    A) Excessive knee flexion
    B) Insufficient knee flexion
    C) Excessive knee extension
    D) Insufficient knee extension

104. What is the definition of a prosthesis?
    A) An artificial substitute for a missing body part
    B) An external device applied to intact body parts to provide support
    C) A brace
    D) A device used to assist with balance

105. Which of the following is **not** an immediate goal of rehabilitation care after amputation?
    A) Wound healing
    B) Edema control
    C) Prevention of contractures
    D) Treadmill training

106. Which of the following is true about joint contractures after amputation surgery?
    A) Prevention is harder than treatment
    B) It is okay to wait to prevent joint contractures until many weeks after amputation surgery
    C) It will not increase the patient's risk of contracture if there is a burn present
    D) In the case of a concomitant nerve injury, passive and assisted range of motion should be implemented to preserve joint mobility

107. Which type of orthotic hand support uses nonelastic components such as hinges, screws, and turn buckles to place a force on the joint to induce change and eventually increase range of motion?
    A) Serial static splint
    B) Static progressive
    C) Continuous passive motion orthosis
    D) Adaptive usage splint

108. Which one of these functions are monkeys **not** able to do?
    A) Palmar prehension
    B) Hook prehension
    C) Cylindrical grasp
    D) Monkeys can perform all the above

109. Which type of ankle-foot orthosis (AFO) is used when clonus is present at the ankle?
    A) Solid AFO
    B) Posterior assist
    C) Anterior assist
    D) Floor reaction brace

110. A patient presents with knee pain. She tells you she just started running again recently. You find that she has patellar tracking disorder. What orthotic do you suggest she use while she is running?
    A) Moon boots
    B) Cho-Pat strap
    C) Lenox Hill derotation orthosis
    D) Bledsoe brace

111. Which lumbar segment is the most mobile?
    A) L2 to L3
    B) L4 to L5
    C) L3 to L4
    D) L1 to L2

112. Which of these orthoses is used to decrease kyphosis from a stable vertebral anterior compression fracture by applying an anterior crossbar to the torso?
    A) Taylor's brace
    B) Jewett brace
    C) Cruciform anterior spinal hyperextension (CASH) brace
    D) Boston brace

113. Which anatomic structure should be used as a reference point in order to determine the proper backrest height for a standard wheelchair?
    A) Iliac crest
    B) Posterior 12th rib
    C) Scapula
    D) T1 vertebrae

114. In patients aged 15 to 50 years, what is the most common cause of lower extremity amputation?
    A) Trauma
    B) Cancer
    C) Infection
    D) Vascular disease

115. Which of the following options for a prosthetic foot is the most affordable?
    A) Multi-axis foot
    B) Solid ankle cushion heel (SACH)
    C) Energy storing
    D) Single-axis foot

116. A patient with which type of amputation will expend the most energy compared with normal walking?
    A) Transfemoral-transtibial
    B) Bilateral transtibial
    C) Transfemoral with use of crutch
    D) Transfemoral

117. What is the leading cause of acquired amputation in the upper extremity?
    A) Cancer
    B) Diabetes
    C) Trauma
    D) Burns

**118.** In order to increase the likelihood of prosthetic use, how soon after surgery should an upper limb amputee patient be fitted with a prosthesis?
   A) Immediately after surgery, within the first week
   B) 3 to 6 months after surgery
   C) 12 months after surgery
   D) At least 2 years after surgery

**119.** Which of the following is **not** a type of terminal device in upper limb prosthetics?
   A) Mechanical
   B) Electrical
   C) Passive
   D) Piston

**120.** Which hand pattern is useful for carrying heavy objects?
   A) Power grasp
   B) Oppositional pinch
   C) Hook pattern
   D) Precision grasp

**121.** This splint is useful after repair of the flexor hand tendons and allows for passive flexion of the digits at rest and active finger extension at the distal interphalangeal (DIP) and proximal interphalangeal (PIP) joints:
   A) Dynamic finger flexion splint forearm based
   B) Dynamic finger flexion splint hand based
   C) Kleinert splint
   D) Duran splint

**122.** Which one of these is an indication for using an ankle-foot orthosis (AFO) to improve a patient's gait?
   A) Amputation of the great toe
   B) Weak push off at late stance phase
   C) Anteroposterior instability at the ankle
   D) Foot fracture

**123.** Where is the ground reaction force (GRF) placed with an offset knee joint on a knee-ankle-foot orthosis (KAFO)?
   A) Medial
   B) Lateral
   C) Anterior
   D) Posterior

**124.** Where does the greatest amount of cervical flexion occur?
   A) C2 to C3
   B) C3 to C4
   C) C5 to C6
   D) C6 to C7

**125.** Which of these braces is used for low-thoracic scoliosis?
   A) Jewett brace
   B) Milwaukee brace
   C) Knight brace
   D) Williams' brace

126. When measuring a patient for a wheelchair, how many inches should the wheelchair width be in relation to the widest part of the buttocks?
    A) 0 in.
    B) 1 in. greater
    C) 2 in. greater
    D) 3 in. greater

*Match the following adaptive equipment labels to its associated photograph:*

127. Reacher

128. Dressing stick

129. Bottle or jar stabilizer

130. Rocker utensil

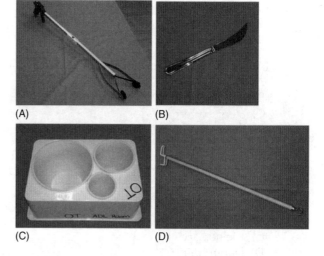

(A)  (B)

(C)  (D)

131. During which phase of the gait cycle is the center of gravity highest in walking?
    A) Midswing
    B) Midstance
    C) Terminal stance
    D) Terminal swing

132. A 60-year-old female complains of left hip pain with ambulation due to osteoarthritis of the left hip. You prescribe a single-point cane to
    A) Improve balance and stability
    B) Compensate for weakness of hip abductors
    C) Decrease weight-bearing forces across the painful arthritic hip
    D) Increase walking speed

133. Which of the following is **not** a cause of an abducted gait (wide-based gait)?
    A) Excessively long prosthesis
    B) Inguinal hernia
    C) Quadriceps weakness
    D) Hip arthritis

134. At what percentage of incline will the energy expenditure of walking double?
    A) 10% incline
    B) 20% incline
    C) 30% incline
    D) 40% incline

135. In which phase of the gait cycle are the calf muscles undergoing eccentric contraction?
    A) Initial contact
    B) Loading response
    C) Midstance
    D) Terminal stance

136. While evaluating a patient's gait, you note a shuffling gait with short step length and decreased arm swing. This best describes which of the following gait patterns?
    A) Hemiplegic gait
    B) Crouched gait
    C) Antalgic gait
    D) Parkinsonian gait

137. At how many degrees of knee flexion contracture do all of the phases of the gait cycle become abnormal and significantly interfere with ambulation?
    A) 5°
    B) 10°
    C) 20°
    D) 30°

138. Which of the following is **not** one of the three main events that consume energy during ambulation?
    A) Controlled deceleration at the end of swing phase
    B) Unloading the stance limb and transferring body weight to the contralateral limb in pre-swing phase
    C) Shock absorption with heel strike
    D) Forward propulsion of the center of mass at push-off

139. What percentage of the gait cycle consists of stance phase and swing phase during normal walking speed?
    A) 40% stance phase and 60% swing phase
    B) 50% stance phase and 50% swing phase
    C) 60% stance phase and 40% swing phase
    D) 70% stance phase and 30% swing phase

140. Which of the following is **not** one of the six determinants of gait?
    A) Pelvic tilt
    B) Knee extension
    C) Foot/ankle motion
    D) Lateral displacement of the pelvis

141. On average, at what age is an infant able to walk with support?
    A) 6 months
    B) 12 months
    C) 15 months
    D) 18 months

142. At what speed is normal walking on level surfaces most energy efficient?
    A) 1 mph
    B) 2 mph
    C) 3 mph
    D) 4 mph

143. Which crutch gait describes **both** crutches and involved limb (eg, lower extremity fracture) advancing together, then the uninvolved limb advancing forward?
   A) Two-point gait
   B) Three-point gait
   C) Swing-through gait
   D) Swing-to gait

*Match each of the following adaptive equipment labels to its associated photograph:*

144. Long-handled bath sponge

145. Pot stabilizer

146. Elongated utensil

147. Pronged cutting board

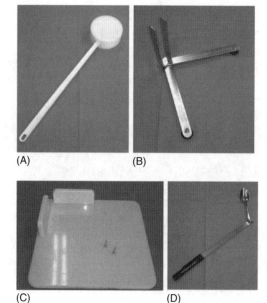

(A)      (B)

(C)      (D)

148. All of the following are typical components of a prosthesis **except**:
   A) Socket
   B) Liner
   C) Terminal device
   D) Computer-aided design (CAD) system

149. A patient is noted to have excessive hip and knee flexion on the right side during swing phase of the right limb. This best describes which of the following gait deviations?
   A) Circumduction
   B) Steppage gait
   C) Vaulting
   D) Trendelenburg gait

150. During gait evaluation of a patient, you observe a right genu recurvatum during the stance phase. Which of the following could be the cause?
   A) Right-ankle plantar flexion contracture
   B) Right hamstring weakness
   C) Right-ankle dorsiflexion contracture
   D) Right gluteus medius weakness

151. In the anatomic position, where is the usual center of mass in the human body?
    A) Directly through the second sacral vertebra
    B) 2 cm anterior to the second sacral vertebra
    C) Directly through the fifth lumbar vertebra
    D) 2 cm anterior to the fifth lumbar vertebra

152. Which crutch gait describes one crutch and opposite extremity moving together followed by the opposite crutch and extremity?
    A) Two-point gait
    B) Three-point gait
    C) Swing-through gait
    D) Swing-to gait

153. When measuring crutch length from the anterior axillary fold to the ground, how many inches span between the rubber end lateral to the fifth toe?
    A) 2 in.
    B) 4 in.
    C) 6 in.
    D) 8 in.

154. On physical examination, a patient is found to have knee extension strength of 2/5. Which of the following gait deviations will likely be present?
    A) Antalgic gait
    B) Extensor lurch gait
    C) Back knee gait
    D) Trendelenburg gait

155. Which of the following amputations requires the highest amount of energy to ambulate with prosthesis?
    A) Unilateral traumatic transtibial amputation
    B) Unilateral vascular transtibial amputation
    C) Unilateral vascular transfemoral amputation
    D) Bilateral transtibial amputation

156. Which of the following is **not** one of the four primary components of quantitative gait analysis?
    A) Kinematics
    B) Kinetics
    C) Equilibrium
    D) Energetics

157. Which crutch gait describes two crutches in contact with the floor and moving both limbs almost to the crutches?
    A) Two-point gait
    B) Three-point gait
    C) Swing-through gait
    D) Swing-to gait

158. Regarding points of contact with the body, what is the difference between a crutch and a cane?
    A) Cane has one point of contact with the body, whereas crutch has two points of contact with the body
    B) Cane has one point of contact with the body, whereas crutch has three points of contact with the body

    C) Cane has two points of contact with the body, whereas crutch has one point of contact with the body

    D) Cane has two points of contact with the body, whereas crutch has three points of contact with the body

159. Which of the following gait abnormalities would you likely see in a patient with chronic right hip osteoarthritis?
    A) Circumduction of the right hip
    B) Circumduction of the left hip
    C) Lateral trunk lean over the right hip
    D) Prolonged stance phase on right lower extremity

160. Walking is more costly in energy than wheelchair ambulation on level ground.
    A) True
    B) False

161. While observing the gait of a 45-year-old right transfemoral amputee patient, you notice exaggerated left plantar flexion during the swing phase of the prosthesis. This gait deviation may be due to which of the following?
    A) Inadequate suspension
    B) Prosthesis is too short
    C) Prosthesis is aligned in abduction
    D) Too much toe out

162. Which crutch gait describes two crutches in contact with the floor and moving both limbs past the crutches?
    A) Two-point gait
    B) Three-point gait
    C) Swing-through gait
    D) Swing-to gait

163. An individual with mildly impaired balance would require which of the following assistive devices?
    A) Single-point cane
    B) Quad cane
    C) Standing walker
    D) Rolling walker

164. The following description illustrates which phase of the gait cycle: From flat foot position until the contralateral foot is off the ground for swing?
    A) Loading response
    B) Mid-stance
    C) Terminal stance
    D) Preswing

165. During which phase of the gait cycle is the center of gravity the lowest while running?
    A) Mid-stance
    B) "Flight" phase
    C) Initial contact
    D) Preswing

166. A 33-year-old male with history of traumatic right transfemoral amputation is observed to have a right medial whip on gait evaluation. What is a possible cause of the medial whip?
    A) Insufficient friction in knee joint
    B) Heel is too firm
    C) Excessive external rotation of the knee
    D) Excessive internal rotation of the knee

167. What is another term commonly used for Lofstrand crutches?
    A) Hand crutches
    B) Wrist crutches
    C) Forearm crutches
    D) Axillary crutches

168. A platform-forearm orthosis would be beneficial in a patient with which of the following conditions?
    A) Cerebral palsy
    B) Ankylosing spondylitis
    C) Parkinson's disease
    D) Arthritis

169. The time from initial contact on the right foot to the following initial contact in the right foot describes which of the following?
    A) Step length
    B) Cadence
    C) Stride length
    D) Stride period

170. You are evaluating the gait of a 10-year-old female with spastic diplegia type cerebral palsy. Which of the following gait abnormalities is most likely to be observed?
    A) Initial contact with the heel
    B) Lack of full knee extension at midstance
    C) Wide base of support
    D) Increased stride length

171. Canes are prescribed by health care providers in various disabilities for which of the following reasons?
    A) Decrease ataxia
    B) Decrease pain and weight-bearing forces of injured structures
    C) Improve spasticity
    D) When the patient is non–weight bearing in the lower extremities

172. A 50-year-old male with a history of recent right transfemoral amputation is found to have a lateral trunk lean over the prosthetic limb in midstance. To what is this gait pattern likely due?
    A) Right hip adductor weakness
    B) Right hip abductor weakness
    C) Right hip extensor weakness
    D) Right hip flexor weakness

173. In which phase of the gait cycle is the gluteus maximus most active?
    A) Initial contact
    B) Midstance

C) Terminal stance

D) Midswing

174. A 55-year-old female with a history of left transfemoral amputation is found to have a circumduction gait pattern on the prosthetic side. Which of the following could be causing this gait pattern?

A) Left hip adduction contracture

B) A short prosthetic limb

C) Short stance phase on prosthetic limb

D) Excessive prosthetic knee friction

175. Individuals with which of the following conditions would most benefit from a black-and-white cutting board, as seen here?

A) Low vision

B) Essential tremor

C) Presbycusis

D) Ageusia

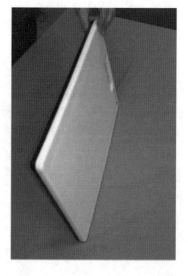

176. Which muscle(s) are normally active during quiet standing?

A) Gastroc-soleus

B) Tibialis anterior

C) Hamstrings

D) Quadriceps

177. As depicted here, which nerve would be affected in an individual who has decreased pincer grasp, hindering the ability to turn on the stove and requiring use of the adaptive device in the picture at left?

A) Median

B) Musculocutaneous

C) Ulnar

D) Radial

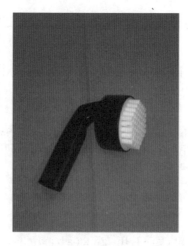 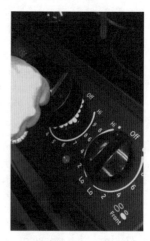

# Prosthetics, Orthotics, Assistive Devices, and Gait

## ANSWERS

1. **A)** The pretibial muscles are a pressure-tolerant area. Nevertheless, pressure should be equally distributed over this area. Hamstring tendons, patella, distal tibia, and fibula as well as the fibular head, tibial crest, tibial tubercle, and femoral condyles are all pressure-sensitive areas.

2. **B)** A transfemoral amputation increases energy expenditure by about 99%, whereas transtibial, bilateral transtibial, and wheelchair use increase energy expenditure by approximately 23%, 41%, and 9%, respectively.

3. **A)** Terminal transverse radial limb deficiency on the left side is the most common congenital upper limb deficiency.

4. **C)** Myoplasty refers to suturing agonist-antagonist muscles to each other. Myodesis refers to directly suturing residual muscle or tendon to bone/periosteum. It is important to retain the maximum amount of functioning muscle to ensure strength, shape, and circulation. The remaining distal muscles at the site of amputation must be secured and stabilized, and this is done with both myodesis and myoplasty.

5. **A)** Dermatological problems are common in patients who use a prosthetic device. Common problems include hyperhidrosis, folliculitis, allergic dermatitis, and skin breakdown. Appropriate hygiene can help to prevent these problems.

6. **A)** The goal for hand positioning is to prevent the development of a "claw" hand deformity. The wrist should be placed in slight extension. This helps the MCP collateral ligaments with maximum stretch, preserving the anatomic arches of the hand, and improving future function of the hand. This position also helps foster the weaker intrinsic muscles, which is difficult to obtain.

7. **A)** This splint is an immobilizing splint that holds the elbow in 45° of flexion to help prevent impingement of the ulnar nerve at the cubital tunnel. Choices (C) and (D) are both mobilization splints. A flail arm splint is used for someone with a brachial plexus injury.

8. **C)** Stops are devices that inhibit certain movements, whereas springs assist certain movements. Anterior stops inhibit dorsiflexion, whereas posterior stops inhibit plantar flexion. Anterior springs aid with plantar flexion, whereas posterior springs help with dorsiflexion.

9. **D)** Lenox Hill derotation orthosis prevents anterior translation of the tibia on the femur.

10. **A)** Forty-five percent of cervical rotation occurs at the atlanto-axial joint, where the atlas rotates around the odontoid process of the axis.

11. *C, only clamshell is indicated for UNstable*

11. **D)** The Taylor's brace is only used for stable compression fractures.

12. **B)** With complete elbow extension, the patient should be able to raise the body 1 to 2 in. This is important when determining crutch length. Crutches are not designed to fit snugly under the arms as support for the body's weight. This would lead to constant compression into the axilla, increasing the likelihood for compressive radial neuropathies or plexopathies. Radial nerve compression at the axilla is termed *crutch palsy* because it is commonly caused by improper spacing between the axilla and the top of the crutch with complete elbow extension. Radial nerve palsy or crutch palsy would result in decreased ability to extend the arm at the elbow, decreased ability to supinate the arm, and difficulty extending the wrist (wrist drop) and fingers. Two to three inches and 3 to 4 in. would be incorrect because there would be too much distance between the axilla and the top of the crutch, which could lead to instability.

13. **A)** A rocker knife is a useful adaptive tool when functional skills in one upper limb are impaired. Just as the name suggests, a rocker knife is used by pushing the knife down into food and rocking the knife until the food is cut. Patients with functional use of one upper extremity would benefit. For example, individuals with unilateral hemiparesis after a stroke, unilateral wrist fracture with a cast or brace, or with no motor strength in one extremity would be able to cut food without the use of another functional hand to stabilize.

14. **C)** The fibular head is a pressure-sensitive area. Therefore, reliefs must be built into this area in order to ensure that skin breakdown or damage to the peroneal nerve does not occur.

15. **C)** Phantom pain is defined as an awareness of pain in the portion of the extremity that has been amputated. The pain is classically described as burning, aching, and cramping. Narcotics are not used in the treatment of phantom limb pain. In addition to the other answers, norepinephrine reuptake inhibitors, calcitonin, capsaicin, and propranolol are reasonable pharmacologic medical interventions.

16. **B)** In a Syme's amputation there is preservation of the articular cartilage covered by the heel pad, which allows direct weight bearing on the residual limb. In long and short transtibial amputations the residual limb is not long enough. A hemicorporectomy is an amputation of both lower limbs and pelvis below the L4, L5 level.

17. **B)** Prehensile refers to grasp by wrapping around, as in the human hand gripping objects by wrapping around them.

18. **B)** In the first 5 years of life, a prosthetic device should be replaced every 12 months. From age 5 to 12 years, the prosthetic can be replaced every 18 months. From age 12 to 21 years, the prosthetic can be replaced every 2 years.

19. **C)** The natural position of the hand at rest is the wrist in flexion. This pulls on the extrinsic extensor tendons causing them to flatten/extend, and extend the MCP joints. The extrinsic finger flexor tension is maintained forcing PIP and DIP joints into flexion.

20. **D)** This splint uses cords running from the wrist across the palm and attaching between the index and the ring fingers. The cords are lax when the wrist is released and tighten when the wrist is extended helping bring the fingers closer to the immobilized thumb.

21. **C)** Foot orthotics for diabetic patients also help to provide support for bony structures, provide relief for bony prominences, and absorb perspiration, keeping the foot dry to prevent fungal infections.

22. **B)** KAFOs are meant to be an adjunct to locomotion for paraplegic patients. They are not meant to replace the use of a wheelchair.

23. **A)** The cervical spine has the greatest range of motion including flexion, extension, side bending, and rotation.

24. **C)** The clamshell orthosis is a custom-molded body thoracolumbosacral (TLS) body jacket that provides the greatest lower truncal immobilization. It is usually used after thoracolumbar fixations. It is effective only as high as T8.

25. **B)** Greater trochanter is the anatomic landmark to which a health care provider measures the height of the top of the walker. When measuring for walkers, the patient should be standing upright, knees in neutral extension, and hips in neutral extension. The level at which the hand grips will be placed is based on the location of the greater trochanter when the elbows are in 20° of flexion and the walker is 12 in. in front of the patient. This positioning will ensure proper support and comfort for the patient. Walkers are useful for hemiplegic and ataxic patients. The xiphoid process, pubic symphysis, and iliac crests are not considered when measuring for walkers.

26. **B)** A rotor is not a component of the transtibial prosthesis. All of the others are components of a transtibial (below-knee) prosthesis.

27. **D)** This is the definition of phantom sensation. It usually diminishes over time, yet is a normal occurrence after amputation of a limb. Allodynia is a painful response to a stimulus that normally does not elicit pain, whereas hyperalgesia is increased pain from a stimulus that normally provokes pain. Phantom pain is defined as an awareness of pain in the portion of the extremity that has been amputated. The pain is classically described as burning, aching, and cramping.

28. **A)** This describes a hemipelvectomy. A hip disarticulation is the surgical removal of the entire lower limb by transection through the hip joint, whereas Boyd's and Pirogoff's amputations are horizontal calcaneal and vertical calcaneal amputations, respectively.

29. **D)** A forequarter amputation, also known as an *interscapulothoracic disarticulation*, involves removal of the scapula, part or all of the clavicle, as well as the entire humerus, radius, ulna, carpal bones, metacarpals and phalanges. It is less common because of recent surgical advances for limb-sparing techniques, but is still used as a treatment for removal of malignant tumors.

30. **A)** The accepted and preferred term for the remaining portion of the limb after amputation is *residual limb*.

31. **A)** The child with a congenital limb deficiency views the prosthesis as an aid rather than a replacement. The child also does not experience the sense of loss as it was absent from birth. The child with a congenital limb deficiency will typically participate in the same activities as other children. The child typically does not put limitations on oneself, but limitations are usually placed by adults.

32. **C)** An ulnar gutter splint helps immobilize the fourth and fifth metacarpal bones to allow for healing. This splint extends from the proximal forearm to beyond the distal interphalangeal (DIP) joint. A stax splint is for mallet finger and helps hold the DIP in full extension. Resting hand splints are used for stroke patients to help prevent contractures of the hand.

33. **B)** The peroneus longus muscle helps with pronation of the foot. Thus, if this muscle was weak, a patient will be prone to supination of the foot. Placing a lateral wedge would help this. A medial wedge is used for patients with weak tibialis posterior who have the opposite problem and have difficulty supinating.

34. **A)** The medial T-strap attaches onto the shoe over the medial side and attaches onto the lateral upright of the double metal upright. Answer choice (B) (lateral T-strap) would be used for a varus deformity/laxity.

35. **B)** Other complications include soft tissue contractures, skin ulcers, physical dependence, psychological dependence, increased movement at the ends where the spine is not immobilized, and osteopenia.

36. **C)** Also known as a *sacroiliac orthosis*, these bands fit between the iliac crests and the greater trochanters of the femur. It avoids application of pressure on the pelvis while providing support to the sacroiliac (SI) joint as well as the ligaments around it that are strained during pregnancy.

37. **C)** This ADL splint is used for many injuries, including for patients with radial nerve palsy or "wrist drop." The radial nerve innervates the extensor muscles of the forearm, which include extensor carpi ulnaris, extensor digiti minimi, extensor digitorum, extensor indicis, extensor pollicis longus, extensor pollicis brevis, extensor carpi radialis brevis, extensor carpi radialis longus, supinator, and abductor pollicis longus. This ADL splint can assist a patient with ADLs as depicted in the photograph to the right. This modified version of the dorsal wrist immobilizer with a universal cuff allows for various utensils to be placed in order to assist patients to function independently. Median (C5–T1) is incorrect because median nerve palsy would result in an inability to abduct and oppose the thumb. Ulnar nerve (C8–T1) entrapment usually occurs by compression of the ulnar nerve at the elbow, resulting in cubital tunnel syndrome. Patients will complain of numbness in the fifth digit and partial to full numbness in the fourth digit. Over time, this will lead to weakness and curling of the affected digits. Musculocutaneous nerve (C5–C6) palsy would cause weakness in flexion at the elbow.

38. **A)** Sitting with the knee extended would be the only acceptable option here. All others would lead to either knee flexion or hip flexion contractures.

39. **B)** Verrucous hyperplasia may result from a chronic choke syndrome. By relieving the proximal constriction and reestablishing total contact within the socket, this condition can be treated successfully. Tinea corporis mainly results from sweating and can be prevented and treated with good socket hygiene and antifungal medications. Hyperhidrosis may cause maceration of the skin, which predisposes the skin to infection. Folliculitis is an infection of the hair root resulting from poor hygiene, sweating, and either pistoning or poor socket fit.

40. **D)** Too much adduction built into the prosthesis will result in an abducted gait. Such a gait is a very wide-based gait with the prosthesis held away from the midline at all times. A circumducted gait is where the prosthesis swings laterally in a wide arc during the swing phase.

41. **B)** The most common upper extremity acquired amputation in the United States (excluding fingers) is below the elbow or transradial amputation. Upper extremity amputation is much less common than lower extremity amputation, accounting for only about 10% of amputation overall. It is frequently caused by trauma in a young worker and is usually work related involving the dominant limb.

42. **D)** Removal of the radius, ulna, carpals, metacarpals, and phalanges is termed elbow disarticulation. This amputation spares the humerus. The term *midelbow* is not used.

43. **B)** The following actions can activate a terminal device on an upper extremity prosthesis: scapular abduction, chest expansion, and humeral flexion.

44. **B)** This position helps keep the oblique retinacular ligament and terminal extensor tendon lengthened, preventing boutonniere deformities during healing.

45. **B)** The outer sole should be approximately half of the required heel elevation. If a patient needed a 2-in. heel lift, the outer sole would be 1 in. tall. The lift should taper from the ball of the shoe to the toe.

46. **B)** T-straps are placed on the ankle with double metal upright AFOs to enhance mediolateral stability at the ankle.

47. **B)** Thomas heel extends anteriorly under the navicular bone and provides support to the medial longitudinal arch for patients with pes planus.

48. **A)** The Jewett brace applies pressure to the manubrium, midback, and pubic symphysis, which allows for extension, but limits flexion.

49. **B)** A rolling walker would be the most appropriate assistive device from the answer choices. Answer choice (A) is a standard walker, answer choice (C) is a pair of crutches, and answer choice (D) is a quad cane (narrow-based). Bradykinesia is a hallmark finding in Parkinson's disease. Affected individuals have difficulty initiating first steps making a rolling walker advantageous versus a standard walker. A standard walker must be picked up after a completed step before taking a new step. This restarts the initiation of first steps, which is already a difficult task. A rolling walker facilitates walking without having to lift up the walker in between steps along with providing the necessary stability.

50. **A)** The amputee patient should wear a shrinkage device 24 hours a day. The only exception should be when bathing. Shrinkers are easy to apply and provide uniform compression. Typically, patients are fitted after the sutures/staples are removed. Close monitoring should be undertaken to avoid constriction and skin damage, which may occur if not properly fitted.

51. **D)** These findings are consistent with choked-stump syndrome. This may result when the residual limb becomes too large to fit properly in the total contact socket. The socket will become too tight proximally and therefore obstruct venous outflow. An edematous distal residual limb will result. Folliculitis, cysts, and dermatitis are all potential complications of a prosthesis, yet do not result in edema and induration.

52. **C)** This problem would be caused by the foot being too plantar flexed. The foot being too dorsiflexed would cause too much knee flexion or toe off of the floor as the patient stands. If the foot is too far anterior or posterior, it can result in limited knee flexion after heel strike or a drop-off at the end of stance phase, respectively.

53. **B)** A terminal deficiency describes a limb that has developed normally to a certain level but is abnormally missing distal skeletal elements (eg, terminal transverse radial limb deficiency). An intercalary deficiency describes a limb deficiency in the long axis where normal skeletal elements may be present distal to the affected segment (eg, partial reduction of the ulna with normal radius and hand elements).

54. **B)** In the acute postop period following an amputation, important aspects of care include wound healing, pain management, activities of daily living (ADL) training, mobility, range of motion, strengthening, skin desensitization, prosthetic consult, and psychological counseling. The prosthesis should not be fit until swelling resolves and the wound heals.

55. **D)** The key functions of the prosthetic socket are comfortable residual limb-prosthesis interface, efficient energy transfer, secure suspension of the prosthesis, and adequate cosmesis. The ability to grasp objects is a function of the terminal device.

56. **C)** Lateral epicondylitis is due to excessive motion involving extension of the hand. Pain is due to inflammation of the hand extensor muscles close to their common origin at the lateral epicondyle. Provocative testing includes resisted extension and pronation.

57. **B)** Minor leg-length discrepancies of up to 1/2 in. may be left uncompensated or treated by placing a 1/4-in. heel pad in the shoe.

58. **A)** The goal of bracing in LCP is to maintain the femoral head completely within the acetabulum to maintain its sphere shape. This is achieved by positioning the hip in hyperabduction and external rotation.

59. **A)** A cushioned heel helps promote plantar flexion. This would promote knee extension rather than knee flexion.

60. **C)** The Taylor's brace is a thoracolumbosacral orthosis (TLSO) that limits flexion and extension. It is used to prevent worsening of kyphosis from a stable anterior compression fracture of the vertebra.

61. **C)** The SOMI has three posters with an anterior chest plate that extend over the shoulder. One of the posters extends from the chest plate to the chin and the other two extend to the occiput. It is useful in bedridden patients as it has no posterior posters. However, this also limits its effectiveness for restricting extension. It is very effective in limiting flexion, lateral bending, and rotation.

62. **D)** In shaping a transtibial residual limb, the ideal shape of the limb for eventual prosthetic fitting is cylindrical. Conical is best after a transfemoral amputation. Pyramidal and rectangular are not correct.

63. **C)** There is improved knee stability with the stance control knee. However, activities that require knee motion under weight-bearing (step-over-step stair descent) are not compatible with this knee. Moreover, it cannot be used in bilateral transfemoral amputee patients. As the knees will not bend with loading, the patient will not be able to bend both knees at the same time to sit down.

64. **D)** The solid ankle cushioned heel (SACH) foot is light, durable, inexpensive, and stable. It is the most commonly used prosthetic foot.

65. **B)** It is important to preserve the epiphyses because they contain the growth plates, which will allow maximum growth of the residual limb. It will also help to avoid bony overgrowth as the bone is not being cut.

66. **B)** The earlier the patient is introduced to the rehabilitation physician and the prosthetic team the better. The rehabilitation physician or prosthetist may be able to advise the surgeon about the most functional level of amputation as well as provide therapy for strengthening and conditioning prior to surgery.

67. **A)** The benefits of IPORD are to control edema, promote healing, protect the limb from trauma, decrease postoperative pain, desensitize the residual limb, prevent contractures, and allow early mobilization and rehabilitation.

68. **D)** The patient has de Quervain's tenosynovitis. The thumb spica splint substitutes for the actions of the abductor pollicis longus and extensor pollicis brevis tendons, permitting their relaxation. This helps promote healing and decrease inflammation around the tendon sheath that surrounds them. The thumb spica splint also extends to the forearm immobilizing the wrist, carpometacarpal joint, and the metacarpophalangeal joint.

69. **C)** Tenodesis splints are a special class of orthosis prescribed mainly in tetraplegic patients. They employ wrist extension to tighten the finger flexor tendons causing the hand to close.

70. **D)** This patient is having his peroneal nerve compressed at the fibular head. The AFO should have a 1- to 2-in. clearance from the upper brim to the fibular head.

71. **A)** The rocker bottom relieves pressure from the metatarsal heads and assists in rollover when plantar flexors are weak.

72. **B)** The Philadelphia collar limits flexion, extension, and sidebending. It is used for cervical ligament ruptures and relatively stable cervical fractures. It is also used after cervical surgery when strict neck immobilization is not necessary.

73. **D)** The chairback brace is used on patients with low-back pain from disk herniations by preventing extension of the lumbar spine. It also helps decrease lumbar lordosis by increasing intra-abdominal pressure by tightening the anterior straps. It is also used as an immobilizer after a lumbar laminectomy.

74. **A)** Weighted utensils assist by compensating for limited hand control, as in the case of movement disorders such as Parkinson's disease. Affected individuals have a tremor that could hinder the ability to eat properly. The additional weight on the utensil allows for less involuntary movement of the hand. Hemiplegic individuals will have one functioning hand that could use conventional utensils without obstacles. Paraplegic individuals have impairment in motor or sensory function of bilateral lower extremities. Osteoarthritis can affect the hands, but it is not associated with a tremor or loss of hand control. There may be pain associated in the affected joints when carrying a weighted utensil.

75. **C)** An amputation at the tarsometatarsal junction is known as a Lisfranc amputation. The tarsometatarsal joint is known as the Lisfranc joint. A transmetatarsal amputation is through the midsection of all metatarsals. A Syme's amputation is an ankle disarticulation with attachment of heel pad to distal end of the tibia. A midtarsal amputation where only the talus and calcaneus remain is called a Chopart amputation.

76. **B)** These are types of suspension for a transfemoral prosthesis. Other suspension systems for the transfemoral prosthesis include the suction socket (total suction versus partial suction) and gel liners with a pin or strap.

77. **A)** Level 0 indicates those individuals who are unable, or do not have potential to ambulate or transfer with or without assistance. Being fit for a prosthesis will not enhance their mobility. They may also have moderate to severe cognitive impairments and/or exercise-limiting cardiopulmonary disease and therefore not benefit from prosthetic rehabilitation. Level 1 are patients with the ability or potential to use a prosthesis for transfers and ambulation on level surfaces (household ambulator). Level 2 patients have the ability to become limited community ambulators with a prosthesis (negotiate curbs, stairs and uneven surfaces). As for level 3, the patient has the ability or potential to ambulate with variable cadence and traverse environmental barriers.

78. **B)** The figure 8 or "O ring" harness is the most commonly used below-elbow harness. It suspends the prosthesis from the shoulder so the socket is held firmly on the residual limb. This uses the body motions as sources of power and transmits this force via cables to operate the terminal device. The figure 8 contains an axilla loop, which is worn on the sound side, and an anterior suspension strap on the involved side, which attaches more distally via cuffs and straps to the terminal device.

79. **C)** Phantom pain is best treated with low dose TCA taken orally. Patients can be started on nortriptyline or amitriptyline 10 to 25 mg every night at bedtime.

80. **C)** Edema is a common complication after amputation surgery. It can be prevented by soft dressings and elastic wrapping done in a figure 8 pattern every 4 to 6 hours. The ideal shape of the upper extremity residual limb is cylindrical, not conical.

81. **A)** Static motion blocking splints permit motion in one direction, but block motion in the other direction. The swan-neck splint allows for flexion at the proximal interphalangeal joint and the distal interphalangeal joint, but prevents hyperextension at these sites.

82. **A)** Airplane splints hold the arm out like a wing and are an example of static shoulder orthoses. However, they are poorly tolerated, and it is difficult for patients to comply with wearing these splints.

83. **C)** Answer choice (A) would be good for a foot drop, but would not address the weak quadriceps. Answer choice (B) is useful for pain with ankle motion. Answer choice (D) is useful for weak plantar flexors.

84. **B)** Medial heel flares resist valgus motion at the ankle, whereas lateral heel flares resist varus motion.

85. **C)** The Halo Vest is usually worn for about 12 weeks to allow for adequate bone healing. Complications of this orthosis include pin loosening, infection, ring migration, pressure sores, and pin scars.

86. **A)** The Williams' brace is a short lumbosacral brace that helps with spondylolisthesis as well as spondylolysis by restricting extension.

87. **B)** This adaptive equipment enables food to be stabilized against a raised edge thus allowing individuals with functional use of one hand the ability to eat. A scoop dish or plate guard helps hemiplegic patients, stroke patients with hemiparesis, or those with temporary use of one hand after injury to gain functional independence. Parkinson's disease consists of four symptoms: postural instability, bradykinesia, rigidity, and resting tremor. When a person with Parkinson's disease moves, the tremor subsides. A scoop dish may be of benefit in this instance but most beneficial in a patient with functional use of just one hand. Paraplegic individuals have impairment in motor or sensory function of bilateral lower extremities. A scoop dish may not be necessary because only the lower extremities are affected. Osteoarthritis is caused by wear and tear on joints leading to degradation of the joint including articular cartilage and subchondral bone. Individuals with this condition notice stiffness and tenderness in the joints.

88. **B)** A standard transtibial amputation is 20% to 50% of the tibial length. A long transtibial amputation is more than 50% of the tibial length, whereas a short transtibial amputation is less than 20% of the tibial length.

89. **D)** These are all problematic issues involving the quadrilateral transfemoral socket. The other choices are examples of sockets for the transfemoral amputee patient which are more comfortable and energy efficient and provide greater medial-lateral control of the pelvis when compared with the quadrilateral socket.

90. **C)** The level described is level 3. Level 1 are patients with the ability or potential to use a prosthesis for transfers and ambulation on level surfaces (household ambulator). Level 2 patients have the ability to become limited community ambulators with a prosthesis (negotiate curbs, stairs and uneven surfaces). Level 4 has the potential for ambulation that exceeds basic skills and exhibits high impact or energy levels.

91. **C)** The voluntary opening terminal device is the most common and practical type. It is held in the closed position at rest and opens with voluntary movement. This allows grasp with less effort than a voluntary closing device.

92. **C)** Phantom pain is pain perceived in the missing part of the limb. Phantom sensation is normal and eventually resolves. Phantom pain must be treated aggressively.

93. **A)** Elbow disarticulation surgery is typically shorter and has less blood loss than transradial. Major disadvantages include marginal cosmetic appearance and a large, bulky elbow joint mechanism.

94. **C)** Gel shell splint is used after carpal tunnel release to help prevent hypertrophy of the scar tissue by applying pressure over the healing scar. It is nonarticular as it does not cross over the joint and restrict its range of motion. Nonarticular orthotics help provide support and protect bones or a body part.

95. **B)** Monkeys can do a cylindrical grip so they can hold onto a rail. As they lack opposing thumbs, giving an "okay" sign (fingertip pinch) and turning a key (lateral pinch) would be difficult. They also are unable to do a spherical grip making holding a ball difficult.

96. **D)** This orthosis has a band of material on the top of the orthosis that helps transfer the extension moment from plantar flexing to the patellar tendon. This helps stabilize the knee during heel strike.

97. **D)** Posterior stops limit plantar flexion and would actually promote knee flexion rather than extension.

98. **C)** The Aspen collar limits cervical flexion and lateral bending. However, it does not limit rotation. The Halo Vest, Minerva, and SOMI also limit flexion and sidebending.

99. **C)** The Minerva brace is an alternative to the Halo Vest and is used for cervical spine fractures below C2. It restricts flexion/extension, sidebending, and rotation similar to the Halo Vest. However, it is not used for fractures at C1/C2.

100. **B)** The item in the photograph is a sock aide. It is used to facilitate donning of socks in patients with limited bending motion due to pain, decreased range of motion, or strength. First, a sock is placed over the sock holder. Next, the foot is slid into the sock holder and then the attached rope is used to pull the sock over the person's foot. This allows a person to put on a sock without introducing increased stress on the body.

101. **C)** The most common type of amputation is a transtibial or below-knee amputation (BKA). Transfemoral or above-knee amputations are approximately half as common as BKA, whereas Syme's (ankle disarticulation) and hip disarticulation are very uncommon.

102. **A)** The flex-foot allows for running, jumping, and most vigorous sports, all while conserving energy. The pylon and foot are incorporated into one unit. The single-axis foot permits movement of the foot and ankle complex in the plantar flexion/dorsiflexion axis, whereas the multi-axis foot allows some controlled movement in the normal anatomic planes (plantar flexion, dorsiflexion, inversion, eversion, and rotation).

103. **B)** A heel cushion that is too soft, or a prosthetic foot in excessive plantar flexion will result in insufficient knee flexion. In addition, the plantar bumper being too soft, the socket too far posterior over the foot, or quadriceps weakness may result in insufficient knee flexion as well.

104. **A)** A prosthesis fits over the existing part of the remaining limb to substitute for a missing body part. An example would be someone with a transradial amputation fitted with a device below the elbow, which functions as a forearm and hand in some fashion and can perform some of the same maneuvers. Choices (B) and (C) refer to braces or orthoses.

105. **D)** The main goals of rehabilitation after amputation include wound healing, edema control, prevention of contractures, and prevention of deconditioning. This is done through various means. Treadmill training is neither an immediate goal nor a long-term goal for amputees.

106. **D)** Joint contractures are a common complication that can occur after amputation and before prosthetic fitting. Prevention is much easier than treatment of joint contracture. Range of motion, positioning, and aggressive rehabilitation should be implemented immediately postop to prevent contracture formation. Burn and nerve injuries can complicate the situation and put the patient at increased risk of developing a joint contracture.

107. **B)** Static progressive splints have components allowing continued adjustment so the splint does not have to be changed like a serial static splint. Serial static splints are remolded to help alter the joint angle for prolonged gentle stretch. Continuous passive motion uses an electrically powered device that moves the joint to the desired range of motion. Adaptive usage splints promote functional use of the upper limb. An example is the universal cuff where one can attach small items such as forks or spoons.

108. **A)** Monkeys cannot perform palmar prehension (three-jaw chuck) as they lack opposing thumbs. They would also not be able to do a finger pinch or lateral pinch for the same reason.

109. **A)** Springs may worsen ankle clonus. Therefore, using a solid AFO helps lock the ankle and control clonus.

110. **B)** This padded strap goes around the knee just below the patella and helps control the tracking of the patella during activities.

111. **B)** About 80% to 90% of lumbar motion occurs at L4 to L5 and L5 to S1. This also makes these segments the most susceptible to degenerative changes.

112. **C)** The cruciform anterior spinal hyperextension (CASH) orthosis uses an anterior cross with padding at the four ends of the cross to prevent further progression of kyphosis from compression fractures by limiting flexion while allowing extension. The brace is adjusted posteriorly with Velcro straps.

113. **C)** Generally, the backrest should be low enough to provide truncal support and still allow the upper limbs access to the pushrims. The scapula, particularly the inferior angle of the scapula, is used to determine the proper backrest height on a standard wheelchair. The scapula connects

the humerus with the clavicle. There are 18 muscles that attach to the scapula, which are indirectly related to the movement of the upper limbs. These include pectoralis minor, long head of triceps brachii, short head of biceps brachii, long head of biceps brachii, coracobrachialis, serratus anterior, subscapularis, rhomboid major, rhomboid minor, levator scapulae, trapezius, deltoid, supraspinatus, infraspinatus, omohyoid, latissimus dorsi, teres minor, and teres major. It is essential, if no cervical pathology is involved, that the backrest be measured below the inferior angle of the scapula in order to avoid any somatic restriction of scapula.

114. **A)** In this age group, trauma is the most common cause for amputation. Cancer is one of the most common between the ages of 5 to 15 years, whereas infection and vascular disease are prominent causes in those older than 50 years.

115. **B)** The SACH foot is an inexpensive option when it comes to prosthetic feet. It is light, durable, and reliable. The other options are more expensive. Energy-storing feet can be quite costly. The single-axis foot permits movement of the foot-ankle complex in the plantar flexion/dorsiflexion axis, whereas the multi-axis foot allows some controlled movement in the normal anatomic planes (plantar flexion, dorsiflexion, inversion, eversion, and rotation).

116. **A)** A transfemoral-transtibial amputation increases energy expenditure by about 118%, whereas bilateral transtibial, transfemoral with use of a crutch, and unilateral transfemoral increase energy expenditure by approximately 41%, 92%, and 99%, respectively.

117. **C)** Trauma is the most common cause of acquired upper limb amputation accounting for approximately 75% of all upper limb amputations and is followed by cancer/tumors and vascular pathology.

118. **B)** The optimum time for fitting an amputee patient with a prosthesis is within a 3- to 6-month window. This will increase the likelihood of long-term prosthetic use. Once a person becomes independent with activities of daily living (ADLs) with the preserved residual limb, the chance of fully incorporating the prosthesis into routine activities is reduced. Within the first week after surgery, the amputated extremity is not ready for prosthetic fitting. Edema reduction and wound healing must take place before the patient is measured for a prosthesis.

119. **D)** A terminal device is a device used to mimic the function of the human hand and is located at the distal end of the prosthetic device. Types of terminal devices include: mechanical (voluntary opening or voluntary closing), electrical (electrical or myoelectrical), and passive.

120. **C)** Power grasps are useful for holding a ball or cylindrical object. Oppositional pinch is a good compromise for fine precision pinch and lateral pinch. Hook pattern is useful for carrying heavy objects such as weights or bags.

121. **C)** Kleinert and Duran splints are used after flexor tendon repair of the fingers. Kleinert is a dynamic motion blocking splint in that it prevents flexion contractures of the PIP and DIP by allowing active extension at the digits but blocks extension at the MCP to prevent pulling of the flexor tendons. The Duran splint is a static splint that holds the IP joints in extension and the MCP joints in flexion. Both prevent wrist extension.

122. **B)** Other indications for using an AFO include foot drop during swing phase, mediolateral instability at the ankle, and foot slap during heel strike due to weak ankle dorsiflexors.

123. **C)** The hinge is placed posterior to the knee's axis of rotation so that the GRF is anterior. This helps with extension of the knee for stability during early stance phase.

124. **C)** The greatest amount of cervical flexion occurs at C5 to C6. C4 to C5 accounts for the second most amount of cervical flexion.

125. **B)** The Milwaukee brace consists of three uprights (two posterior and one anterior) that attach onto a ring around the neck and pelvic girdle. Straps with pressure pads are mounted onto the brace to help improve spinal alignment.

126. **B)** The wheelchair seat width should be approximately 1 in. wider than the width of the widest part of the buttocks. If the distance is too narrow, as in answer choice (A), pressure injuries may develop from the pelvic bony prominences being in close contact to the sides of the chair. Answer choices (C) and (D) are incorrect because if the distance is too wide, the individual will have to markedly abduct the shoulders making it more difficult to push the chair.

127. **A)** A reacher, as seen in photo choice (A), is an adaptive and versatile tool for retrieving items of clothing when a person has limited reach and mobility. A reacher is an extended stick with a grasping unit at the end. When the handle is squeezed the opposite end of the grasping unit closes. It only opens when the squeeze is released. This is most beneficial for patients with limited range of motion in forward bending at the lumbar spine or in the upper extremities while reaching for items at an elevated level. A reacher is also indicated in patients with proximal upper extremity muscle weakness.

128. **D)** A dressing stick, as seen in photo choice (D), is an adaptive tool for dressing used by individuals with decreased range of motion in upper extremities, limitations with reach, or arthritis. Assistance with pulling up pants and socks can be solved with this adaptive tool. Not only can this aid with dressing, but can provide assistance as a reacher to hook onto items on the floor to pick up.

129. **C)** A bottle or jar stabilizer, as seen in photo choice (C), is an adaptive tool used by patients with functional use of one upper extremity. With three different choices for bottle or jar size, individuals can place a bottle into the cylindrical aperture and hold it in place while opening the bottle. The cylindrical shape allows the bottle or jar to be stabilized and opened with the same unaffected upper extremity.

130. **B)** A rocker utensil, as seen in photo choice (B), is a useful adaptive tool when functional skills in one upper limb are impaired. For example, individuals with unilateral hemiparesis after a stroke would be able to cut food without the use of the other functional hand to stabilize. Just as the name suggests, a rocker knife is used by pushing the knife down into food and rocking the knife until the food is cut.

131. **B)** The body has the highest center of gravity with walking during midstance phase of the gait cycle. The body has the lowest center of gravity with walking during the loading response phase.

132. **C)** A cane can be used to take some weight off of a painful hip. A cane is usually held on the patient's unaffected side, and it can decrease the force exerted on the pathologic hip. A cane can assist in decreasing the forces generated across the affected hip joint by decreasing the work of the gluteus medius-minimus complex by minimizing the pelvic drop on the contralateral side to the weight-bearing limb. A disadvantage of using a cane is that it can be associated with decreased walking speed.

133. **C)** An abducted gait (wide-based gait) is defined as a distance greater than 10 cm between the heels. Common causes of an abducted gait include perineal discomfort, excessively long prosthesis, abduction contracture, poor balance, hip arthritis, hip dislocation, and inguinal hernia. A cane can help minimize lateral bending and wide-based walking.

134. **A)** Walking on a 10% to 12% incline will double the energy expenditure.

135. **C)** The calf muscles are inactive in initial contact and loading response phase. They undergo eccentric contraction in midstance phase, and concentric contraction in terminal stance phase. Midstance phase is the period from lift off of the contralateral extremity from the ground to the point where the ankles of both extremities are aligned in the frontal plane.

136. **D)** Common signs and symptoms of Parkinson's disease are resting tremor, bradykinesia, cogwheel rigidity, masked facies, postural instability, freezing phenomena, and festinating (shuffling) gait. While ambulating, the patients have a characteristic shuffling gait with short step length and increasing speed with decreased arm swing. Hemiplegic gait is seen with an extensor synergy pattern in the lower extremity (knee extension, ankle plantarflexion, and inversion). Toe clearance is typically achieved with a circumduction gait pattern. Crouched gait is seen in cerebral palsy patients. The hips and knee are flexed and internally rotated with standing. When ambulating, there is scissoring due to increased adductor tone. Antalgic gait develops as a way to avoid pain while ambulating. Antalgic gait presents as a decrease in stance phase on the affected side, a reduced step length on the unaffected side, and a prolonged double support period.

137. **D)** At 30° of knee flexion contracture all of the phases of the gait cycle become abnormal. Knee flexion contractures of 30° or more essentially produce a leg-length discrepancy.

138. **B)** The three main events that consume energy during walking are controlled deceleration at the end of swing phase, shock absorption at heel stroke, and forward propulsion of the center of mass at push-off.

139. **C)** The gait cycle is divided into the stance phase (while the foot is in contact with the ground) and swing phase (while the foot is in the air). Stance phase makes up 60% of the gait cycle and swing phase makes up 40% during normal walking speed. Walking faster decreases the time spent in stance phase and increases the time spent in swing phase. The stance phase of gait is decreased from 60% while walking to 30% while running, and 20% while sprinting. When gait becomes fast enough that there is no longer a double-support phase, that is the definition of running.

140. **B)** The six determinants of gait are the following:
    1. Pelvic rotation
    2. Pelvic tilt
    3. Knee flexion (Not knee extension)
    4. Foot/ankle motion
    5. Knee motion
    6. Lateral displacement of the pelvis

141. **B)** At 6 months the infant is usually able to sit and roll both ways. At 12 months the infant is able to walk with support (hand held). At 15 months the infant is able to walk independently. At 18 months the infant can run.

142. **C)** Normal walking on level surfaces is most energy efficient at a walking speed of 3 mph (1–1.3 m/s).

143. **B)** This crutch gait pattern is employed when there is unilateral lower extremity pathology, for example, a lower extremity fracture or amputated extremity. The motion is both crutches and involved leg advancing together, then the uninvolved/stronger extremity advancing forward last. This eliminates weight bearing on the affected lower limb. For this pattern to be successful, good balance and coordination are required.

144. **A)** A long-handled bath sponge is used for reaching the back or lower extremities in the shower when range of motion is limited or when bending is contraindicated because of lack of balance.

145. **B)** Pot stabilizer, as seen here in action, would help individuals with functional use of one extremity, as in the case of hemiparesis or hemiplegia, gain independence with cooking. This serves also as a safety precaution to prevent spills, especially with hot items.

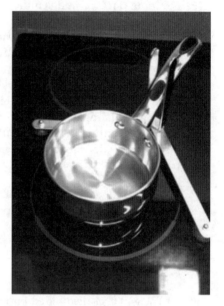

146. **D)** An elongated utensil can help an individual with decreased range of motion in either upper extremity with feedings.

147. **C)** A pronged cutting board is a useful adaptive tool when upper limb functional skills are impaired. For example, individuals with unilateral hemiparesis after a stroke or fractures of the forearm, wrist, or hand, would be able to cut food without the use of another functional hand to stabilize. As seen in the photo here, a vegetable can be inserted onto the prongs to help stabilize while the unaffected hand is used to slice.

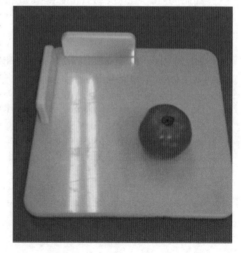

148. **D)** Answer choices (A), (B), and (C) are components of a prosthesis. CAD stands for computer aided design (not to be confused with CAT-CAM or contour adducted trochanteric controlled alignment system, a type of transfemoral prosthesis design). This is a type of design and not a prosthetic component.

149. **B)** Steppage gait. Ankle dorsiflexion weakness leads to a foot drop during swing phase. Patients may clear the foot by different compensatory mechanisms. They may accomplish this by vaulting on the contralateral limb, circumducting the affected side, or by hyperflexing the knee and hip on the affected side (steppage gait). Vaulting describes a gait pattern in which the affected limb is advanced by pelvis elevation and plantar flexion of the unaffected (stance) leg. Trendelenburg gait is seen in cases of hip abductor weakness where the contralateral pelvis drops during stance phase (uncompensated Trendelenburg gait).

150. **A)** Right-ankle plantarflexion contracture. Possible causes of genu recurvatum (knee hyperextension) during stance phase include ankle plantar flexion contracture, plantar flexion spasticity, quadriceps weakness, and quadriceps spasticity.

151. **B)** The center of mass tends to be located 2 cm in front of the second sacral vertebra in the anatomic position. The center of mass moves in a sinusoidal pattern with an average of 5 cm vertical and horizontal displacement while walking.

152. **A)** In this crutch pattern, one crutch and opposite extremity move together simultaneously followed by the opposite crutch and extremity. For example, the left crutch and right foot would be the first movement followed by the right crutch and the left foot and so on. The advantage with this gait pattern is stability and reduction of weight bearing on both lower extremities. Two canes or crutches would be necessary for this gait pattern. This mirrors natural arm and leg motion during gait. This pattern would be indicated in patients with poor coordination and/or weakness in lower extremities.

153. **C)** With the patient standing upright, crutch length is determined by measuring the distance from the anterior axillary fold to a point 6 in. lateral to the fifth toe. After this initial crutch length is determined, hand piece location can be determined by moving the crutch 3 in. lateral to the foot and flexing the elbow to 30° with complete wrist extension.

154. **C)** Quadriceps weakness leads to a quadriceps (back knee) gait. Patient may compensate in various ways to prevent knee buckling. They may use their hands to force the knee into extension, lurch their trunks forward at initial contact and strongly contract their ankle plantar flexors to bring the center of gravity anterior to the knee and force it into extension, or the patient may externally rotate the leg at initial contact to bring the medial collateral ligament anteriorly and prevent buckling. Antalgic gait develops as a way to avoid pain while ambulating. Antalgic gait presents as a decrease in stance phase on the affected side, a reduced step length on the unaffected side, and a prolonged double support period. Gluteus maximus (extensor lurch) gait is seen in cases of hip extensor weakness where the patient has difficulty decelerating the forward momentum of the body at heel strike. The patient develops a posterior lean and locks the hip joint into extension, which maintains the center of gravity posterior to the hip joint. Gluteus medius (Trendelenburg) gait is seen in cases of hip abductor weakness where the contralateral pelvis drops during stance phase (uncompensated Trendelenburg gait).

155. **C)** Traumatic transtibial amputation requires an approximately 7% increase in energy cost, vascular transtibial amputation requires an additional 13%, traumatic transfemoral amputation requires an additional 33%, vascular transfemoral amputation requires an additional 87%, and bilateral transtibial amputations require an additional 33%.

156. **C)**. Equilibrium is not a primary component of quantitative gait analysis. Gait can be studied through the collection of a wide range of information in a gait laboratory. The four primary components of quantitative gait analysis include kinematics (analysis of motion and resulting temporal and stride measures), kinetics (analysis of forces that produce motion), polyelectromyography or dynamic electromyography (EMG) (analysis of muscle activity), and energetics (analysis of metabolic and mechanical energy).

157. **D)** In this crutch pattern, both crutches are equally advanced forward together. The individual's body weight is shifted onto the hands for support and both legs are swung forward up to the point of crutch placement. This pattern requires the use of two crutches or a standard, non-rolling walker. This pattern is easy to learn and expends less energy in comparison with swing-through gait pattern. Paraplegic individuals would benefit from this gait pattern.

158. **A)** An essential difference between a crutch and a cane is the number of points of contact with the body. A cane has one point of contact with the body, which is the hand. A crutch, on the other hand, has two points of contact, one being at the hand and the other being either below the elbow (forearm crutches) or below the axilla (axillary crutches).

159. **C)** With hip osteoarthritis, an antalgic gait and abductor lurch (swaying of the trunk over the side of the affected hip) may be noted. A trunk lean toward the painful hip brings the center of mass over the joint and decreases the mechanical stress across the joint. Circumduction is seen in a long limb, abductor muscle contracture, and stiff knee.

160. **A)** Walking requires a greater amount of energy than wheelchair ambulation because the body's center of mass has to rise and fall with each step of walking, while with wheelchair ambulation the center of mass remains horizontal. The work done with walking can be estimated by multiplying the vertical displacement of the center of mass by the body weight and then by the number steps.

161. **A)** *Vaulting* refers to exaggerated plantar flexion on the contralateral (intact) leg during swing phase of the prosthesis. Vaulting increases the distance between the prosthetic foot and the ground. Causes of vaulting include the prosthesis being too long, inadequate suspension, and excessive knee stability.

162. **C)** In this gait pattern, both crutches are equally advanced forward together. The individual's body weight is shifted onto the hands for support and both legs are swung forward beyond the point of crutch placement. This pattern requires the use of two crutches. This is the fastest gait pattern with two crutches, but it expends a large amount of energy. Paraplegic individuals can use this gait pattern, but it requires strong upper body muscles.

163. **A)** Individuals with mildly impaired balance would only require a single point cane. For moderately impaired balance, a quad cane would be indicated because of its increased support compared with the single point canes. Quad canes come in narrow-based quad cane and wide-based quad canes. Hemiplegic patients would most benefit from quad canes, but slow gait is the compromise in comparison with a single point cane. For severely impaired balance, a standing or rolling walker would be indicated for controlled bilateral arm support.

164. **A)** Loading response occurs immediately following initial contact from flat foot position until the opposite foot is off the ground for swing. Midstance is from the time the opposite foot is lifted until the ipsilateral tibia is vertical. Terminal stance is from heel rise until the opposite foot contacts the ground. Preswing is from initial contact of the opposite foot and finishes with ipsilateral toe-off.

165. **A)** The lowest center of gravity while running is in midstance of single limb support, and the highest center of gravity is in the "flight" phase. However, with walking, the highest center of gravity is in the midstance phase of single limb support.

166. **C)** A whip is a sudden rotation of the prosthesis that occurs at the end of stance phase as the knee flexes to begin swing phase. If the prosthetic heel moves medially on initial flexion at the start of swing phase it is called a medial whip, and if the prosthetic heel moves laterally it is called a lateral whip. A medial whip can result from excessive external rotation of the knee with respect to the socket. A lateral whip can occur due to excessive internal rotation of the knee with respect to the socket.

167. **C)** Lofstrand crutches, or forearm crutches, consist of a forearm cuff with narrow anterior opening with a molded hand piece. The forearm piece is adjustable, which can extend to two inches below the elbow. These crutches place the weight of one's body on the forearms and hands, while still leaving the hand available to use if necessary. In order to use forearm crutches, the user must have better trunk balance and needs more strength and skill.

168. **D)** A platform forearm orthosis is very helpful for patients with a weak handgrip as in the case of arthritis. It is also indicated in patients with weak handgrip because of pain and deformities of the hands and wrists. A patient's body weight can be displaced onto the forearm instead of the hand with a platform forearm orthosis. A platform is placed on the top level of the crutch, and a vertical handgrip is placed at the distal end of the platform.

169. **D)** Stride period is the time from the occurrence of an event in one foot until the recurrence of the same event in the same foot (ie, initial contact to initial contact in the same foot). Stride length is the distance between the same foot during one stride. Step length is the distance between the same part of both feet during one step. Step period is the time from an event in one foot to the occurrence of the same event in the other foot. Cadence is the number of steps in a period of time.

170. **B)** Common gait abnormalities seen in cerebral palsy are initial contact with the forefoot, exaggerated knee extension moment, lack of full knee extension at midstance, a narrow base of support with scissoring, and shortened stride length.

*[handwritten annotation: Not in the crouch gait tho; "knee extension moment" underlined]*

171. **B)** Canes are prescribed to improve balance, decrease pain, decrease the weight-bearing forces of injured structures, and assist in compensating for weak muscles by shifting the weight on the healthier side, and can be used as a tool to survey the surrounding environment during ambulation. The purpose of canes is to decrease the loading and demand on the lower limbs and to assist with acceleration and deceleration during locomotion. There are many types of canes including C-handle cane, functional grip cane, small-based quad cane, and wide-based quad cane depending on the level of support an individual requires.

172. **B)** A lateral trunk lean over the prosthetic limb in midstance is a compensated Trendelenburg gait. A Trendelenburg gait occurs due to hip abductor muscle (gluteus medius and gluteus minimus) weakness. As the patient ambulates, he or she swings his or her body to the right to compensate for a left hip drop, thus keeping the center of gravity over the stance leg. However, if this patient was noted to have a left hip drop as he or she ambulated, it would be called an *uncompensated right Trendelenburg gait*.

173. **A)** The gluteus maximus is inactive in all phases of the gait cycle except the initial contact phase. The gluteus maximus is eccentrically contracting during initial contact, which occurs the instant the foot touches the ground.

174. **D)** A circumduction gait pattern can be caused by either prosthetic issues or the amputee patient's compensatory maneuvers. Some causes of a circumduction gait pattern are hip abductor contracture or overuse, long prosthetic limb, and excessive prosthetic knee friction (making it difficult to flex the knee).

175. **A)** A black-and-white cutting board is designed for use by individuals with low vision. The two options of color provide the individual with contrast, making it easier to see light-colored food. This option allows for functional independence while cooking. Essential tremor is a rhythmic tremor that is present when in use. For this reason, patients should refrain from using knives in the kitchen if the essential tremor is severe or unless there is supervision. Presbycusis is a progressive bilateral symmetrical age-related sensorineural hearing loss. Ageusia is loss of taste functions.

176. **A)** The gastroc-soleus complex (primarily the soleus muscle) is the only muscle normally active during quiet standing. Ligaments and bony articulations help maintain the stability of other joints (knees, hips, and spine) during quiet standing.

177. **A)** The motor part of the median nerve is involved for fine control of pincer grasp (for example, when attempting to turn a knob). The median nerve innervates the thenar muscle and two radial lumbricals necessary to grip onto the handle. The musculocutaneous nerve innervates the anterior compartment of the arm. The ulnar nerve innervates the flexor carpi ulnaris, flexor digitorum profundus, lumbrical muscles, opponens digiti minimi, flexor digiti minimi, abductor digiti minimi, interossei, and adductor pollicis. These muscles are found along the ulnar side of the arm and not directly involved with the pincer grasp. The radial nerve is involved with the supination necessary to adjust the temperature of the gas stove.

# 10

# Joint and Connective Tissue Disorders

## QUESTIONS

1. What tendons are affected by de Quervain's synovitis?
   A) Extensor carpi radialis longus (ECRL) and extensor carpi radialis brevis (ECRB)
   B) Abductor pollicis longus (APL) and extensor pollicis brevis (EPB)
   C) Extensor pollicis longus (EPL) and EPB
   D) Extensor digiti minimi (EDM) and extensor carpi ulnaris (ECU)

2. Which of the following is **not** a common disease complication of ankylosing spondylitis (AS)?
   A) Iritis/uveitis
   B) Inflammatory bowel disease
   C) Osteoporosis
   D) Dementia

3. Which of the following is **not** a typical severe side effect leading to rehabilitation hospitalization in patients with rheumatic diseases?
   A) Decline in activities of daily living (ADLs)
   B) Steroid myopathy
   C) Vasculitis
   D) Pressure injury

4. Later stage of rheumatoid arthritis affects which type of joint?
   A) Amphiarthrodial joint
   B) Synarthrodial
   C) Diarthrodial joint
   D) Triarthrodial joint

5. Which of the following radiographic features is **not** seen in patients with rheumatoid arthritis?
   A) Narrowing of the joint space
   B) Increased bone density
   C) Marginal erosion of bone
   D) Joint fusion

6. Which of the following is elevated in Paget's disease?
   A) Calcium
   B) Phosphate
   C) Aminotransferase
   D) Alkaline phosphatase

ANSWERS TO THIS SECTION CAN BE FOUND ON PAGE 323

7. Which of the following pulmonary conditions is often seen in patients with systemic sclerosis?
   A) Interstitial lung disease
   B) Pneumothorax
   C) Aspiration pneumonia
   D) Chronic obstructive pulmonary disease (COPD)

8. There is strong evidence to support the use of the following nonpharmacologic therapies in the treatment of fibromyalgia **except**:
   A) Patient education
   B) Cognitive behavioral therapy
   C) Massage therapy
   D) Exercise

9. Which of the following is an acute phase protein seen in response to tissue injury?
   A) Antinuclear antibody (ANA)
   B) C-reactive protein (CRP)
   C) Cytoplasmic antineutrophil cytoplasmic antibodies (C-ANCA)
   D) Anticentromere

10. What causes a Boutonnière deformity?
    A) Rupture of the extensor hood at the proximal interphalangeal joint (PIP), which causes subluxation of the lateral bands of the extensor hood
    B) Flexor synovitis
    C) Ligamentous laxity
    D) Rupture of the flexors with subluxation causing hyperextension at the PIP

11. Which of the following is **not** true about ankylosing spondylitis (AS)?
    A) Onset is usually late adolescence or early adulthood
    B) It is three times more common in men than in women
    C) It can be associated with human leukocyte antigen (HLA)-B27
    D) The sacroiliac joint is usually not involved

12. What is the name for an abnormal fibrous hyperplasia and contracture of the palmar fascia that causes a flexion contracture of the metacarpophalangeal (MCP) and proximal interphalangeal (PIP) joints?
    A) Charcot joint
    B) Dupuytren's contracture
    C) De Quervain's tenosynovitis
    D) Trigger finger

13. Gout commonly involves which of the following areas?
    A) Knee
    B) Toe
    C) Elbow
    D) Fingers

14. Which of the following sports would be contraindicated in a patient with ankylosing spondylitis?
    A) Archery
    B) Badminton
    C) Bicycling
    D) Table tennis

15. Which of the following is **not** a seronegative arthritis?
    A) Psoriatic arthritis
    B) Rheumatoid arthritis
    C) Reactive arthritis
    D) Ankylosing spondylitis

16. Which of the following antibodies is tested in patients suspected of having systemic lupus erythematosus (SLE)?
    A) Anticentromere
    B) Antigliadin
    C) Perinuclear antineutrophil cytoplasmic antibodies (P-ANCA)
    D) Anti-Smith

17. What is the most common cause of neuropathic arthropathy?
    A) Osteoarthritis
    B) Septic arthritis
    C) Systemic lupus
    D) Diabetes

18. Fibroblast growth factor receptor 3 (FGFR3) mutation causes which of the following conditions?
    A) Paget's disease
    B) Achondroplasia
    C) Osteogenesis imperfecta
    D) Osteoporosis

19. Which of the following are characteristic of rheumatoid arthritis (RA)?
    A) Morning stiffness
    B) Asymmetric arthritis
    C) Arthritis of the elbow joints
    D) Normal x-rays

20. Which joint/area of the body is affected first in ankylosing spondylitis (AS)?
    A) Lumbar spine
    B) Sacroiliac joint
    C) Cervical spine
    D) Thoracic spine

21. Which of the following is **not** a characteristic symptom or sign in systemic lupus erythematosus (SLE)?
    A) Asymmetric joint pain
    B) Pain disproportionate to swelling
    C) Fatigue and fever
    D) Erosive arthritis

22. Pseudogout commonly involves which of the following areas?
    A) Knee
    B) Toe
    C) Elbow
    D) Fingers

23. The Wright-Schober test is used in which of the following conditions?
    A) Ankylosing spondylitis (AS)
    B) Systemic lupus erythematosus
    C) Reiter's syndrome
    D) Dermatomyositis

24. In Duchenne muscular dystrophy, which protein is absent?
    A) Fibrillin
    B) Dystrophin
    C) Huntingtin
    D) Sarcoglycan

25. Which of the following is the leading cause of morbidity and mortality in patients with Marfan syndrome?
    A) Arachnodactyly
    B) Pneumothorax
    C) Ectopia lentis
    D) Aortic disease

26. Which of the following organisms has been identified as the cause of Lyme disease?
    A) *Borrelia burgdorferi*
    B) *Streptococcus pyogenes*
    C) *Neisseria meningitidis*
    D) *Babesia microti*

27. Antihistone antibodies are present in which of the following conditions?
    A) Rheumatoid arthritis
    B) Sjögren's syndrome
    C) Polymyositis
    D) Drug-induced lupus

28. Which of the following is **true** about rheumatoid arthritis (RA)?
    A) Asymmetric and nonerosive
    B) Symmetric and erosive
    C) Asymmetric and erosive
    D) Symmetric and nonerosive

29. Which of the following is **not** associated with human leukocyte antigen (HLA)-B27 (+) serology?
    A) Reiter's syndrome (reactive arthritis)
    B) Ankylosing spondylitis
    C) Psoriatic arthritis
    D) Osteoarthritis

30. Which of the following is characteristic of pseudogout?
    A) Negative birefringence
    B) Affects primarily the spine
    C) Caused by calcium pyrophosphate crystals
    D) Is usually associated with a rash

31. Long-term use of which of the following class of medications has been associated with poor outcomes in fibromyalgia?
    A) Dual-reuptake inhibitors
    B) Nonsteroidal anti-inflammatory drugs
    C) Anticonvulsants
    D) Opioids

32. What type of hypersensitivity reaction is noted in systemic lupus erythematosus (SLE)?
    A) Type I
    B) Type II
    C) Type III
    D) Type IV

33. Which of the following conditions is associated with formation of abnormal fibrillin?
    A) Osteogenesis imperfecta
    B) Scleroderma
    C) Marfan syndrome
    D) Ehlers-Danlos syndrome

34. Which of the following is the most common benign tumor composed of adipocytes?
    A) Focal nodular hyperplasia
    B) Neuroblastoma
    C) Hemangioma
    D) Lipoma

35. Which of the following vitamin deficiencies can cause scurvy?
    A) Vitamin A
    B) Vitamin B
    C) Vitamin C
    D) Vitamin D

36. In rheumatoid arthritis, which of the following is considered to be the most destructive element?
    A) Infiltration of T-lymphocytes
    B) Formation of pannus
    C) Activation of synoviocytes
    D) Increased blood flow to the tissues

37. Which of the following is **true** of gouty arthritis?
    A) Calcium pyrophosphate dihydrate crystals are found in joint fluid
    B) Female predominance
    C) Allopurinol can be used during an attack
    D) Tophi (deposits of uric acid crystals) may be present

38. Which of the following is a characteristic of gout?
    A) Negative birefringence crystals noted on microscopy of joint aspiration
    B) Positive birefringence crystals noted on microscopy of joint aspiration
    C) Chondrocalcinosis
    D) Affects hyaline cartilage

39. Which of the following is **not** a subtype of juvenile rheumatoid arthritis?
    A) Chronic
    B) Systemic
    C) Pauciarticular
    D) Polyarticular

40. A Boutonnière deformity is noted in your patient. Which condition is most likely, and which area would have a hyperflexion deformity?
    A) Osteoarthritis, proximal interphalangeal joint (PIP)
    B) Rheumatoid arthritis, PIP
    C) Osteoarthritis, distal interphalangeal joint (DIP)
    D) Rheumatoid arthritis, DIP

41. Reiter's syndrome, or reactive arthritis, is made up of a triad of symptoms. Which of the following is **not** involved in Reiter's syndrome?
    A) Urethritis
    B) Conjunctivitis
    C) Arthritis
    D) Pericarditis

42. What type of collagen deficiency is present in osteogenesis imperfecta?
    A) Type 1 collagen
    B) Type 2 collagen
    C) Type 3 collagen
    D) Type 4 collagen

43. A painful joint is aspirated and is found to contain calcium pyrophosphate dihydrate crystals. These joint crystals are pathognomonic of which of the following conditions?
    A) Gout
    B) Pseudogout
    C) Psoriatic arthritis
    D) Osteoarthritis

44. In which of the following disorders would patients have a negative rheumatoid factor (RF)?
    A) Mixed connective tissue disease
    B) Rheumatoid arthritis
    C) Scleroderma
    D) Sjögren's syndrome

45. Which physical modality has demonstrated improvement in patients with rheumatic diseases by increasing activity of synovial collagenase in the joint?
    A) Ultrasound
    B) Superficial heat
    C) Diathermy
    D) Massage

46. All of the following are true in systemic lupus erythematosus (SLE) **except**:
    A) Avascular necrosis typically occurs in small joints
    B) Low-dose steroids can be used to manage SLE
    C) Arthritis is not necessary to diagnose SLE
    D) Antimalarial drugs can be used for symptom control

**47.** What is the most common form of childhood arthritis?
  A) Osteoarthritis
  B) Juvenile rheumatoid arthritis
  C) Rheumatic fever
  D) Ankylosing spondylitis

**48.** What is a characteristic finding in polymyositis?
  A) Skin abnormalities
  B) Proximal muscle weakness
  C) Distal muscle weakness
  D) Ligamentous laxity

**49.** A swan-neck deformity is noted in your patient. Which condition is most likely, and which area would have a hyperflexion deformity?
  A) Osteoarthritis, proximal interphalangeal joint (PIP)
  B) Rheumatoid arthritis, PIP
  C) Osteoarthritis, distal interphalangeal joint (DIP)
  D) Rheumatoid arthritis, DIP

**50.** Which of the following synovial fluid laboratory values is **not** consistent with an inflammatory arthritis?
  A) White blood cell (WBC) count higher than 3,000
  B) 70% polymorphonuclear leukocytes
  C) Decreased erythrocyte sedimentation rate (ESR)
  D) Low viscosity

**51.** Which specific autoantibody is associated with systemic lupus erythematosus (SLE)?
  A) Anti-Smith
  B) Anti-Scl-70
  C) Anticentromere
  D) Anti-Jo-1

**52.** A patient presenting with flexion contracture of the metacarpophalangeal (MCP) joint, hyperextension of the proximal interphalangeal (PIP) joint, and the flexion of the distal interphalangeal (DIP) joint is seen in which of the following diseases?
  A) Osteoarthritis
  B) Gout
  C) Psoriatic arthritis
  D) Rheumatoid arthritis

**53.** Which of the following is **not** part of the CREST syndrome?
  A) Telangiectasia
  B) Scleroderma
  C) Raynaud's phenomenon
  D) Calcinosis

**54.** What is the typical position of a swan-neck deformity of the finger in rheumatoid arthritis?
  A) Hyperextension of the proximal interphalangeal joint (PIP) with hyperextension of the distal interphalangeal joint (DIP)
  B) Hyperextension of the PIP with flexion of the DIP
  C) Flexion of the PIP with flexion of the DIP
  D) Flexion of the PIP with hyperextension of the DIP

55. A reasonable first-line of treatment in osteoarthritis (OA) of the knee is:
    A) Intra-articular injections
    B) Oral steroids
    C) Acetaminophen and/or nonsteroidal anti-inflammatory drugs (NSAIDs)
    D) Colchicine

56. Which of the following is **not** a characteristic radiographic finding in rheumatoid arthritis (RA)?
    A) Erosion of the ulnar styloid
    B) Marginal bony erosions
    C) Asymmetric joint involvement
    D) Uniform joint-space narrowing

57. Which of the following is **not** a part of rehabilitation of the hand in a patient with rheumatoid arthritis?
    A) Resting the involved joints
    B) Heavy exercise of the involved joints
    C) Joint protection instructions
    D) Splinting regimens

58. What is the most serious complication of osteoarthritis (OA) of the cervical spine?
    A) Radiculopathy
    B) Myelopathy
    C) Osteoporosis
    D) Chronic pain

59. Which of the following is **not** a criterion for rheumatoid arthritis according to the American College of Rheumatology (ACR)?
    A) Involvement of three or more joints
    B) Nodules present
    C) Asymmetric involvement
    D) Morning stiffness

60. All of the following are true regarding rheumatoid arthritis **except**:
    A) 85% of cases are rheumatoid factor (+)
    B) Rheumatoid nodules are present
    C) More common in males
    D) Inflammation of the synovial capsule

61. Symmetric erosive destruction of multiple joints is more likely to be seen in which of the following arthropathies?
    A) Osteoarthritis
    B) Reactive arthritis
    C) Rheumatoid arthritis (RA)
    D) Gout

62. Which of the following pediatric conditions leads to fragile bones resulting in multiple fractures?
    A) Juvenile rheumatoid arthritis
    B) Sickle-cell disease
    C) Osteogenesis imperfecta
    D) Osteoarthritis

63. Which of the following exercises is recommended for rheumatoid arthritis?
    A) Isotonic
    B) Concentric
    C) Isokinetic
    D) Isometric

64. Rheumatoid arthritis (RA):
    A) Is primarily a noninflammatory disorder of weight-bearing joints
    B) Primarily affects the distal interphalangeal (DIP) joints
    C) Is more prevalent in females than in males
    D) Is also known as "wear and tear" arthritis

65. Which of the following is **not** a characteristic radiographic finding in osteoarthritis (OA)?
    A) Asymmetric narrowing of the joint space
    B) Erosive changes seen on x-ray
    C) Subchondral bony sclerosis
    D) Osteophytosis

66. What is the gold standard for diagnostic imaging in rheumatoid arthritis (RA)?
    A) Ultrasound
    B) MRI
    C) Plain radiograph
    D) Bone scan

67. What is the most appropriate treatment for pain relief for osteoarthritis of the base of the thumb (carpometacarpal and metacarpophalangeal joints)?
    A) Massage
    B) Transcutaneous electrical nerve stimulation (TENS)
    C) Range of motion exercises
    D) Thumb spica splint

68. Where are Bouchard's nodes found?
    A) Distal interphalangeal joint (DIP)
    B) Proximal interphalangeal joint (PIP)
    C) Metacarpophalangeal joint (MCP)
    D) Intermediate phalanges

69. Which condition is associated with the following features: heliotrope rash, Gottron's papules, and shawl sign?
    A) Dermatomyositis
    B) Inclusion body myositis
    C) Osteoarthritis
    D) Fibromyalgia

70. Pain on ulnar deviation of the wrist with the thumb grasped in the fist is a positive sign for which of the following conditions?
    A) Carpal tunnel syndrome
    B) Rheumatoid arthritis
    C) Medial epicondylitis
    D) De Quervain's tenosynovitis

71. Which of the following is the most destructive element of rheumatoid arthritis?
    A) Joint erosion
    B) Pannus formation
    C) Crystalline formation
    D) Rheumatoid nodules

72. All of the following are common in idiopathic osteoarthritis (OA) of the knee **except**:
    A) Age is over 50 years
    B) Bony tenderness
    C) Stiffness
    D) Erythrocyte sedimentation rate (ESR) is higher than 40

73. All of the following are common in idiopathic osteoarthritis (OA) of the knee **except**:
    A) Palpable warmth
    B) Negative rheumatoid factor (or low titer)
    C) Bony enlargement
    D) Bony tenderness

74. Which of the following are characteristics of osteoarthritis (OA)?
    A) Dull, aching pain that does not remit
    B) Joint stiffness lasting less than 30 minutes and improving as the day progresses
    C) Typically involves the metacarpophalangeal (MCP) joints in the hands
    D) Infrequently involves the spine

75. What is the earliest radiographic sign of rheumatoid arthritis?
    A) Diffuse periarticular osteopenia
    B) Ulnar deviation of the phalanges at the metacarpophalangeal joints (MCP)
    C) Periarticular erosions
    D) Pencil-in-cup deformity

76. Which of the following is associated most strongly with obesity in women?
    A) Hip osteoarthritis
    B) Rheumatoid arthritis
    C) Knee osteoarthritis
    D) Lupus

77. All of the following statements are true **except**:
    A) Pseudogout is caused by a buildup of uric acid in the bloodstream
    B) Pseudogout is caused by the formation of calcium pyrophosphate
    C) The big toe is the most common joint involved in gout
    D) Swelling, warmth, pain, and redness of the joint are common symptoms of gout

78. Massage, manipulation, and traction are all examples of which type of therapy?
    A) Relaxation
    B) Hydrotherapy
    C) Mobilization
    D) Immobilization

79. Which contracture is caused by forearm injuries leading to lack of blood supply to the region?
    A) Dupuytren's contracture
    B) Capsular contracture

    C) Volkmann's contracture

    D) Immobilization contracture

80. Which of the following organisms is commonly responsible for inflammatory polyarthritis?

    A) Parvovirus B-19

    B) *Haemophilus influenzae*

    C) *Streptococcus pneumoniae*

    D) *Neisseria gonorrhoeae*

81. How long must symptoms be present to diagnose fibromyalgia according to the 2010 American College of Rheumatology (ACR) fibromyalgia classification criteria?

    A) 1 month

    B) 3 months

    C) 6 months

    D) 1 year

82. A 52-year-old female with fibromyalgia who you have been following for several months complains of difficulty sleeping and generalized muscle pain. You are considering starting her on cyclobenzaprine at night. Which of the following side effects is commonly seen with cyclobenzaprine?

    A) Dry mouth

    B) Diarrhea

    C) Weight loss

    D) All of the above

83. A 43-year-old female with rheumatoid arthritis presents to you during an acute flare. Which of the following types of exercise would you recommend for this patient to maintain strength while minimizing further joint pain?

    A) Isotonic exercise

    B) Isometric exercise

    C) Isokinetic exercise

    D) Plyometric exercise

84. Which of the following vasculitides commonly affects small arteries, and is associated with necrotizing granulomatous vasculitis affecting the respiratory tract and focal segmental glomerulonephritis?

    A) Wegener's granulomatosis

    B) Polyarteritis nodosa

    C) Behcet's syndrome

    D) Temporal arteritis

85. What is the term given to the enlargement of the gastrocnemius-semimembranosus bursa?

    A) Baker's cyst

    B) Septic arthritis

    C) Gout

    D) Pseudogout

86. Which of the following conditions should be excluded prior to making the diagnosis of fibromyalgia?

    A) Rheumatoid arthritis

    B) Osteoarthritis

    C) Hypothyroidism

    D) All of the above

87. Which of the following is **not** seen in cases of rheumatoid arthritis?
    A) Heberden nodes
    B) Swan-neck deformity
    C) Ulnar deviation of metacarpal phalangeal joints
    D) Adduction of first metatarsal

88. Which of the following vasculitides commonly affects large arteries and is associated with ery-thema nodosum of the legs?
    A) Temporal arteritis
    B) Takayasu's arteritis
    C) Behcet's syndrome
    D) Wegener's granulomatosis

89. Heberden's nodes are a common feature in which of the following disease processes?
    A) Rheumatoid arthritis
    B) Septic arthritis
    C) Osteoarthritis
    D) Gouty arthritis

90. A 44-year-old female with a 6-month history of diffuse muscular pain presents to you for evalu-ation. After taking further history and performing a physical exam, you suspect that the patient has fibromyalgia. Which of the following must be checked to confirm your working diagnosis according to the 2010 American College of Rheumatology (ACR) diagnostic criteria?
    A) Check the 18 specific tender points
    B) Check a brain MRI
    C) Check antinuclear antibodies
    D) Check widespread pain index and symptom severity scale

91. Which of the following findings are you **least** likely to see in a case of long-standing rheumatoid arthritis?
    A) Erosion of the ulnar styloid
    B) Hallux valgus
    C) Volar subluxation at the metacarpophalangeal joint
    D) Chondrocalcinosis

92. Which of the following is **not** classically part of the triad of disorders that are associated with reactive arthritis?
    A) Conjunctivitis
    B) Uveitis
    C) Urethritis
    D) Arthritis

93. Which of the following is **not** a feature of Scheuermann's kyphosis?
    A) Vertebral body wedging of at least 5°
    B) Flattening of curvature with extension
    C) Involvement of at least three vertebral bodies
    D) Anterior wedging

94. There appears to be a close relationship between fibromyalgia and which of the following disorders?
    A) Obsessive compulsive personality disorder
    B) Complex regional pain syndrome
    C) Systemic exertion intolerance disease/chronic fatigue syndrome
    D) Chronic Lyme disease

95. Which of the following is an example of classic radiographic changes seen with osteoarthritis?
    A) Bony erosions, syndesmophytes, and "pencil-in-cup" deformity
    B) Erosions, bony decalcification, and symmetric joint-space narrowing
    C) Sclerosis of facet joints, anterior osteophytes, and loss of intervertebral space in the spine
    D) Erosion and periosteal changes at the insertion of the plantar fascia and Achilles tendon.

96. A decrease in 2 BMI units over a 10-year period in females above the median BMI may decrease the odds of developing osteoarthritis by:
    A) 5%
    B) 15%
    C) 25%
    D) 50%

97. Ankylosing spondylitis is associated with which of the following human leukocyte antigen (HLA) allele?
    A) HLA-B47
    B) HLA-B27
    C) HLA-DR4
    D) HLA-B72

98. The muscle stiffness associated with fibromyalgia typically increases as the day progresses.
    A) True
    B) False

99. Which of the following is an example of classic radiographic changes seen with rheumatoid arthritis?
    A) Osteophytes, subchondral cysts, and loss of articular space
    B) Erosions, bony decalcification, and symmetric joint-space narrowing
    C) Sclerosis of facet joints, anterior osteophytes, and loss of intervertebral space in the spine
    D) Erosion and periosteal changes at the insertion of the plantar fascia and Achilles tendon

100. Polymyositis is characterized by which of the following?
    A) Weakness of shoulder and hip girdle muscles
    B) Weakness of anterior neck flexors
    C) Weakness of pharyngeal muscles
    D) All of the above

101. Pain relieved by activity is a feature of which of the following types of arthritis?
    A) Osteoarthritis
    B) Rheumatoid arthritis
    C) Septic arthritis
    D) Gouty arthritis

102. When compared to the general population, how much higher is the chance of developing fibromyalgia in someone with a family history of fibromyalgia?
    A) No difference
    B) Two times higher
    C) Five times higher
    D) Eight times higher

103. Which of the following joints is **least** likely involved in rheumatoid arthritis?
    A) Distal interphalangeal
    B) Proximal interphalangeal
    C) Wrist
    D) Ankle

104. Up to 16% of patients with polymyalgia rheumatica (PMR) develop which of the following vasculitides?
    A) Wegener's granulomatosis
    B) Polyarteritis nodosa
    C) Temporal arteritis
    D) Takayasu's arteritis

105. What is the most common cause of acute nontraumatic monoarthritis in young adults?
    A) Septic arthritis
    B) Gonococcal arthritis
    C) Gout
    D) Rheumatoid arthritis

106. Fibromyalgia most commonly affects people in which of the following age groups?
    A) 13 to 20 years
    B) 20 to 35 years
    C) 30 to 55 years
    D) 55 to 70 years

107. Which of the following is **not** one of the major theories of the cause of rheumatoid arthritis?
    A) Genetic predisposition
    B) Immunogenetic
    C) Trauma
    D) Environmental causes

108. A 23-year-old male presents to you complaining of insidious onset low-back pain for the last 5 months which is worse in the morning, and improves with exercise. Additionally, the patient reports fatigue and blurry vision. You suspect that the patient has ankylosing spondylitis. Which of the following maneuvers can evaluate spinal mobility?
    A) Crossed straight-leg raise
    B) Schober's test
    C) Bowstring sign
    D) Slump test

109. Which of the following conditions causes calcification of connective tissue?
    A) Fibrodysplasia ossificans progressiva
    B) Hajdu-Cheney syndrome
    C) Fetal hydantoin syndrome
    D) Hurler disease

110. A patient with fibromyalgia is likely to experience all of the following symptoms **except**:
    A) Nausea and vomiting
    B) Sleep disturbances
    C) Mood disturbances
    D) Fatigue

111. Which of the following disease processes is characterized by chronic symmetric erosive synovitis in joints which causes articular damage?
   A) Osteoarthritis
   B) Rheumatoid arthritis
   C) Diffuse idiopathic skeletal hyperostosis
   D) Gout

112. Which of the following is **not** one of the four major seronegative spondyloarthropathies?
   A) Behcet's disease
   B) Reactive arthritis
   C) Ankylosing spondylitis
   D) Psoriatic arthritis

113. Which of the following is **not** a type of connective tissue fiber?
   A) Ependymal
   B) Collagen
   C) Elastic
   D) Reticular

114. Which of the following medications is **not** approved by the U.S. Food and Drug Administration (FDA) for the treatment of fibromyalgia?
   A) Milnacipran
   B) Pregabalin
   C) Duloxetine
   D) Percocet

115. Which of the following nonpharmacologic treatment options may be effective and complementary in the management of fibromyalgia?
   A) Aerobic exercise program
   B) Muscle-strengthening exercise program
   C) Tai chi
   D) All of the above

116. Which of the following joints is most commonly affected in an obese patient with primary osteoarthritis?
   A) Hip
   B) Knee
   C) Spine
   D) Metatarsophalangeal

# Joint and Connective Tissue Disorders

## ANSWERS

1. **B)** The first compartment of the wrist contains the APL and EPB tendons and they are affected in de Quervain's synovitis.

2. **D)** Common potential complications of AS include iritis or uveitis, inflammatory bowel disease, aortic insufficiency and aortic root dilatation, osteoporosis, and spine fracture. Dementia is not a common complication of AS.

3. **D)** Typical reasons for hospitalizing rheumatic disease patients include a decline in ADLs, steroid myopathy, tetraparesis, vasculitis, severe anemia, uncontrolled inflammation, and amputation. Pressure injury is not common in rheumatic disease patients.

4. **C)** Diarthrodial joints are freely moveable joints that are held together by a joint capsule. The composition of diarthrodial joints includes type 2 hyaline cartilage, subchondral bone, synovial membrane, synovial fluid, and joint capsule. Examples include the knee and shoulder. Rheumatoid arthritis first commonly affects the small joints of the hands. In later stages, it affects larger joints such as the knee and shoulder, both of which are diarthrodial joints. An amphiarthrodial joint is a slightly movable joint, such as the spinal joints. A synarthrodial joint is an immoveable joint such as sutural joints.

5. **B)** Radiographic findings of rheumatoid arthritis include osteopenia. All of the other answer choices can be seen in radiographs of patients with rheumatoid arthritis. Patients with osteoarthritis show no signs of osteopenia on radiographs.

6. **D)** Paget's disease is a disease of the bone. The bones are broken down and regenerated, causing them to weaken. Arthritic pain is common near sites of bone weakening, especially when subchondral bone is involved. Paget's disease commonly involves the pelvis, vertebrae, skull, tibia, and femur. Patients are usually asymptomatic; diagnosis is made by increased alkaline phosphatase levels or patchy appearance of bones on x-ray. The skull can become enlarged and patients may complain of increased hat size over time. In addition, if the temporal bone is involved, headaches and hearing loss can occur from cranial nerve palsies.

7. **A)** Interstitial lung disease is reported in more than 75% of patients with systemic sclerosis. A fivefold increase in lung neoplasm is also noted in patients with systemic sclerosis.

8. **C)** There is strong evidence to support the use of patient education, cognitive behavioral therapy, and exercise in the treatment of fibromyalgia. Patients should be informed that fibromyalgia is not a life-threatening disease and be educated on the various treatment options. Understanding fibromyalgia may improve a patient's response to treatments. Education, behavior modification, exercise, and stretching may help patients manage their symptoms.

9. **B)** CRP is an acute phase reactant that plays a role in host defense with both inflammatory and anti-inflammatory actions. Serum CRP levels increase within 4 to 6 hours and normalize in 7 days.

10. **A)** A Boutonnière deformity is characterized by weakness or rupture of the terminal portion of the extensor hood, which holds the lateral bands in place at the PIP joint. There is initially PIP synovitis then a downward slippage of the lateral bands, causing flexion at the PIP joint.

11. **D)** In ankylosing spondylitis, the sacroiliac joint is usually the first joint to be involved, and both sides are affected. It can be associated with HLA-B27. It is much more common in men than in women, and the onset is usually late adolescence to early adulthood.

12. **B)** Dupuytren's contracture is an abnormal fibrous hyperplasia and contracture of the palmar fascia that causes a flexion contracture of the MCP and PIP joints. It is more common in White men age 50 to 70 years. It is associated with alcoholism, pulmonary tuberculosis, epilepsy, and diabetes mellitus. It is painless, but can cause functional problems.

13. **B)** Gout is an inflammatory arthritis most commonly found in the metatarsophalangeal joint at the base of the big toe, also termed *podagra*. Gout is caused by elevated levels of uric acid in the blood, which crystallizes into monosodium urate monohydrate crystals. These crystals are deposited into joints, most commonly the great toe. Causes include genetic predisposition, medications such as diuretics, increased alcohol consumption, and high-purine diets. During an acute gouty attack, the great toe can become red, tender, and swollen. Acute gouty attacks can be treated with nonsteroidal anti-inflammatory drugs (NSAIDs), colchicine, and steroids. For long-term prevention, xanthine oxidase inhibitors, such as allopurinol, would be indicated.

14. **C)** Owing to the loss of joint and spinal motion in patients with ankylosing spondylitis, these patients should engage in range of motion exercises, including stretching and strengthening. Spinal extension exercises help decrease the severity of the condition. Sports that promote spinal extension are favored, including archery, badminton, and table tennis. Sports that require spinal flexion should be avoided in this group, including golf, bicycling, and bowling. Ninety percent of patients with ankylosing spondylitis are HLA-B27 positive.

15. **B)** A seronegative arthritis is an arthritis in which the rheumatoid factor is negative. Of the choices, psoriatic arthritis, reactive arthritis, and ankylosing spondylitis are all rheumatoid factor negative. Psoriatic arthritis is often a milder inflammatory arthritis that develops in approximately 30% of patients who already suffer with psoriasis. During flares, the arthritic symptoms may worsen. Reactive arthritis is an autoimmune condition developed in response to a recent infection, particularly after a genital infection with *Chlamydia trachomatis* or after an episode of gastroenteritis by *Campylobacter* species. The triad of symptoms includes urethritis, conjunctivitis, and arthritis. Ankylosing spondylitis is a chronic inflammatory condition of the spine and sacroiliac joint with osseous formation. Rheumatoid arthritis is an autoimmune disease, usually with a positive rheumatoid factor, resulting in inflammation in tissue and joints.

16. **D)** SLE is a chronic inflammatory disorder involving multiple organs of the body, including skin, lungs, kidneys, and joints. Antibody testing for SLE usually includes antinuclear antibodies (ANA), antiphospholipid, anti–double stranded DNA, and anti-Smith antibodies. Complement levels C3 and C4 are monitored for response to therapy.

17. **D)** Most commonly seen in patients with diabetes mellitus, *Charcot foot* is a term given to neuropathic arthropathy causing painless soft-tissue swelling, bony fragments, and joint effusion in the ankle. Although the pathophysiology of this process is unknown, current theories suggest that diabetic neuropathy causes lack of proprioception and results in ligamentous laxity.

18. **B)** Achondroplasia is an autosomal dominant genetic disorder caused by a mutation in FGFR3. It is the most common form of dwarfism. This mutation leads to impaired cartilage matura-tion in the growth plate, resulting in shortened bone, shortened stature, and a prominent fore-head. The frequency is approximately 1 case in 15,000 to 40,000 births worldwide. No evidence of receptor mutation is linked with Paget's disease of bone, a disease where bone is broken down and regenerated, causing bones to weaken. Osteogenesis imperfecta, or brittle-bone disease, is an autosomal dominant disorder caused by a mutation in the gene producing type 1 collagen. Osteoporosis is caused when there is an imbalance between bone formation and bone resorption, leading to weak and fragile bones.

19. **A)** Morning stiffness lasting more than 1 hour, arthritis of three or more joints simultaneously affected with soft-tissue swelling, arthritis of the hand joints including the wrist/metacarpopha-langeal joint/proximal interphalangeal joint, symmetric arthritis of the same joints on both sides of the body, rheumatoid nodules (subcutaneous nodules over the extensor surfaces), positive serum rheumatoid factor, and radiographic changes, such as erosions/joint-space narrowing, are all characteristics of rheumatoid arthritis. Not all are necessary for diagnosis.

20. **B)** In AS, the typical order of progression is that the sacroiliac joint is affected first, followed by the lumbar spine, thoracic spine, and lastly cervical spine. This is distal to proximal progression.

21. **D)** SLE is associated with a nonerosive arthritis.

22. **A)** Pseudogout commonly involves the knee and wrist as opposed to gout, which usually affects the big toe (termed *podagra*). Pseudogout is inflammation caused by calcium pyrophosphate crystals. Gout is inflammation caused by monosodium urate monohydrate crystals. Both can be diagnosed with aspirated synovial fluid. Pseudogout presents with acute joint swelling and pain commonly in the knee, but can also affect the wrist, shoulders, and hip.

23. **A)** The Wright-Schober test is used to measure the ability to flex the lower back in a patient with AS. AS is a chronic inflammatory condition of the spine and sacroiliac joint that leads to osse-ous formation in the spine. The test is conducted with the examiner identifying the fifth lumbar vertebrae (L5), marking 5 cm below this point, and another point 10 cm above L5. The examiner instructs the patient to attempt to touch his or her toes. Lumbar flexion should increase the dis-tance between the two points by more than 5 cm. If the distance between the two points does not increase by 5 cm, flexion is limited and the test is considered positive.

24. **B)** Duchenne muscular dystrophy is an X-linked recessive muscle disease caused by an absence of the muscle protein dystrophin, leading to rapid muscle weakness. The first sign and symptom of Duchenne muscular dystrophy is progressive muscle weakness in the proximal muscles of the lower extremities. This can result in a positive Gower's sign (the child has to use hands and arms to stand up because of weakness of hip and thigh muscles). Levels of creatine kinase are very elevated. The prognosis is poor, with affected individuals having life expectancy of less than 25 years of age. A less severe form of muscular dystrophy is Becker's muscular dystrophy, which is caused by deficient dystrophin production, causing a slower progression of proximal muscle weakness. Fibrillin is deficient in patients with Marfan syndrome. Fibrillin is normally found in connective tissue and is necessary for formation of elastic fibers.

25. **D)** Aortic root disease causing aortic dilatation, aortic dissection, and regurgitation is the main cause of morbidity and mortality in patients with Marfan syndrome. Approximately 60% to 80% of adult patients with Marfan syndrome have aortic root dilatation, and the American Heart Association recommends an echocardiogram at the time of diagnosis.

26. **A)** Lyme disease is a tick-borne illness caused mostly by *B. burgdorferi* in the United States. The early stage of Lyme disease involves formation of erythema migrans, a characteristic skin lesion that develops within 2 weeks to a month of exposure. Later stages can involve neurological and cardiac symptoms along with persistent arthritis involving large joints such as the knee.

27. **D)** Drug-induced lupus is a lupus-like syndrome without involvement of the central nervous system or kidneys. Certain drugs, including hydralazine, procainamide, isoniazid, chlorpromazine, methyldopa, and quinidine, have been linked to drug-induced lupus. Upon discontinuing the offending drug, symptoms usually resolve. Antihistone antibodies are present, which can help identify the problem. Rheumatoid arthritis is an autoimmune disease resulting in inflammation in tissue and joints. Sjögren's syndrome is an autoimmune disease involving lymphocyte infiltration and destruction of lacrimal and salivary glands. Patients with Sjögren's syndrome usually have dry eyes and dry mouth. Polymyositis is an inflammatory myopathy that results in symmetrical proximal muscle weakness.

28. **B)** Rheumatoid arthritis is a systemic autoimmune inflammatory disorder of unknown etiology that affects multiple organ systems. It affects the musculoskeletal system and specifically the synovial lining of diarthrodial joints. Diarthrodial joints contain type II hyaline cartilage, subchondral bone, synovial membranes, joint capsule, and synovial fluid. It is a chronic, symmetric, erosive synovitis that develops in the joints and leads to joint destruction. Erosions are specific to RA.

29. **D)** All of the choices **except** osteoarthritis are associated with HLA-B27 (+) serology. They are called seronegative arthropathies. Other HLA-B27 (+) diseases include enteropathic arthropathy and pauciarticular juvenile rheumatoid arthritis.

30. **C)** Pseudogout is caused by calcium pyrophosphate crystals and exhibits positive birefringence when a polarizer is used. The crystals line up parallel to the polarizer and are yellow.

31. **D)** Observational studies have demonstrated that patients who receive opioids have poorer outcomes than those who do not. Dual-reuptake inhibitors (milnacipran and duloxetine) inhibit norepinephrine and serotonin reuptake, and they improve fatigue, pain, and the general well-being of those with fibromyalgia. Nonsteroidal anti-inflammatory drugs (NSAIDs) used alone and steroids are generally not effective in treating fibromyalgia as there is no tissue inflammation. NSAIDs may be beneficial when used in combination with other medications. Anticonvulsants, such as pregabalin, may alleviate pain and improve sleep in those with fibromyalgia.

32. **C)** Type I hypersensitivity reaction is immediate with IgE as a mediator. Examples include asthma and anaphylaxis. Type II is also known as cytotoxic, or antibody dependent, with IgM or IgG as mediators. Examples of type II hypersensitivity reaction include thrombocytopenia and erythroblastosis fetalis. Type III is also known as immune complex with IgG as a mediator. Examples include rheumatoid arthritis and systemic lupus erythematosus. SLE is an autoimmune connective tissue disease. The immune system attacks the patient's own cells and tissues causing inflammation and damage to the tissue. Type IV is also known as delayed type or cell mediated, with T-cells as a mediator. Examples include multiple sclerosis and chronic transplant rejection.

33. **C)** Marfan syndrome is an autosomal dominant condition caused by FBN1 gene mutation located on chromosome 5. There is a defect in the fibrillin protein. Fibrillin is normally found in connective tissue and is necessary for formation of elastic fibers. Excess linear growth of long bones, arachnodactyly, and joint laxity are common skeletal findings. Cardiac conditions such as aortic root dilation and mitral valve pathology may be noted. Patients with Marfan syndrome exhibit

long fingers and toes (arachnodactyly), dislocation of the lens in either or both eyes (ectopia lentis seen in 50%–80% of patients with Marfan syndrome), and skeletal deformities such as pectus excavatum and scoliosis. The most potentially fatal effect is cardiac involvement, especially with aortic root dilatation and aortic dissection.

34. **D)** Lipomas are lobules of adipocytes found in subcutaneous tissue, deep soft tissue, or surfaces of bone. These lesions are usually painless, unless compressing against adjacent tissue or nerves resulting in neurological or functional deficits.

35. **C)** Vitamin C deficiency leads to impaired collagen synthesis, resulting in pathological manifestations in tissues and organs containing collagen.

36. **B)** Rheumatoid arthritis is an inflammatory disorder that primarily affects synovial joints. Inflammation of the capsule around the joints, known as the synovium, is the first step in this destructive disease. Over time, synovial cells are destroyed, causing hyperplasia. Neutrophils, macrophages, and B- and T-cell lymphocytes are activated to increase the inflammatory response. Pannus develops when the inflammation-causing fibrin deposits and develops into granulation tissue.

37. **D)** Tophi can be seen in gout. Calcium pyrophosphate dihydrate crystals are seen in pseudogout. Gout has a male predominance. Allopurinol is used to lower serum uric acid and prevent or decrease attacks, but is not used for an acute attack.

38. **A)** Gout is inflammation caused by monosodium urate crystals. Gout is characterized by needle-shaped crystals seen under microscopy after joint aspiration. If a polarizing filter is used, the crystals are yellow when they align parallel but turn blue when aligned across the direction of the polarizer (negative birefringence).

39. **A)** The subtypes of juvenile rheumatoid arthritis are systemic, pauciarticular, and polyarticular. Pauciarticular involves one to four joints, polyarticular involves five or more joints, and systemic is characterized by a systemic onset.

40. **B)** Rheumatoid arthritis is an autoimmune disease resulting in inflammation in tissue and joints. The disease affects the digits of the hand. Boutonnière deformity is caused when the PIP is slowly forced into flexion by chronic synovitis of the joint from rheumatoid arthritis. This causes an elongation of the central slip, ultimately leading to rupture. Subsequent volar displacement of the lateral bands below the axis of the PIP rotation creates increased tension on the DIP extensor mechanism, leading to hyperextension and limited flexion of the DIP. Osteoarthritis results from generalized wear and tear on the body with progressive degeneration of joints, including cartilage, bone, synovium, muscles, and ligaments. Rheumatoid arthritis is more commonly found in women, whereas osteoarthritis has more equal sex distribution. Rheumatoid arthritis is commonly diagnosed as early as age 20 years, whereas osteoarthritis affects those above age 40 years. Answer choices (A) and (C) are incorrect because Boutonnière deformity is seen in rheumatoid arthritis. Answer choice (D) is incorrect because hyperflexion of the DIP would result in swan-neck deformity.

41. **D)** Reactive arthritis is an autoimmune condition developed in response to a recent infection, particularly after a genital infection with *Chlamydia trachomatis*, or after an episode of gastroenteritis caused by *Campylobacter* species. The triad of symptoms includes urethritis, conjunctivitis, and arthritis. The mechanism of action is unknown, but it is assumed to involve the migration of bacterial antigens into the affected triad sites, which proceed to cause an inflammatory response.

This syndrome is usually self-limiting, but if symptoms are more severe, a course of steroids and immunosuppressants may be indicated. Of the answer choices, pericarditis is not a finding in Reiter's syndrome. Patients with rheumatic fever, an inflammatory disease after a streptococcal infection affecting the heart, joint, skin, and brain, can develop pericarditis. Patients with systemic lupus erythematosus can develop antigen-antibody complexes in the pericardium, causing inflammation or pericarditis.

42. **A)** Osteogenesis imperfecta, or brittle-bone disease, is an autosomal dominant disorder caused by a gene mutation producing type 1 collagen. Type 1 collagen is the most abundant collagen in the body found in scar tissue during healing. The bone mass in individuals with this disorder is diminished. Patients classically have blue sclera because of the lack of type 1 collagen formation in the eye allowing the choroidal veins to be seen.

43. **B)** Pseudogout is an arthropathy caused by a collection of positively birefringent crystals of calcium pyrophosphate dihydrate crystals. Symptoms are usually noted in the knee, but can be present in other joints as well. Inflammation and limited range of motion of the involved joint are noted.

44. **C)** RFs are antibodies against the Fc part of the IgG and are not commonly seen in patients with scleroderma. Although the sensitivity of rheumatoid factor in rheumatoid arthritis is close to 90%, it is nonspecific because elevated levels of RF are found in Sjögren's syndrome, mixed connective tissue disease, systemic lupus erythematosus, and myositis.

45. **B)** Heating the joint to therapeutic levels increases the activity of synovial collagenase obtained from a rheumatoid joint. Superficial heat is commonly used by patients for self-treatment in those with rheumatic diseases.

46. **A)** Avascular necrosis typically affects large joints. Although joint pain is common, arthritis is not necessary to diagnose SLE and is not always present. The other choices are true.

47. **B)** Juvenile rheumatoid arthritis is the most common form of childhood arthritis and is characterized by onset at under 16 years of age, persistent arthritis of one or more joints for at least 6 weeks, and exclusion of other types of childhood arthritis, and type of onset of disease during the first 6 months classified as polyarthritis, oligoarthritis, or systemic arthritis with intermittent fever.

48. **B)** Polymyositis is characterized by proximal muscle weakness (hips are affected first, then the shoulders), dysphagia, and elevated muscle enzymes. Dermatomyositis has dermatological abnormalities in addition to the other listed symptoms.

49. **D)** Rheumatoid arthritis is an autoimmune disease resulting in inflammation in tissue and joints. The disease affects the digits of the hand. Swan-neck deformity is caused by a rupture of the lateral retinaculum of the extensor tendon at the proximal interphalangeal joint, resulting in hyperextension of the proximal interphalangeal joint and hyperflexion of the distal interphalangeal joint. Osteoarthritis results from generalized wear and tear on the body with progressive degeneration of joints, including cartilage, bone, synovium, muscles, and ligaments. Rheumatoid arthritis is more commonly found in women, whereas osteoarthritis has more equal sex distribution. Rheumatoid arthritis is commonly diagnosed as early as age 20 years, whereas osteoarthritis affects those above age 40 years. Answer choices (A) and (C) are incorrect because swan-neck deformity is seen in rheumatoid arthritis. Answer choice (B) is incorrect because hyperflexion of the PIP would result in Boutonnière deformity. This is caused by chronic synovitis of the joint, resulting in elongation and eventual rupture of the central slip tendon.

50. **C)** Joint fluid analysis in a patient with an inflammatory arthritis would consist of a white blood cell count greater than 3,000 cells/mm³, greater than 70% polymorphonuclear leukocytes, lower viscosity due to its inflammatory nature, and elevated ESR. ESR is a sign of inflammation and, as such, ESR would be elevated in inflammatory arthritis. The differential diagnosis for inflammatory arthritis includes rheumatoid arthritis, systemic lupus erythematosus, gouty arthritis, Reiter's disease, pseudogout, and psoriatic arthritis. Decreased ESR would be found in noninflammatory arthritis, most commonly in osteoarthritis. Inflammatory arthritis patients usually have an acute onset, whereas noninflammatory arthritis patients usually have a slow, progressive, and degenerative course.

51. **A)** Indirect immunofluorescence pattern assists in determining the type of antibody present in the serum. Anti–double stranded DNA and anti-Smith antibodies are specific for SLE. Anti-Scl-70 or antitopoisomerase and anticentromere antibodies are specific for scleroderma. Anti-Scl-70 or antitopoisomerase antibody is specific for diffuse scleroderma. Anticentromere antibody is specific for limited scleroderma. Anti-Jo-1 antibody is associated with polymyositis and/or dermatomyositis.

52. **D)** Swan-neck deformity is commonly seen in patients with rheumatoid arthritis, but can also be seen in patients with Ehlers-Danlos syndrome.

53. **B)** The CREST syndrome comprises calcinosis, Raynaud's phenomenon, esophageal dysmotility, sclerodactyly, and telangiectasia.

54. **B)** A swan-neck deformity can be seen in the hands of rheumatoid arthritis patients and is a hyperextension of the PIP with flexion of the DIP. There is also flexion at the metacarpophalangeal joint (MCP). It is caused by chronic inflammation at the PIP, which causes a stretch of the volar plate. The PIP joint then moves into hyperextension. At the DIP, there is elongation or rupture of the extensor hood at the base of the phalanx.

55. **C)** The other choices are used in inflammatory arthritis, or as treatments for refractory OA, but not as a first-line treatment. OA is not an inflammatory arthritis.

56. **C)** In patients with RA, characteristic changes on x-ray are as follows: uniform joint-space narrowing, symmetric joint involvement, marginal bony erosions, juxta-articular osteopenia, ulnar deviation of phalanges, radial deviation of the radiocarpal joint (carpals and metacarpals), erosion of the ulnar styloid, atlantoaxial subluxation, and small joint involvement, including metacarpophalangeal joints, proximal interphalangeal joints, and carpal joints.

57. **B)** In rheumatoid arthritis, it is important to rest the involved joints. Heavy exercise of the involved joints is contraindicated as it could cause more damage. Other important rehabilitation measures include modification of activities that stress the joints, joint protection, work simplification instructions, splinting regimens, heat modalities followed by active range of motion exercise, and resistive exercise.

58. **B)** Cervical myelopathy (spinal cord compression) is the most serious complication of OA of the cervical spine. Although nerve roots can become impinged because of osteophytes (radiculopathy) as well, it is not as serious as spinal cord compression. Cervical myelopathy from OA usually requires surgical intervention. Chronic pain can be associated with OA, but is not as serious as myelopathy.

59. **C)** The ACR criteria state that rheumatoid arthritis involves the same area on both sides of the body. Involvement of three or more joints, presence of nodules, and morning stiffness are all seen in rheumatoid arthritis. Morning stiffness, arthritis of three or more joints, arthritis of the hand joints, and symmetric arthritis must be present for more than 6 weeks to qualify under the ACR guidelines. Radiographic changes and serum rheumatoid factor are included in the criteria. Four of the above mentioned criteria must be present.

60. **C)** Rheumatoid arthritis is more common in females than in males. Rheumatoid arthritis is an inflammatory disorder that primarily affects synovial joints. Inflammation of the capsule around the joints, known as the synovium, is the first step in this destructive disease. Nodules are present in about 50% of patients with rheumatoid arthritis and are located most commonly over the pressure points of joints.

61. **C)** RA usually presents as morning stiffness in multiple joints. RA is caused by autoimmune destruction of unknown etiology. Current American College of Rheumatology criteria for rheumatoid arthritis include morning stiffness lasting for at least 1 hour, involvement of three or more joints, involvement of at least one joint in the hand, symmetric involvement of joints, rheumatoid nodules, positive rheumatoid factor, and radiographic evidence of erosions or decalcification of joints. At least four of the seven criteria must be met for diagnosis.

62. **C)** Osteogenesis imperfecta, also known as brittle-bone disease, is caused by gene mutations of alpha-1 and alpha-2 chains of type 1 collagen and posttransitional modification of type 1 collagen. Type 1 collagen is an important structural protein for ligament, tendon, sclera, and bone. Dysfunctional type 1 collagen results in defective quality and fragility of bone seen in patients with osteogenesis imperfecta.

63. **D)** Isometric contraction of a muscle does not cause a change in muscle length or joint angle and is ideal for rheumatoid arthritis because it allows the joint to rest.

64. **C)** RA has a 3:1 female:male predominance. The other choices describe OA.

65. **B)** In patients with OA, characteristic changes on x-ray are as follows: asymmetric narrowing of the joint space, no erosive changes on x-ray, joint involvement that does not have to be symmetric, no osteoporosis or osteopenia, osseous cysts, subchondral bony sclerosis, osteophytosis, and loose bodies. Common joints involved include the first carpometacarpal joint, distal interphalangeal joints, knees, and hips.

66. **C)** Plain radiograph remains the gold standard for diagnostic imaging in rheumatoid arthritis.

67. **D)** A thumb spica splint immobilizes the two joints of the thumb. Although it may interfere with some activities of daily living (ADLs), it does provide consistent pain relief.

68. **B)** The DIP is the location for Heberden's nodes. Bouchard's nodes and Heberden's nodes are formed when osteophytes, also known as calcific spurs, develop in the cartilage of the articular joint. Bouchard's and Heberden's nodes are seen in osteoarthritis. Metacarpophalangeal (MCP) joints are joints formed between the metacarpal bones and the proximal ends of the phalanges. Arthritis in the MCP joint is commonly found in patients with rheumatoid arthritis.

69. **A)** *Dermatomyositis* is a term used to describe polymyositis with the addition of a characteristic heliotrope rash, Gottron's papules, and shawl sign. A heliotrope rash is a butterfly rash around the eyes, bridge of the nose, and cheeks. Gottron's papules are papular, erythematous, scaly lesions over the metacarpophalangeal joints, proximal interphalangeal joints, and distal interphalangeal joints. Shawl sign is a rash on the shoulders and upper back, elbows, and knees. Similar to polymyositis, there is symmetric proximal muscle weakness sparing the distal musculature. Creatine kinase (CK) levels are markedly elevated, indicating muscle breakdown. The rash usually precedes the muscle weakness.

70. **D)** A positive Finkelstein's test (as described earlier) is suggestive of de Quervain's tenosynovitis, which is a tendonopathy of the extensor pollicis brevis and abductor pollicis longus tendons. This syndrome is commonly seen in new mothers and repetitive movements that involve repetitive ulnar or radial deviation of the wrist. De Quervain's tenosynovitis may also be seen in patients with rheumatoid arthritis.

71. **B)** Pannus is a tissue derived from synovial membrane that causes destruction of cartilage and bone. Multinucleated cells with osteoclastic characteristics have been identified in the pannus-bone interface. This destruction can lead to instability of joints and eventual fibrosis, becoming the leading cause of morbidity in patients with rheumatoid arthritis.

72. **D)** OA is not associated with an elevated erythrocyte sedimentation rate as there is no inflammatory response. It is commonly characterized as "wear and tear arthritis." The other choices are common in OA.

73. **A)** OA is not typically associated with inflammation or warmth. The other choices are common.

74. **B)** Osteoarthritis is characterized by joint stiffness that is worse in the morning, lasting less than 30 minutes, and improving as the day goes on.

75. **A)** Diffuse periarticular osteopenia is the earliest radiographic sign of rheumatoid arthritis. Joint-space narrowing and periarticular erosions may be observed later (usually within 2 years of the disease). Other deformities such as ulnar deviation of the MCP, radial deviation of the wrist, and swan-neck deformities are later findings.

76. **C)** Osteoarthritis (OA) of the knee is associated with obesity in women. OA has not been shown to be the result of osteochondritis dissecans or athletic activity.

77. **A)** Hyperuricemia is found in gout, not pseudogout. Pseudogout is inflammation caused by calcium pyrophosphate crystal deposition. The exact mechanism is unknown, but aging is the only true risk factor. The onset is between ages 60 and 70 years. Gout is inflammation caused by monosodium urate monohydrate crystals. Both can be diagnosed with aspirated synovial fluid. Pseudogout is an acute form of the broader calcium pyrophosphate dihydrate deposition disease, presenting with acute joint swelling and pain commonly in the knee, but can also affect the wrist, shoulders, hip, elbows, and metacarpophalangeal (MCP) joints.

78. **C)** Mobilization therapy aids in pain control and range of motion of joints and muscles. It includes massage, manipulation, and traction. Manipulation involves moving the stiff joints in their normal range of motion. Traction is the constant, steady pull of the joint or muscle. Relaxation therapy involves techniques that are taught to help release the tension formed in the muscles and joints of the body. Hydrotherapy consists of patients relaxing the muscles and joints in warm water.

79. **C)** Volkmann's contracture is contracture of the flexor muscles owing to ischemia in the volar aspect of the forearm. It usually occurs after a forearm injury. Forearm fractures and supracondylar fractures leading to compartment syndrome secondary to swelling can lead to ischemia of the affected region. Extended episodes of ischemia will cause necrosis of the muscle fibers causing them to scar and shorten. Usually, the deep muscles of the forearm, flexor digitorum profundus, and flexor pollicis longus are involved. Capsular contracture is the formation of capsular collagen fibers owing to an abnormal immune response to artificial materials in the body (such as breast implants or prosthetic devices). Dupuytren's contracture is a flexion contracture caused by thickening of the connective tissue in the palmar fascia resulting in flexion of the fingers, particularly the fourth and fifth digits.

80. **A)** Acute inflammatory polyarthritis is a self-limiting viral arthritis that presents with morning stiffness and symmetrical joint involvement of the upper extremities lasting a few weeks. Viruses commonly noted to cause polyarthritis include parvovirus B-19, Rubella, alphavirus, and hepatitis B and C viruses.

81. **B)** According to the 2010 ACR classification criteria, the patient must meet three of the following conditions: (a) widespread pain index (WPI) of 7 or more, and symptom severity (SS) scale score of 5 or more, or WPI 3 to 6 and SS scale score of 9 or more; (b) symptoms have been present **for at least 3 months**; and (c) the patient does not have a disorder that would otherwise explain the pain.

82. **A)** Cyclobenzaprine is a muscle relaxant, and its chemical structure, mechanism of action, and side-effect profile is similar to tricyclic antidepressants (TCAs). TCAs given at bedtime may improve sleep and relieve muscle pain. Common side effects of TCAs and cyclobenzaprine include difficulty concentrating, fatigue, somnolence, constipation, weight gain, fluid retention, and dry mouth.

83. **B)** Muscle contractions can be divided into two categories: static and dynamic. Isometric exercise uses static muscle contractions, while isotonic and isokinetic exercises use dynamic muscle contractions. Plyometric exercise is a form of isotonic exercise which involves quick, powerful movements that start with an eccentric muscle contraction immediately followed by a concentric muscle contraction. Isometric exercises are most useful during an acute rheumatoid arthritis (RA) flare as it causes the least amount of periarticular bone destruction and joint inflammation while helping to maintain strength. Isotonic and isokinetic exercises should be avoided in an acute flare of RA as they can exacerbate symptoms.

84. **A)** Wegener's granulomatosis is a small-artery vasculitis that commonly affects middle-aged males. Wegener's granulomatosis is associated with "saddle-nose" deformity, necrotizing granulomatous vasculitis affecting the respiratory tract, and focal segmental glomerulonephritis.

85. **A)** The gastrocnemius-semimembranosus bursa is found between the tendons of the medial head of the gastrocnemius and the semimembranosus muscles. The distention of this bursa is called a Baker's cyst. Although usually asymptomatic, the rupture of a Baker's cyst can cause acute pain in the back of the knee.

86. **D)** Many disease processes may mimic fibromyalgia as they can also present with generalized muscle aches and fatigue. Some examples of conditions that must be ruled out prior to diagnosing fibromyalgia include rheumatoid arthritis (RA), systemic lupus erythematosus (SLE), osteoarthritis (OA), ankylosing spondylitis (AS), polymyalgia rheumatica (PMR), hypothyroidism, myositis, and metabolic myopathy. RA typically presents as joint pain and swelling; however, RA causes inflammation of the synovial membranes which can help differentiate it from fibromyalgia. OA typically presents as joint stiffness, tenderness and pain; however, degenerative changes on radiographs will be seen with OA which can help differentiate it from fibromyalgia. Hypothyroidism can cause generalized body aches, sleep disturbances, and fatigue; therefore, thyroid function tests are routinely checked prior to diagnosing fibromyalgia.

87. **A)** Heberden's and Bouchard's nodes are seen in osteoarthritis. Heberden's nodes affect the distal interphalangeal joint, while Bouchard's nodes affect the proximal interphalangeal joint. Bouchard nodes may also be seen in rheumatoid arthritis. Swan-neck deformities, Boutonnière deformities, ulnar deviations, metatarsal phalangeal subluxation, and adduction of the first metatarsal are

seen in cases of rheumatoid arthritis. Swan-neck deformities (MCP flexion, PIP hyperextension, and DIP flexion) are caused by rupture of the lateral retinaculum of the extensor tendon at the proximal interphalangeal joint (PIP). Boutonnière deformities (MCP hyperextension, PIP flexion, and DIP hyperextension) are caused by rupture of the extensor hood, which holds the lateral bands in place. This causes the lateral bands of the extensor hood to sublux, which turns them into flexors of the PIP joint. Ulnar deviations are caused by rupture of the radial retinaculum and the pull of the long finger flexors.

88. **B)** Takayasu's arteritis is a large-vessel vasculitis that commonly affects Asian females. Takayasu's arteritis is associated with pulselessness, arm claudication, and erythema nodosum on the lower extremities. It can lead to hypertension, heart failure, stroke, myocardial infarction, and aneurysm of the aorta.

89. **C)** Heberden's nodes are osteoarthritis enlargements in the distal interphalangeal joints and appear in more than half of patients with osteoarthritis. Repeated trauma causes these osteophyte formations to develop and may cause joint stiffness and tenderness.

90. **D)** According to the 2010 ACR classification criteria, the patient must meet three of the following conditions: (a) widespread pain index (WPI) of 7 or more and symptom severity (SS) scale score of 5 or more, or WPI 3 to 6 and SS scale score of 9 or more; (b) symptoms have been present for at least 3 months; (c) the patient does not have a disorder that would otherwise explain the pain. Tenderness in at least 11 out of the 18 specific sites was used to diagnose patients with fibromyalgia according to the 1990 ACR classification criteria. The 2010 guidelines do not require a tender point examination.

91. **D)** Chondrocalcinosis is seen in pseudogout (not rheumatoid arthritis) when calcium pyrophosphate dihydrate (CPPD) crystals are deposited in articular cartilage, synovial lining, ligaments, and tendons. Chondrocalcinosis commonly occurs in the menisci of the knee causing narrowing of the tibial-femoral joint. Typical radiographic findings in rheumatoid arthritis include erosion of the ulnar styloid, hallux valgus, ulnar deviation and volar subluxation at the metacarpophalangeal (MCP) joint, axial migration of the hip (protrusion acetabuli), juxta-articular osteopenia (bone washout), cervical atlantoaxial (A-A) subluxation, erosion of the metatarsal head, and radial deviation of the radiocarpal joint.

92. **B)** The triad of disorders that are associated with reactive arthritis are arthritis, urethritis, and conjunctivitis. Reactive arthritis typically follows a 2- to 4-week period of diarrhea or urethritis. Uveitis, along with skin rashes, psoriasis, and aortitis, are common extra-articular symptoms of spondyloarthropathies.

93. **B)** Scheuermann's kyphosis occurs in early adolescence and is defined as anterior wedging of at least 5° involving at least three vertebral bodies. Forward bending, extension, or lying supine does not resolve this rigid kyphosis that usually involves the thoracic or thoracolumbar spine.

94. **C)** There is a close relationship between fibromyalgia and systemic exertion intolerance disease (SEID), also known as chronic fatigue syndrome (CFS). SEID/CFS is characterized by debilitating chronic fatigue, and up to 70% of those with fibromyalgia also fulfill the diagnostic criteria for SEID/CFS. Common symptoms of SEID/CFS include unrefreshing sleep, brain fog, muscle and joint pain, headache, light sensitivity, abdominal pain, bloating, nausea, swollen glands, tender lymph nodes, and sore throat.

95. **C)** Classic radiographic changes seen in rheumatoid arthritis include erosions, bony decalcification in and next to the involved joints, and symmetric joint-space narrowing (due to loss of articular cartilage). Classic radiographic changes seen in osteoarthritis (OA) include asymmetric joint-space narrowing, osteophyte formation, subchondral bony sclerosis, osseous cysts, and loose bodies. Sclerosis of facet joints, anterior vertebral body osteophytes, and loss of intervertebral space in the spine is commonly seen in OA of the spine. Erosion and periosteal changes at the insertion of the plantar fascia and Achilles tendon ("lover's heel") is typically seen with reactive arthritis. Bony erosions, syndesmophytes, and "pencil-in-cup" deformity of the distal interphalanx (DIP) are typically associated with psoriatic arthritis.

96. **D)** A reduction of 2 BMI units over a 10-year period in females with a BMI above the median BMI can decrease the chances of developing osteoarthritis by over 50%.

97. **B)** The human leukocyte antigen is synonymous with the major histocompatibility complex and describes a group of genes on chromosome 6. Ankylosing spondylitis is a chronic inflammatory disease of the axial skeleton commonly associated with HLA-B27.

98. **B)** The primary symptom of fibromyalgia is diffuse and chronic pain. The pain may fluctuate in intensity and can be aggravated by anxiety, poor sleep, exertion, or exposure to cold temperatures. The pain may be described as aching, sore, stiff, throbbing, or burning. Typically the muscle stiffness tends to improve as the day progresses.

99. **B)** Classic radiographic changes seen in rheumatoid arthritis include erosions, bony decalcification in and next to the involved joints, and symmetric joint-space narrowing (due to loss of articular cartilage). Classic radiographic changes seen in osteoarthritis (OA) include asymmetric joint-space narrowing, osteophyte formation, subchondral bony sclerosis, osseous cysts, and loose bodies. Sclerosis of facet joints, anterior vertebral body osteophytes, and loss of intervertebral space in the spine is commonly seen in OA of the spine. Erosion and periosteal changes at the insertion of the plantar fascia and Achilles tendon ("lover's heel") is typically seen with reactive arthritis.

100. **D)** Inflammatory muscle disorders, such as polymyositis, dermatomyositis and inclusion body myositis, commonly affect striated muscles. Polymyositis and dermatomyositis classically present with significant symmetrical proximal muscle weakness involving the shoulder and hip girdle, anterior neck flexors, and pharyngeal muscles (which can lead to dysphagia). Characteristic electrodiagnosis (EMG) findings in polymyositis and dermatomyositis include complex repetitive discharges, abnormal spontaneous resting activity, and myopathic motor unit action potentials with early myopathic motor unit recruitment.

101. **B)** Morning stiffness is a feature of nearly all types of arthropathies, but rheumatoid arthritis has classically been noted to have morning stiffness lasting longer than an hour and relieved by movement.

102. **D)** The likelihood of developing fibromyalgia is increased eightfold in someone if they have a family history of fibromyalgia.

103. **A)** According to the American College of Rheumatology criteria for the classification of rheumatoid arthritis (RA), the patient is said to have RA if they meet four out of the seven criteria. The seven criteria include morning stiffness, arthritis of three or more joint areas, arthritis of hand joints, symmetric arthritis, rheumatoid nodules, serum rheumatoid factor, and radiographic changes. The 14 possible joint areas are bilateral proximal interphalangeal (PIP),

metacarpophalangeal (MCP), wrist, elbow, knee, ankle, and metatarsal phalangeal (MTP) joints. Unlike osteoarthritis, RA typically does not involve the distal interphalangeal (DIP) joints.

104. **C)** Temporal arteritis, also known as giant cell arteritis, involves the large arteries. Temporal arteritis presents as headaches, tenderness of the scalp region, and sudden visual loss. Up to 16% of patients with polymyalgia rheumatica (PMR) develop temporal arteritis, and 50% of patients with temporal arteritis have symptoms of PMR. Common symptoms of PMR include sudden myalgias/arthralgias, malaise, weight loss, fever, and muscle pain/stiffness around the neck, shoulder, and pelvis.

105. **B)** Disseminated gonococcal infection can lead to gonococcal arthritis. This may present initially as tenosynovitis and eventually lead to destruction of the articular cartilage and fibrosis of the joint. Culture from synovial fluid is important for early diagnosis and to determine sensitivity to antibiotic therapy.

106. **C)** Most people begin to develop symptoms of fibromyalgia between 30 and 55 years of age. In the United States, 2% of people are affected by fibromyalgia by age 20 years, and 8% of people are affected by age 80 years. Fibromyalgia is more common in women than men. Fibromyalgia is the most common cause of generalized muscular pain in females between the ages of 20 and 55 years.

107. **C)** Rheumatoid arthritis (RA) affects about 1% of the adult population, and affects females two to three times more often than males. The exact etiology of RA is unknown; however, there are three major theories: environmental causes (infections), genetic predisposition, and immunogenic. Some factors that may contribute to the development of osteoarthritis (OA) include genetics, age, previous trauma or surgery to the joint, increased body weight, and increased stress on the joint.

108. **B)** The Schober's test is commonly used to evaluate for decrease in lumbar flexion motion seen in ankylosing spondylitis. The Schober's test is performed by marking the first sacral spinous process and then making another mark 10 cm above the first mark. The patient is instructed to flex forward at the lumbar spine and the increased distance between the two marks is measured. An increase of less than 5 cm is considered a restriction. The straight-leg raise, crossed straight-leg raise, bowstring sign, and slump test are all used to evaluate for lumbar disc herniation.

109. **A)** Fibrodysplasia ossificans progressiva is an autosomal dominant disorder of connective tissue characterized by bone formation within connective tissue. Trauma usually precipitates the ossification of connective tissue, including minor trauma such as intramuscular injections or bruises. Attempts to remove the calcified bone from the connective tissue result in further ossification.

110. **A)** Fibromyalgia is a chronic condition that causes diffuse muscle pain and tenderness. Many patients with fibromyalgia will also experience fatigue, headaches, sleep disturbances, mood and cognitive disturbances such as depression and anxiety, as well as bowel and bladder irritability.

111. **B)** Rheumatoid arthritis (RA) is a systemic autoimmune inflammatory condition, which primarily affects the synovial lining of diarthrodial joints. The pathognomonic erosions of RA are caused by chronic symmetric erosive synovitis, which leads to joint destruction. Osteoarthritis (OA) is generally a noninflammatory condition that affects weight-bearing joints. OA is characterized by degeneration of the joint, cartilage, bone, synovium, muscles, and ligaments. Diffuse

idiopathic skeletal hyperostosis (DISH) is a variant form of primary OA in which spinal fusion occurs owing to osteophytes, which extend the length of the spine. DISH most commonly affects the thoracic or thoracolumbar spine. The hallmark of DISH is ossification across three or more intervertebral disks. Gout is characterized by acute or intermittent inflammation due to deposition of crystals in or around joints.

112. **A)** The seronegative spondyloarthropathies (SEAs) are a group of multisystem inflammatory diseases that affect multiple joints. Most of the SEAs are human leukocyte antigen (HLA)-B27 positive and rheumatoid factor (RF) negative. The four major SEAs are ankylosing spondylitis, reactive arthritis, psoriatic arthritis, and arthritis of inflammatory bowel disease. Behcet's disease is a rare immune-mediated small-vessel vasculitis that commonly presents with oral ulcers, genital ulcers, and uveitis.

113. **A)** Collagenous fibers are the most abundant of the connective tissue fibers and are found in vessels, cartilage, gut, skin, bone, tendons, and ligaments. Elastic fibers form the extracellular matrix and can stretch up to 1.5 times their length. Reticular fibers provide a framework and are found in the liver, marrow, and lymphatic organs.

114. **D)** Tricyclic antidepressants, serotonin-norepinephrine reuptake inhibitors, and alpha-2-delta ligands have demonstrated efficacy in the treatment of fibromyalgia. The FDA has approved duloxetine, milnacipran, and pregabalin for the treatment of fibromyalgia.

115. **D)** Regular cardiovascular exercise for a minimum of 30 minutes three times a week may be helpful in reducing muscle pain in those with fibromyalgia. Muscle-strengthening exercise programs also reduce pain and number of tender points. Some fibromyalgia patients have benefited from tai chi, which merges mind-body practice with graceful movement exercises. Additionally, relaxation therapies, such as stress-reduction programs, relaxation techniques, hypnosis, biofeedback, and cognitive behavioral therapy (CBT) may improve fibromyalgia symptoms.

116. **B)** Primary osteoarthritis (OA) most commonly affects the following joints: knee, metatarsophalangeal, distal interphalangeal, carpometacarpal, hip, and spine. Obesity most commonly leads to OA of the knees (most commonly the medial compartment). Secondary OA (when there is a recognizable underlying cause) commonly affects the elbows and shoulders.

# 11

# Exercise/Modalities

## QUESTIONS

1. Which of the following is a physiologic result of wound treatment with ultraviolet radiation?
   A) Decreased vitamin D production
   B) Increased bacterial growth
   C) Increased vascularization of wound margins
   D) Decreased calcium metabolism

2. Which of the following is best defined as repeated, rapid stretching, such as bouncing?
   A) Ballistic stretching
   B) Plyometric stretching
   C) Passive stretching
   D) Static stretching

3. Which of the following best describes eccentric contractions?
   A) They cause more tissue damage than concentric contractions
   B) They have high metabolic cost
   C) They are muscle shortening contractions
   D) Slow eccentric contractions generate the least amount of force

4. All of the following are contraindications for ultrasound **except**:
   A) Malignancy
   B) Amyotrophic lateral sclerosis
   C) Skeletal immaturity
   D) Proximity to a pacemaker

5. Which of the following is **not** an effect of ultraviolet radiation?
   A) Increased vascularization
   B) Decreased muscle spasm
   C) Cell protein changes
   D) Bactericidal

6. Which of the following types of massage involves rhythmic alternating contact of varying pressure between the hands and the body's soft tissue?
   A) Pétrissage
   B) Effleurage
   C) Tapotement
   D) Friction

7. Which of the following types of cold modalities use evaporation as the main form of energy transfer?
   A) Cold packs
   B) Vapocoolant spray
   C) Ice massage
   D) Whirlpool baths

ANSWERS TO THIS SECTION CAN BE FOUND ON PAGE 347

8. Which of the following is **not** a goal of massage?
   A) Produce relaxation
   B) Improve arterial insufficiency
   C) Reduce pain
   D) Improve circulation

9. Phonophoresis involves:
   A) The use of ultrasound to facilitate transdermal mitigation of topically administered medications
   B) The use of an imposed electric field to mitigate charged particles across biologic membranes
   C) The use of ultraviolet radiation to mitigate charged particles across biologic membranes
   D) The use of ultraviolet radiation to facilitate transdermal mitigation of topically administered medications

10. Which of the following mechanisms is best described as transfer of heat by fluid circulation over the surface of a body?
    A) Convection
    B) Conduction
    C) Conversion
    D) Circumduction

11. Which of the following best describes a gradual stretch over 15 seconds?
    A) Ballistic stretching
    B) Plyometric stretching
    C) Passive stretching
    D) Static stretching

12. Which of the following best describes concentric contractions?
    A) Low metabolic cost
    B) Produces greater force than eccentric contraction
    C) Muscle lengthens against resistance
    D) High metabolic cost

13. All of the following are indications for ultrasound **except**:
    A) Bursitis
    B) Tendinitis (calcific tendinitis)
    C) Degenerative arthritis and contracture
    D) Deep tissue inflammation

14. Which of the following is **not** an indication for cold therapy?
    A) Acute sprains
    B) Spasticity
    C) Arterial insufficiency
    D) Chronic muscle spasm

15. Which of the following stretching techniques requires a trainer or a partner?
    A) Static
    B) Ballistic
    C) Passive
    D) Active

16. Which of the following is a physiologic effect of cold?
    A) Slowing of conduction velocity
    B) Increase in muscle strength reflexes
    C) Increase muscle fatigue
    D) Decreased joint stiffness

17. Whirlpool baths are typically used for treatment of a limb or localized lesion. Which of the following describes the thermal energy transfer of whirlpool baths?
    A) Convection
    B) Conduction
    C) Evaporation
    D) Radiation

18. Which of the following is **not** a contraindication to massage?
    A) Areas of trauma
    B) Areas of known deep vein thrombosis (DVT)
    C) Areas of malignancy
    D) Areas of osteoarthritis or osteoporosis

19. Which of the following mechanisms is best described as the transfer of energy between two bodies at different temperatures through direct contact?
    A) Convection
    B) Conduction
    C) Conversion
    D) Circumduction

20. Which of the following is an appropriate therapeutic ultrasound frequency?
    A) 100 MHz
    B) 1,000 MHz
    C) 1 MHz
    D) 20 MHz

21. Which of the following is a cardiovascular effect of conditioning exercises?
    A) Increased resting heart rate
    B) Decreased stroke volume during maximal exercise
    C) Increased myocardial oxygen consumption at rest
    D) Decreased blood pressure at rest

22. Deep heat modalities include all of the following **except**:
    A) Ultrasound
    B) Shortwave diathermy
    C) Microwave diathermy
    D) Hydrotherapy

23. What is an effect of cryotherapy?
    A) Decreased nerve conduction velocity
    B) Increased muscle-spindle activity
    C) Increased tissues metabolism
    D) Decreased nerve-pain threshold

24. Which of the following is **not** a component of an exercise prescription?
    A) Mode
    B) Intensity
    C) Isometric
    D) Progression

25. Which of the following is a general precaution for the use of cryotherapy (cold modalities)?
    A) Hypothyroidism
    B) Hyperthyroidism
    C) Raynaud's disease
    D) Spasticity

26. What is the typical duration when applying cold packs?
    A) 1 to 2 hours
    B) 40 to 60 minutes
    C) 20 to 30 minutes
    D) As long as the patient can tolerate

27. Which is **not** an indication for ultraviolet radiation therapy?
    A) Psoriasis
    B) Septic wounds
    C) Acne treatment
    D) Eczema

28. Which of the following theories is commonly accepted as the mechanism of action of transcutaneous electrical nerve stimulation (TENS)?
    A) Electric theory
    B) Blast theory
    C) Desensitization theory
    D) Gate theory

29. Which of the following is the most effective type of transcutaneous electrical nerve stimulation (TENS) stimulator?
    A) High frequency, high intensity
    B) High frequency, low intensity
    C) Low frequency, high intensity
    D) Low frequency, low intensity

30. Which contraction generates the **least** force?
    A) Slow eccentric
    B) Fast eccentric
    C) Slow concentric
    D) Fast concentric

31. What is the main mechanism of deep heat transfer via diathermy?
    A) Conversion
    B) Convection
    C) Conduction
    D) None of the above

32. In which of the following areas could microwave diathermy be used?
    A) Edematous tissue
    B) Fluid-filled cavities
    C) Reproductive organs
    D) Muscle with spasm

33. At similar oxygen consumptions,
    A) Heart rate (HR), systolic blood pressure (SBP), and diastolic blood pressure (DBP) are lower during arm work because arm work is less mechanically efficient than leg work
    B) HR, SBP, and DBP are higher during arm work because arm work is less mechanically efficient than leg work
    C) HR, SBP, and DBP are lower during arm work because arm work is more mechanically efficient than leg work
    D) HR, SBP, and DBP are higher during arm work because arm work is more mechanically efficient than leg work

34. Which of the following is **not** a contraindication for ultrasound use?
    A) Skeletal immaturity
    B) Over a pacemaker
    C) Over a laminectomy site
    D) Near metal

35. Which of the following is **not** a risk for acupuncture?
    A) Cardioversion
    B) Infection
    C) Organ puncture
    D) Needle shock

36. What is an effect of ultrasound in the pulsed mode?
    A) Standing waves
    B) Cavitations
    C) Media motion
    D) All of the above

37. Hot packs are typically maintained in water baths at what temperature?
    A) 40°C to 50°C
    B) 60°C to 70°C
    C) 70°C to 80°C
    D) 80°C to 90°C

38. Which of the following best describes the placebo effect on the mechanism of pain control in transcutaneous electrical nerve stimulation (TENS)?
    A) There is no placebo effect in TENS
    B) Placebo effect accounts for 90% of pain relief in TENS
    C) Placebo effect accounts for 50% of pain relief in TENS
    D) Placebo effect accounts for 30% of pain relief in TENS

39. The greatest force is generated with what type of contraction?
    A) Slow eccentric
    B) Fast eccentric

C) Slow concentric

D) Fast concentric

40. What is a contraindication for the use of contrast baths?

A) Rheumatoid arthritis

B) Complex regional pain syndrome

C) Muscular strain

D) Buerger's disease

41. All of the following are indications for microwave diathermy **except**:

A) Increase heat to muscles

B) Resolution of hematomas

C) Multiple sclerosis (MS)

D) Increase heat to joints

42. In the supine position:

A) Gravity has an increased effect on return of blood to the heart so the systolic blood pressure (SBP) is lower

B) Gravity has less effect on return of blood to the heart so the SBP is higher

C) Gravity has an increased effect on return of blood to the heart so the SBP is higher

D) Gravity has less effect on return of blood to the heart so the SBP is lower

43. Paraffin baths are superficial heating agents that utilize which mode or mechanism for heat transfer?

A) Convection

B) Conversion

C) Conduction

D) Radiation

44. Which of the following is **not** a physiologic effect of cold?

A) Immediate cutaneous vasoconstriction

B) Decreased acute inflammation

C) Slowing of conduction velocity

D) Increased spasticity

45. Which one is **not** a therapeutic effect of heat therapy?

A) Increased nerve signal conduction

B) Increased tendon extensibility

C) Increased blood flow

D) Decreased collagen extensibility

46. What is the force recommended for cervical traction?

A) 5 to 10 lb

B) 10 to 15 lb

C) 15 to 20 lb

D) 25 to 30 lb

47. Bed rest or immobilization has what impact on muscle mass?

A) 5% to 10% of muscle mass is lost weekly

B) 10% to 15% of muscle mass is lost weekly

C) 15% to 20% of muscle mass is lost weekly

D) 20% of muscle mass is lost weekly

48. Which of the following best describes type 2 muscle fibers?
    A) Used for high-intensity, short-duration activities
    B) Small muscle fiber diameter
    C) Innervated by small, slow-conducting motor neurons
    D) High in oxidative enzymes

49. Prolonged use of which modality produces erythema ab igne (skin mottling)?
    A) Ultrasound
    B) Hot pack
    C) Shortwave diathermy
    D) Contrast therapy

50. All of the following are contraindications to the use of shortwave diathermy **except**:
    A) Metal implants, including pacemakers
    B) Contact lenses
    C) Skeletal maturity
    D) Gravid or menstruating uterus

51. At rest, 15% to 20% of cardiac output is:
    A) Shunted to the skin
    B) Shunted to the brain
    C) Shunted to the splanchnic vasculature
    D) Shunted to the skeletal muscles

52. Which heating modality is most likely to cause erythema ab igne?
    A) Heating pads
    B) Paraffin baths
    C) Fluidotherapy
    D) Ultrasound

53. Manipulation and body-based therapies affect health by application of passive (massage, spinal manipulation) or active body movement. Which of the following is not a contraindication to utilizing manipulation and mobilization?
    A) Osteoarthritis
    B) Acute fracture/dislocation
    C) Severe osteoporosis
    D) Cauda equina syndrome

54. Which of the following is characteristic of open kinetic chain exercises?
    A) Distal end fixed
    B) Squatting
    C) Less shear stress
    D) Distal end not fixed

55. What is iontophoresis?
    A) Using ultrasound to drive topical medications into tissue
    B) Using electric current to drive medications into tissue
    C) Using massage to drive topical medications into tissue
    D) Using cold spray to numb a painful area

56. Bed rest or immobilization has what type of impact on strength?
    A) Decreases strength by 10% daily
    B) Decreases strength by 10% monthly
    C) Decreases strength by 5% daily
    D) Decreases strength by 1% daily

57. Which of the following best describes type 1 muscle fibers?
    A) Fast twitch, high in oxidative enzymes
    B) Fast twitch, low in oxidative enzymes
    C) Large muscle fiber diameter
    D) Slow twitch, high in oxidative enzymes

58. What is a mechanism of heat transfer?
    A) Conduction
    B) Convection
    C) Conversion
    D) All of the above

59. All of the following are indications for shortwave diathermy **except**:
    A) Chronic prostatitis
    B) Pregnancy
    C) Muscle pain and spasms
    D) Refractory pelvic inflammatory disease

60. Which of the following is not a method where venous return is maintained or increased during exercise:
    A) Contracting skeletal muscle acts as a "pump" against the various structures that surround it, including deep veins, forcing blood back to the heart
    B) Smooth muscles around the venules contracts, causing venoconstriction
    C) Increased heart rate and relaxation of the arterioles leading to increased venous return
    D) Diaphragmatic contraction during exercise creates lowered intrathoracic pressure, facilitating blood flow from the abdominal area to the lower extremities

61. Which of the following pathologies is a general contraindication for utilizing heat modalities?
    A) Osteoarthritis
    B) Diabetes
    C) Malignancy
    D) Hypertension

62. Which of the following is **not** considered a mind-body therapy?
    A) Cognitive behavioral therapy
    B) Aromatherapy
    C) Meditation
    D) Ayurveda

63. Which of the following is a contraindication to heat therapy?
    A) Muscle spasm
    B) Chronic inflammation
    C) Arthritis
    D) Scar tissue

64. What is phonophoresis?
   A) Using ultrasound to drive topical medications into tissue
   B) Using electric current to drive medications into tissue
   C) Using massage to drive topical medications into tissue
   D) Using cold spray to numb a painful area

65. Which of the following best defines a concentric contraction?
   A) Muscle lengthening contraction
   B) Muscle shortening against resistance
   C) Muscle does not change length during contraction
   D) A contraction generating little force

66. What axiom states that "high-intensity, low-repetition exercise builds strength, and low-intensity, high-repetition exercise builds endurance"?
   A) Miranda axiom
   B) Aaron axiom
   C) DeLorme axiom
   D) Fiat axiom

67. Why is heat therapy **not** appropriate for scar tissue?
   A) Scar tissue is rich in collagen fiber
   B) Scar tissue has inadequate vascular supply
   C) Scar tissue has inadequate collagen fiber
   D) Heat decreases tissue metabolism

68. All of the following are indications for phonophoresis **except**:
   A) Tendinitis
   B) Tenosynovitis
   C) Lateral epicondylitis (tennis elbow)
   D) Tinnitus

69. Age-predicted maximal heart rate:
   A) Increases with age
   B) Stays relatively consistent throughout the years
   C) Decreases with age
   D) None of the above

70. Which of the following is **not** a hemodynamic physiological effect from using heat modality?
   A) Increased blood flow
   B) Decreased bleeding
   C) Decreased chronic inflammation
   D) Increased edema

71. Electroejaculation:
   A) Is induced by electrical stimulation via rectal probe
   B) Is known to adversely affect sperm motility
   C) Does not cause retrograde ejaculation
   D) Can cause mucosal injury

72. Therapeutic ultrasound uses which of the following techniques to warm tissue?
   A) Conduction
   B) Convection

C) Conversion

D) Sublimation

73. How long is the average therapeutic ultrasound session?
    A) 0 to 5 minutes
    B) 7 to 15 minutes
    C) 15 to 20 minutes
    D) 20 to 30 minutes

74. Which of the following best defines an eccentric contraction?
    A) Muscle-lengthening contraction
    B) Muscle-shortening against resistance
    C) Muscle does not change length during contraction
    D) A contraction generating little force

75. Which of the following is characteristic of closed kinetic chain exercises?
    A) Distal end fixed
    B) More shear stress created
    C) An example would be leg extensions with free weights
    D) Distal end not fixed

76. All of the following are indications for heat therapy **except**:
    A) Arthritis
    B) Chronic inflammation
    C) Superficial thrombophlebitis
    D) Vascular Insufficiency

77. The technique that uses ultrasound to deliver medications through the skin is:
    A) Phonophoresis
    B) Diathermy
    C) Iontophoresis
    D) Pulsed wave

78. What is a contraindication for spinal traction?
    A) Bursitis
    B) Cervical radiculopathy
    C) Osteopenia
    D) Muscle spasm

79. Which of the following mechanisms involves the transfer of thermal energy between two bodies in direct contact?
    A) Conduction
    B) Convection
    C) Radiation
    D) Conversion

80. Iontophoresis involves:
    A) The use of ultrasound to facilitate transdermal mitigation of topically administered medications
    B) The use of an imposed electric field to mitigate charged particles across biologic membranes
    C) The use of ultraviolet radiation to mitigate charged particles across biologic membranes
    D) The use of ultraviolet radiation to facilitate transdermal mitigation of topically administered medications

# Exercise/Modalities

## ANSWERS

1. **C)** Ultraviolet radiation increases vascularization of wound margins.

2. **A)** Ballistic stretching involves bouncing-type maneuvers.

3. **A)** Eccentric contractions cause more tissue damage than concentric contractions. With eccentric contractions, muscles lengthen with contraction resisting a stretching force. With concentric contractions, muscles shorten against resistance.

4. **B)** Contraindications to the use of ultrasound include malignancy, use in close proximity to some organs (eg, brain, eye, reproductive organs, spine), pregnancy, a menstruating uterus, infection, near metal (pacemaker, arthroplasty), skeletal immaturity, and near a laminectomy site.

5. **B)** Ultraviolet light can be bactericidal, increase vascularization, and alter cell proteins. It has not been shown to help decrease muscle spasm.

6. **C)** Tapotement, or percussion massage, uses rhythmic alternating contact of varying pressure between the hands and the body's soft tissue. Various techniques are used to produce this type of massage, including hacking, clapping, beating, pounding, and vibration. Effleurage involves the gliding of palms, finger tips, and thumbs over the skin in a circular pattern with different forms of pressure. Pétrissage is also known as "kneading massage." It involves compressing the skin between the thumb and fingers. Friction massage is a circular, longitudinal, or transverse pressure applied by the fingers, thumb, or hypothenar region of the hand to small areas.

7. **B)** Vapocoolant spray is the only cold modality listed that utilizes evaporation as the main form of energy transfer. Vapocoolant spray and stretch methods are used by some practitioners to treat myofascial and musculoskeletal pain syndromes. The technique consists of a series of unidirectional applications of Fluori-Methane spray, which has replaced the highly flammable ethyl chloride spray in clinical usage. Treatment begins in the "trigger area" (area of deep myofascial hypersensitivity) and extends over the "reference zone" (area of referred pain) while passively stretching the muscle. Ice massage is the direct application of ice to the skin using gentle stroking motions. It combines the therapeutic effects of cooling with the mechanical effects of massage. Whirlpool baths and Hubbard tanks control water temperature and agitate the water by aeration, dispersing thermal energy by convection.

8. **B)** Massage has multiple effects on the body, including mechanical, reflexive, neurologic, and psychologic effects. The exact therapeutic mechanism by which massage works is not fully understood. The goals of therapeutic massage are to produce relaxation, relieve muscle tension, reduce pain, increase mobility of soft tissues, and improve circulation.

9. **A)** Phonophoresis involves the use of ultrasound to facilitate transdermal migration of topically administered medications. Corticosteroids are the most frequently used phonophoresis agents. The anti-inflammatory effects of ultrasound and corticosteroids are thought to be synergistic. The actual mechanism of transdermal migration has not been well defined but could involve increased cell permeability from the thermal effects of ultrasound.

10. **A)** Convection is best described as the transfer of heat by fluid circulation over the surface of a body. Conduction is the transfer of energy between two bodies at different temperatures through direct contact.

11. **D)** Static stretching keeps a muscle in the same position for some time period, usually 15 to 20 seconds, and is relatively safe.

12. **D)** Concentric contractions have a high metabolic cost compared with eccentric contractions.

13. **D)** Indications for ultrasound include tendinitis (calcific tendinitis), bursitis, subacute trauma, degenerative arthritis, contracture (hip contracture, adhesive capsulitis), and musculoskeletal pain. Ultrasound works best on superficial tissues.

14. **C)** Indications for cryotherapy include musculoskeletal conditions (sprain, strain, tendinitis, tenosynovitis, bursitis, capsulitis), myofascial pain, spasticity, and acute trauma (in the first 24- to 48-hour period, cold therapy can help reduce inflammation and edema). Cold therapy may exacerbate arterial insufficiency.

15. **C)** There are four main methods of stretching: ballistic, static, passive, and neuromuscular facilitation. Ballistic stretching uses repetitive rapid application of force in an active bouncing or jerking maneuver. Passive stretching is performed with a partner who applies a stretch to a relaxed joint or extremity. This method requires the slow and sensitive application of force. Static stretching applies a steady force for a period of 15 to 60 seconds. This method is the easiest and probably the safest type of stretching. The specific activities most frequently used include hold-relax and contract-relax techniques, characterized by an isometric or concentric contraction of the musculotendinous unit followed by a passive or static stretch.

16. **A)** Some effects of cold modalities include increased joint stiffness, decreased muscle fatigue, decrease in muscle strength, slowing of conduction velocity, and decreased muscle strength fibers. Other effects of cold modalities are decreased muscle firing rates, delayed reactive vasodilation, and decreased acute inflammation.

17. **A)** Whirlpool baths disperse thermal energy via convection. Because only a portion of the body is immersed, greater extremes of temperature can be tolerated without significant core body temperature changes.

18. **D)** Special care should be observed in patients who receive massages over areas of severe osteoarthritis or osteoporosis. However, having such diseases is not a contraindication to massage. Areas of trauma or recent bleeding should not be treated with deep tissue massage. Mobilization of these areas can increase the propensity for rebleeding. Massage should not be used over areas of known DVT or atherosclerotic plaques. This could result in dislodgment of these vascular thrombi, resulting in embolic infarcts affecting the pulmonary, cerebral, or peripheral systems. Massage should not be performed in areas of malignancy as it is thought to have the potential to cause mobilization of tumor cells into the vascular lymphatic supply.

19. **B)** Conduction is the transfer of energy between two bodies at different temperatures through direct contact. Convection is best described as the transfer of heat by fluid circulation over the surface of a body.

20. **C)** An appropriate frequency for a therapeutic ultrasound prescription would be 0.8 to 1.1 MHz.

21. **D)** Decreased blood pressure at rest is a cardiovascular effect of conditioning exercise. Resting heart rate is decreased by exercise. Stroke volume is increased during maximal exercise.

22. **D)** Ultrasound, shortwave diathermy, and microwave diathermy are deep heating modalities. The main mechanism of heat transfer from hydrotherapy is convection, and it is considered superficial heating.

23. **A)** The therapeutic effects of cryotherapy include decreased nerve conduction velocity, vaso-constriction, diminished acute inflammatory responses, diminished muscle-spindle activity, and increased nerve-pain threshold.

24. **C)** Isometric is when the joint angle and the muscle length do not change during a contraction. There are five components of an exercise prescription: mode, intensity, duration, frequency, and progression. Mode is the particular type of exercise, intensity is the physiologic difficulty of the exercise, duration is the length of an exercise session, frequency is the number of sessions per day and per week, and progression is the increase in activity during exercise training.

25. **C)** There are no contraindications to cold modalities in patients with hypothyroidism or hyper-thyroidism. Cold modalities actually help decrease spasticity. General precautions for the use of cold modalities should be taken into account in patients with impaired sensation, cold intol-erance, cryoglobulinemia, Raynaud's disease, cognition or communicative deficits, and arterial insufficiency.

26. **C)** Typical duration when applying cold packs is 20 to 30 minutes. Cold packs include hydrocol-lator packs, endothermic chemical gel packs, and ice packs. Hydrocollator packs are cooled in a freezer to −12°C (10°F) and applied over a moist towel. Endothermic chemical gel packs have separate compartments with compounds such as ammonium nitrate and water, which when mixed undergo a heat-absorbing reaction. They are portable, pliable, and easily used in the field. Although many endothermic chemical gel packs are designed for one-time use, some have the advantage that they can be refrozen and reused as a simple cryogel pack.

27. **D)** The indications for ultraviolet radiation therapy include psoriasis, wounds (septic and asep-tic), acne, and folliculitis. Eczema is a contraindication.

28. **D)** The gate theory, in which stimulated large myelinated afferent fibers block the transmission of pain by small unmyelinated fibers at the level of the spinal cord is commonly accepted as the mechanism of action of TENS.

29. **B)** High-frequency, low-intensity stimulation is the most effective type of TENS stimulation.

30. **D)** Fast concentric contractions generate the least amount of force. Greatest force is generated with fast eccentric contractions. However, these types of contractions can result in damage to the muscles. Eccentric contractions are lengthening contractions whereas a concentric contraction is muscle shortening with resistance.

31. **A)** Conversion of electromagnetic energy into radiant heat energy is the main mechanism of heat transfer via diathermy.

32. **D)** Microwave diathermy selectively heats fluid-filled cavities. Therefore, it should be avoided in fluid-filled cavities (blisters, edematous tissue) and some organs (brain, reproductive organs, eyes).

33. **B)** At similar oxygen consumptions, HR, SBP, and DBP are higher during arm work than during leg work. This is because the total muscle mass in the arms is smaller requiring the recruitment of a greater percentage of the available mass to perform the work. In addition, arm work is less mechanically efficient than leg work.

34. **D)** Studies have reported that temperature increases from ultrasound near metal were actually lower than temperature rises near bone, so metal per se should not be a contraindication to ultrasound. Deep heating over an open epiphysis could result in either increased growth (from hyperemia) or decreased growth (from thermal injury). Avoiding ultrasound near pacemakers is reasonable because of potential thermal or mechanical injury to the pacemaker. Ultrasound over laminectomy sites could theoretically result in spinal cord heating. Ultrasound at therapeutic dosage over the peroneal nerve has been shown to produce a reversible conduction block in some patients with polyneuropathy.

35. **A)** The literature regarding acupuncture safety indicates a low rate of complications, even among acupuncture students. Risks for acupuncture include bleeding, infection, and organ puncture (including pneumothorax). Needle shock is an uncommon side effect that typically occurs during the first acupuncture treatment. The description of this event is similar to a vasovagal episode: sweating, flushing, and the sensation that the world is being seen from down a long tunnel. Treatment of needle shock is the immediate removal of the needles.

36. **D)** The pulsed mode of ultrasound produces nonthermal effects including cavitation, media motion, and standing waves.

37. **C)** Hot packs are typically maintained in water baths at 70°C to 80°C. Hot packs should never be applied directly to the skin. There should be towels between the patient and the hot pack to avoid burning the patient's skin.

38. **D)** The placebo effect accounts for about 30% of pain relief in TENS.

39. **B)** Greatest force is generated with fast eccentric contractions. However, these types of contractions can result in damage to the muscles. Eccentric contractions are lengthening contractions whereas a concentric contraction is muscle shortening with resistance.

40. **D)** A contraindication for the use of contrast baths include small vessel disease caused by diabetes or Buerger's disease. The other options are indications for contrast baths.

41. **C)** The indications for the use of microwave diathermy include heating muscle and joints, and decreasing hematomas under the skin. Heat should never be used in MS.

42. **D)** In the supine position, gravity has less of an effect on the return of blood to the heart, so the SBP is lower. When the body is upright, gravity works against the return of blood to the heart so the SBP increases. Diastolic blood pressure does not change significantly with body position in healthy individuals.

43. **C)** A paraffin bath is a superficial heating agent that uses conduction as the primary form of heat transfer. Paraffin wax and mineral oil are mixed in a ratio of 6:1 or 7:1. Treatment temperatures at 52.2°C to 54.4°C (126°F to 130°F) are used. These are tolerated because of the low heat conductivity of the paraffin mixture. Methods of application include dipping, immersion, and brushing. The dipping method involves 7 to 12 dips followed by wrapping in plastic and towels or insulated mitts to retain heat. The immersion method involves several dips to form a thin glove of paraffin, followed by immersion for 30 minutes. The brushing method involves brushing on several coats of paraffin, followed by covering with towels. The brushing method is more cumbersome, and infrequently used in the adult population.

44. **D)** Physiologic effects of cold consist of immediate cutaneous vasoconstriction, decreased acute inflammation, slowing of conduction velocity, reduced spasticity, decreased pain, and generalized relaxation.

45. **D)** Heat increases nerve signal conduction, collagen extensibility, and blood flow; cold decreases all of these physiologic parameters.

46. **D)** The recommended force for cervical traction is 25 to 30 lb.

47. **A)** With immobilization, 5% to 10% of muscle mass is lost weekly.

48. **A)** Type 2 muscle fibers are large muscle fibers, with peak tension and relaxation achieved rapidly. They are primarily used for high-intensity, short-duration activities.

49. **B)** Prolonged usage of hot packs can produce skin mottling (erythema ab igne), which is characterized by reticular pigmentation and telangiectasia.

50. **C)** Shortwave diathermy produces deep heating by the conversion of radiowave electromagnetic energy into thermal energy. Contraindications for shortwave diathermy include metal (pacemakers, intrauterine devices, and implants), contact lenses, pregnancy, menstruating uterus, and skeletal immaturity.

51. **D)** About 15% to 20% of the cardiac output is distributed to the skeletal muscles during rest while the remaining blood is distributed to visceral organs such as the brain and the heart. During exercise, 85% to 90% of the cardiac output is delivered to working muscles, shunted away from the skin and splanchnic vasculature.

52. **A)** Heating pads are most likely to cause erythema ab igne (hot water bottle rash, laptop thigh, fire stains, and toasted skin syndrome). Patients should be advised that leaving heating pads on the skin for prolonged periods of time can lead to hyperpigmentation, scaling, and telangiectasias. The most common reason for erythema ab igne is placing a hotpack on the skin while sleeping.

53. **A)** Osteoarthritis is not a contraindication to using manipulation or mobilization. Acute fracture/dislocation, severe osteoporosis, cauda equina, active inflammatory arthropathy, tumor/metastasis, and spinal infection/osteomyelitis are some absolute contraindications to using manipulation and mobilization.

54. **D)** Open kinetic chain exercises have a distal end (usually the foot) that is not fixed, and create more shear stress than closed kinetic chain exercises.

55. **B)** Iontophoresis is a technique that uses electric current to drive electrically charged medications into tissue.

56. **D)** Immobilization decreases strength by about 1% daily.

57. **D)** Type 1 muscle fibers are slow-twitch, oxidative muscle fibers. They are primarily for low-intensity, long duration activities.

58. **D)** The mechanisms of heat transfer include radiation, conduction (eg, hot water, hot packs), convection (eg, fluidotherapy, hydrotherapy), and conversion (eg, ultrasound, shortwave diathermy, microwave diathermy).

59. **B)** The indications for shortwave diathermy include chronic prostatitis, refractory pelvic inflammatory disease, and muscle pain and spasms.

60. **C)** With exercise, the heart rate increases and arterioles constrict to increase blood flow and venous return. Arterioles do not dilate with exercise. Contraction of the skeletal muscles, constriction of the venules, and diaphragmatic contraction are methods that increase venous return.

61. **C)** Caution should be utilized when using heat over malignancies because of the potential for increased rate of tumor growth. Heat can also exacerbate acute inflammation, but is known to decrease chronic inflammation. In a patient with impaired circulation, increased metabolic activity with heating can exceed the capacity of arterial supply, so heat should be used with caution in those patients. Heat should be avoided in areas of impaired sensation due to the potential for thermal injury. Heat should also not be used in areas of large scars because scars can be relatively avascular and have a reduced ability to dissipate heat.

62. **D)** Ayurveda is an alternative medical approach that encompasses a gamut of herbal and mineral preparations that are prescribed based on the energetic qualities of the preparation. Cognitive behavioral therapy (CBT), aromatherapy, and meditation are mind-body therapies. CBT integrates the cognitive restructuring approach of cognitive therapy with the behavioral modification techniques of behavioral therapy. A therapist typically works with patients to identify thoughts and behaviors that are maladaptive, and attempts to change their thought patterns, leading to a change in behavior. Aromatherapy uses essential oils, distilled from plants, to improve mood, health, or both. Scents can be inhaled or applied in oil during a massage. The acts of meditation is to train, calm, or empty the mind, often by achieving an altered state, as by focusing on a single object.

63. **D)** Heat increases the metabolic demand of scar tissue, which is poorly vascularized. This can result in ischemic necrosis.

64. **A)** Phonophoresis uses ultrasound to drive topical medications into tissue.

65. **B)** A concentric contraction is best defined as a muscle shortening against resistance. In an isometric contraction, the length of the muscle doesn't change during the contraction. An eccentric contraction is a lengthening contraction

66. **C)** The DeLorme axiom states that "high-intensity, low-repetition exercise builds strength, and low-intensity, high-repetition exercise builds endurance."

67. **B)** Scar tissue does not have adequate vascular supply. When metabolic demand is increased by heat, scar tissue is prone to ischemia.

68. **D)** Indications for phonophoresis include tendinitis (Achilles, bicipital), tenosynovitis, and medial, as well as lateral epicondylitis.

69. **C)** Normal resting heart rate (HR) is approximately 60 to 80 beats per minute and HR increases in a linear fashion with the work, rate, and oxygen uptake and exercise. Heart rate response is related to age, body size, disease, medications, type of activity, and environmental factors, such as temperature and humidity. HR during maximal exercise can be calculated in the following formula: HRmax = 220 – age.

70. **B)** Hemodynamic effects from using heat modalities are increased blood flow, decreased chronic inflammation, increased acute inflammation, increased edema, and increased bleeding. Heat can also increase tendon extensibility, increase collagenase activity, and decrease joint stiffness.

71. **A)** Ejaculation induced by electrical stimulation via a rectal probe is one of several standard techniques to collect semen in spinal cord–injured persons with ejaculatory failure. This technique does not adversely affect sperm motility, but retrograde and bidirectional ejaculation can occur. In these cases the ejaculate can be retrieved from the bladder with a catheter. Electroejaculation appears safe from the standpoint of mucosal injury and autonomic dysreflexia, but might not be well tolerated in persons with preserved rectal sensation.

72. **C)** Conversion is the change (conversion) of one form of energy to heat energy (in this case, sound wave energy to heat).

73. **B)** The average therapeutic ultrasound session lasts between 7 and 15 minutes.

74. **A)** An eccentric contraction is a lengthening contraction. A common example is the controlled lengthening of the quadriceps while descending stairs. Muscles shortening against resistance is a concentric contraction. In an isometric contraction, the length of the muscle doesn't change during the contraction.

75. **A)** Closed kinetic chain exercises have the distal end fixed. For example, while squatting, the feet are fixed to the ground.

76. **D)** Indications for heat therapy are pain management, muscle spasms, chronic inflammation, superficial thrombophlebitis, contractures, joint stiffness, and arthritis. It is not indicated for vascular insufficiency.

77. **A)** Phonophoresis is a modality that uses ultrasound to deliver medications through the skin. Iontophoresis uses electrical current to drive medication into tissue. Diathermy is a high-frequency electric current that is delivered via shortwave, ultrasound, or microwave to heat deep structures.

78. **C)** Contraindications to the use of spinal traction include metastases to the spine, osteopenia, and congenital spinal deformity. Cervical radiculopathy and muscle spasm are indications for spinal traction.

79. **A)** Mechanisms of heat transfer include conduction, convection, radiation, evaporation, and conversion. Conduction is the transfer of thermal energy between two bodies in direct contact. Convection uses movement of a medium (eg, water, air, or blood) to transport thermal energy, although the actual transfer of thermal energy is ultimately by conduction. Radiation refers to the thermal radiation emitted from any body, the surface temperature of which is above absolute zero (−273.15°C or −459.67°F). Evaporation involves the transformation of a liquid into gas, a process that requires thermal energy. Evaporation is actually a process of heat dissipation, and plays a role in cooling modalities, such as vapocoolant sprays. Conversion refers to the transformation of energy (eg, sound or electromagnetic) to heat.

80. **B)** Iontophoresis is the migration of charged particles across biologic membranes under an imposed electrical field. Its primary use has been in transcutaneous systemic or local delivery of medicines. For systemic drug delivery, it avoids the problems associated with oral or intravenous routes such as gastric irritation, first-pass hepatic metabolism, and variable serum concentrations. Iontophoresis in physical medicine is used to deliver medicines directly to soft tissues, limiting systemic absorption.

# 12

# *Legal and Ethics*

1. Which act is best defined as a wide-ranging civil rights law that prohibits, under certain circumstances, discrimination based on disability?
   A) Americans With Disabilities Act (ADA)
   B) Family Medical Leave Act
   C) Maternity Leave Act
   D) Stark Law

2. Which of the following is/are appropriate step(s) that should be taken when ending a physician-patient relationship?
   A) Providing the patient a written notice
   B) Providing the patient an explanation
   C) Providing resources to help find another physician
   D) All of the above

3. Which of the following is a form of insurance providing wage replacement and medical benefits to employees injured in the course of employment in exchange for mandatory relinquishment of the employee's right to sue?
   A) Workers' compensation
   B) Tort reform
   C) Health Insurance Portability and Accountability Act (HIPAA)
   D) Americans With Disabilities Act

4. Which of the following terms best describes malingering?
   A) An exaggeration of symptoms for secondary gain
   B) Multiple complaints regarding several organ systems
   C) Deliberate production of symptoms
   D) None of the above

5. In the acute rehabilitation unit, which of the following can be a potential barrier to the principle of autonomy?
   A) Feeling of being outnumbered by the interdisciplinary team
   B) Reluctance to decline the recommendations of the team
   C) Anxiety about new techniques
   D) All of the above

ANSWERS TO THIS SECTION CAN BE FOUND ON PAGE 365

6. An 86-year-old female presents for a follow-up appointment for ankle sprain after "falling down some stairs." The patient reveals that her injury was actually sustained after she was pushed by her daughter, with whom she lives. Which of the following is **true** regarding the management of this patient?
   A) Counsel the patient on elder abuse and encourage her to seek help, but do not disclose the new information to anybody because of patient confidentiality laws
   B) Notify the proper authorities of suspected elder abuse
   C) Continue to treat the patient for her sprained ankle and ignore the new information
   D) Ask the patient's family to confirm the means of injury

7. A well-known pharmaceutical company has developed a new pain medication and approaches your practice to take part in clinical research. The study has received Institutional Review Board (IRB) approval and the pharmaceutical company gives you a copy of a consent that the patient must sign. A valid consent process contains all of the following **except**:
   A) Disclosing any conflicts of interest
   B) Answering any questions prospective participants may have
   C) Determination of capacity
   D) Persuading individuals to take part in the study

8. Which act allows eligible employees of covered employers to take unpaid, job-protected leave for specified family and medical reasons with continuation of group health insurance coverage under the same terms and conditions as if the employee had not taken leave?
   A) Americans With Disabilities Act
   B) Family Medical Leave Act (FMLA)
   C) Maternity Leave Act
   D) Stark Law

9. Which of the following best describes breach of confidentiality according to the American Medical Association (AMA)?
   A) Not disclosing a breech fetal position to an expecting mother
   B) Informing a patient of his or her test results
   C) Disclosure of information to a third party without patient permission
   D) Explaining risks and benefits of a procedure

10. Which of the following is defined as intentionally ending a life to provide relief from pain and/or suffering?
    A) Euthanasia
    B) Double effect
    C) Abortion
    D) Advanced directive

11. The Supreme Court case decision, the Daubert standard, established the following precedent:
    A) Individuals with disabilities are entitled to a vocational rehabilitation program to maximize their employment potential
    B) Information given as an expert testimony must be based on evidence-based medicine and widely accepted in the medical community
    C) Public areas and buildings constructed with federal funds must be made accessible for disabled individuals
    D) Handicapped children are provided a free, appropriate education

12. Which of the following are components of decision-making capacity?
   A) Express a choice verbally
   B) Seek the opinion of family members and friends
   C) Understand the risks and benefits related to treatment decisions
   D) All of the above

13. Which of the following is/are potential ethical challenge(s) to conducting research in the population treated by physiatrists?
   A) Lack of decision-making capacity secondary to cognitive deficits from injuries
   B) Difficulty with timing of an injury and subject recruitment
   C) The misconception of equating a therapeutic intervention with a cure
   D) All of the above

14. A 94-year-old female presents for follow-up after undergoing rehabilitation for a total hip arthroplasty. She brings a plate of homemade chocolate brownies for the office staff and a gift certificate for the physician worth $200 to her son's restaurant as a thank-you gesture for the care she has received. Which of the following is **true** regarding patient gifts?
   A) It is the physician's right to accept or reject gifts of monetary value from patients as long as no preferential treatment is given to the patient
   B) The gift certificate is excessive and should be returned to the patient
   C) Physicians should reject all patient gifts no matter what the monetary value may be
   D) The physician should refer the patient elsewhere as there is now a conflict of interest

15. Which of the following best describes beneficence?
   A) Automatically making a decision for a patient
   B) The right of an individual to make his or her own informed decision
   C) Taking action that serves the best interest of the patient
   D) Do not harm the patient

16. Which of the following best describes informed consent according to the American Medical Association (AMA)?
   A) Informing the patient you are going to perform a procedure
   B) Informing the patient you made a mistake
   C) Informing the parent of a minor
   D) Informed consent is a process of communication between a patient and a physician that results in the patient's authorization or agreement to undergo a specific medical intervention

17. Which of the following best defines an action that produces two effects, one positive and one negative?
   A) Beneficence
   B) Autonomy
   C) Double effect
   D) Euthanasia

18. The Americans with Disabilities Act (ADA) ensures equality in which of the following areas?
   A) Education and employment opportunities
   B) Employment, public accommodations/transportation, state/government services, telecommunications
   C) Medical and legal services
   D) Federal but not state services

19. Which of the following refers to a reimbursement model system in which a group of health care providers and facilities provides coordinated high-quality care where cost efficiency is used as a performance measure?
    A) Coordinated health care system
    B) Accountable care organization (ACO)
    C) Quality improvement model
    D) Clinical excellence measures

20. Which of the following was achieved by the Lystedt Law?
    A) Any individual who sustained an injury that resulted in tetraplegia will be approved to receive both a powered and manual wheelchair for his or her mobility
    B) Any individual with an injury or disability is eligible for acute rehabilitation if there is reason to believe that he or she will benefit from the services
    C) Any individual affected by traumatic or nontraumatic amputation is entitled to receive a prosthetic device
    D) A young athlete can be removed from a sport if there is any suspicion of sustaining a concussion and he or she requires medical clearance to return to play

21. A 16-year-old female presents with pain on her left side after a collision during a soccer match. After a thorough history and physical exam, it is suspected that she may have fractured one or more ribs, and an x-ray is ordered for confirmation. During further questioning, the patient discloses that she just found out she is pregnant but is planning on getting an abortion. How should this patient be managed?
    A) Cancel the x-ray and treat the patient for rib fracture
    B) Explain to the patient that she must disclose her pregnancy to her parents so they can consent to the abortion
    C) Order the x-ray of the ribs because the patient is not planning on maintaining her pregnancy
    D) Notify her parents about her likely rib fracture and pregnancy as she is a minor

22. Which of the following best describes autonomy?
    A) Automatically making a decision for a patient
    B) The right of an individual to make his or her own informed decision
    C) Taking action that serves the best interest of the patient
    D) Do not harm the patient

23. Which of the following is a unique 10-digit identification number issued to health care providers by Centers for Medicare and Medicaid Services (CMS)?
    A) Social Security number
    B) Drug enforcement agency (DEA) number
    C) National provider identification (NPI) number
    D) State license number

24. Which of the following is best defined as a contract between physician and employer, preventing the physician from practicing in a geographic location?
    A) Prospective payment
    B) Health care proxy
    C) Restrictive covenant
    D) Palliative care

25. Which of the following statements is **false** regarding the American With Disabilities Act (ADA)?
    A) Employers must make reasonable accommodations to allow disabled employees to perform their jobs
    B) An able-bodied individual with HIV is protected under the ADA
    C) A preemployment physical is required to properly place the individual in the appropriate job
    D) Employers cannot discriminate against individuals with impairments in the workplace

26. What is the name of the legislation that made the practice of physician self-referrals unlawful?
    A) The Stark Law
    B) The Disability Amendment
    C) The Independent Business Act
    D) The Rehabilitation Act

27. Which of the following are ways in which the rehabilitation team can become more culturally competent?
    A) A monthly journal club that discusses articles focused on cultural issues
    B) The utilization of interpreter services during therapies and patient rounds
    C) Attending an international conference
    D) All of the above

28. Medicare pays for inpatient rehabilitation using which of the following payment systems?
    A) Pay for fee service
    B) Medicare does not pay for inpatient rehabilitation
    C) Pay by outcome system
    D) Prospective payment system (PPS)

29. The degree to which a patient follows medical advice is best described as:
    A) Abandonment
    B) Good Samaritan Law
    C) Health Insurance Portability and Accountability Act (HIPAA)
    D) Compliance

30. Which of the following is a palliative care goal?
    A) Treatment of the disease
    B) Preventive care
    C) Comfort and quality of life
    D) Ensuring that a Do Not Resuscitate (DNR) is signed

31. The Individuals With Disabilities Education Act (IDEA) established all of the following **except**:
    A) A mechanism to diagnose pediatric functional disorders
    B) Provision of assistive technology services to school-aged children with disabilities who require them for their continued education
    C) Provision of transportation to and from school for children with disabilities
    D) Provision of early intervention for children before they start schooling if developmental milestones are delayed

32. Which of the following instances will rehabilitation facilities now be required to report to Medicare?
    A) Cases of nosocomial respiratory infections
    B) Cases of surgical site infections

C) Cases of *Clostridium difficile*

D) Cases of new pressure injuries

33. Which of the following statements is **not** true and in compliance with the Health Insurance Portability and Accountability Act (HIPAA)?
    A) A patient's health care information can be shared with police for reporting purposes
    B) Any violation should be addressed to the Office of Civil Rights
    C) Health information is allowed to be shared with those health care professionals directly involved in a patient's care
    D) A patient's health information can be shared with his or her employer

34. Medicare Part D primarily covers which of the following?
    A) Inpatient hospitalization
    B) Outpatient imaging studies
    C) Outpatient physician visits
    D) Prescription drugs

35. Which of the following describes ending a physician-patient relationship when a patient is in need of treatment, without making certain they have continuing care?
    A) Abandonment
    B) Good Samaritan Law
    C) Health Insurance Portability and Accountability Act (HIPAA)
    D) Compliance

36. Which of the following best describes the use of an appointed agent to make medical decisions in case the patient is unable to?
    A) Health Insurance Portability and Accountability Act (HIPAA)
    B) Health care proxy
    C) Living will
    D) Palliative care

37. Which of the following legislative acts prohibits discrimination based on disability?
    A) Americans With Disabilities Act (ADA)
    B) The Rehabilitation and Disability Amendment
    C) The Federal Equality Bill
    D) Justice in Employment Act

38. A patient with a joint replacement would qualify for acute rehabilitation if he or she:
    A) Is above the age of 65 years
    B) Has a body mass index (BMI) of 40
    C) Has a unilateral hip replacement
    D) Has a bilateral knee replacement

39. Recommending a new medication from a pharmaceutical company in which the physician is a member of the board of directors is an example of which concept?
    A) Communication
    B) Bias
    C) Conflict of interest
    D) Principle of double effect

40. Medicare Part A primarily covers which of the following?
    - A) Outpatient physician visits
    - B) Yearly physicals
    - C) Inpatient hospitalizations
    - D) Outpatient surgical procedures

41. Which of the following is best described as protection for the physician from civil punishment in an emergency?
    - A) Abandonment
    - B) Good Samaritan Law
    - C) Health Insurance Portability and Accountability Act (HIPAA)
    - D) Compliance

42. Which of the following conveys your preferences regarding medical care intended to sustain life?
    - A) Health Insurance Portability and Accountability Act (HIPAA)
    - B) Health care proxy
    - C) Living will
    - D) Palliative care

43. A letter of medical necessity should include all of the following **except**:
    - A) The impact of the equipment on the patient's functional abilities
    - B) The current functional limitations of the patient including activities of daily living (ADLs) and mobility
    - C) The amount of money the equipment costs
    - D) Description of the features and all required components of the equipment

44. What percentage case mix of the compliant 13 diagnoses (also known as the compliance threshold) must be met by a unit to receive payment as an inpatient rehabilitation facility (IRF) according to Medicare?
    - A) 50
    - B) 60
    - C) 75
    - D) 80

45. The philosophy of "first, do no harm" is based on which principle?
    - A) Autonomy
    - B) Nonmaleficence
    - C) Dignity
    - D) Beneficence

46. Medicaid is primarily funded by which of the following?
    - A) Federal government
    - B) State government
    - C) Private companies
    - D) Split between federal and state governments

47. What does HIPAA stand for?
    - A) Human Interference Protection and Privacy Act
    - B) Health Insurance Portability and Accountability Act
    - C) Home Insurance Portability and Accountability Act
    - D) Health Income Potential and Protection Act

48. Which best describes a legal document that allows you to convey your decisions about end-of-life care ahead of time?
    A) Advanced directives
    B) Health care proxy
    C) Power of attorney
    D) Palliative care

49. Which of the following is the groundbreaking federal law that became the foundation for the Americans With Disabilities Act?
    A) The National Housing Act Amendments
    B) The Disability Act of 1970
    C) Urban Mass Transportation Act
    D) The Rehabilitation Act of 1973

50. Which of the following diagnoses is **not** compliant with Medicare's guidelines for medical conditions that require intensive acute rehabilitation services?
    A) 87-year-old woman with a total hip replacement
    B) 70-year-old man with coronary artery disease (CAD) who underwent coronary artery bypass graft (CABG)
    C) 60-year-old man with polyneuropathy on electrodiagnosis (EMG)
    D) 55-year-old woman with femur fracture after a fall

51. Informed consent is based on which principle?
    A) Justice
    B) Beneficence
    C) Autonomy
    D) Nonmaleficence

52. Which of the following generally provides health coverage for low-income patients and individuals with disabilities?
    A) Medicare
    B) Americans With Disabilities Act
    C) Medicaid
    D) Welfare

53. Which of the following is best defined as "a branch of philosophy dealing with values pertaining to human conduct, considering the rightness and wrongness of actions, and the goodness or badness of the motives and ends of such actions"?
    A) Ethics
    B) Tort
    C) Stark
    D) Hippocratic oath

54. Medicare is funded by which of the following?
    A) Federal government
    B) State government
    C) Private companies
    D) Split between federal and state governments

55. What criteria must be considered when examining a patient on the medical floor/intensive care unit (ICU) and making recommendations for an acute versus subacute facility?
    A) The patient must need the coordinated care of an interdisciplinary team of therapists, nurses, social workers, and physicians
    B) The patient must be able to participate in and benefit from an intensive program in a reasonable time
    C) The patient must be medically stable and require close medical supervision
    D) All of the above

56. What does the acronym CARF stand for?
    A) The Commission on Accreditation of Rehabilitation Facilities
    B) The Committee on Amputation, Restoration, and Function
    C) The Council for the Administration of Rehabilitation Facilities
    D) The Central Agency for Regulating Function

57. Who is the legally recognized proxy to make medical decisions for a patient with impaired decision-making capacity?
    A) Health care provider
    B) A close friend
    C) A close relative
    D) Health care proxy

58. Which of the following is a federal program providing health coverage for people older than 65 years?
    A) Medicare
    B) Americans With Disabilities Act
    C) Medicaid
    D) Welfare

59. Which of the following governs physician self-referral for Medicare and Medicaid patients?
    A) Americans With Disabilities Act
    B) Family Medical Leave Act
    C) Maternity Leave Act
    D) Stark Law

60. Which of the following does **not** qualify for the Medicare 60% inpatient rule?
    A) Stroke
    B) Hip fracture
    C) Knee replacement
    D) Burns

61. Which of the following is an example of incentives provided by the government for industries that comply with the American With Disabilities Act?
    A) The Targeted Jobs Tax Credit
    B) The Revenue Reconciliation Act
    C) Both (A) and (B)
    D) None of the above

62. Which of the following refers to the federal government's effort to classify the potential functional ability of an individual with an amputation to determine the most appropriate prosthetic components he or she requires?
    A) M-levels
    B) L-levels

    C) P-levels
    D) K-levels

63. All of the following are required to obtain informed consent **except**:
    A) Disclosure
    B) Competency
    C) Agreement of the health care proxy
    D) Understanding

64. A 33-year-old male presents after being referred from orthopedics for "occupational therapy." The referral does not have any further information. The patient reports he injured his hand after falling off his motorcycle and was placed in a brace. During the physical exam, the brace is removed and the patient is put through a series of tests including grip strength and range of motion. Which of the following principles has been violated in this scenario?
    A) Autonomy
    B) Justice
    C) Informed consent
    D) Nonmaleficence

# Legal and Ethics

## ANSWERS

1. **A)** The ADA prohibits discrimination based on disability. It was signed into law in 1990.

2. **D)** According to the American Medical Association (AMA) guidelines, appropriate steps to terminate a patient-physician relationship typically include giving the patient written notice, preferably by certified mail, return receipt requested; providing the patient with a brief explanation for terminating the relationship (this should be a valid reason, for instance, noncompliance, failure to keep appointments); agreeing to continue to provide treatment and access to services for a reasonable period, such as 30 days, to allow the patient to secure care from another person (a physician may want to extend the period for emergency services); providing resources and/or recommendations to help a patient locate another physician of like specialty; and offering to transfer records to a newly designated physician upon signed patient authorization to do so.

3. **A)** Workers' compensation is a form of insurance providing wage replacement and medical benefits to employees injured in the course of employment in exchange for mandatory relinquishment of the employee's right to sue the employer.

4. **A)** The secondary gains may include financial compensation, avoiding work/school, and legal incentives. All of these can be categorized as fraudulent activity. Somatization disorder is characterized by multiple complaints resulting in the individual making numerous visits to the doctor. In factitious disorder, an individual also magnifies and even fabricates symptoms but without the intent of a secondary gain.

5. **D)** All of the answer choices can be potential obstacles to the self-determination of a patient.

6. **B)** Although laws vary from state to state, most have enacted statutes mandating the reporting of suspected elder abuse. Types of elder abuse may include physical, emotional, neglect, verbal, and financial. The elderly population often underreports cases of abuse.

7. **D)** Informed consent protects an individual's right to autonomy. Answer choice (D) is not part of this process. Although the significance of a study grows with increased participation, researchers should not attempt to persuade individuals who may be wavering. Aspects of informed consent include disclosure of materials, drugs, procedures, conflicts of interest, risks, hazards, benefits, alternatives, nature of the research plan; making sure the study is understood by potential participants; determining capacity; answering any questions; avoiding unrealistic expectations; and documenting voluntary consent.

8. **B)** The FMLA protects eligible employees and allows them to take job-protected leave while keeping group health insurance.

9. **C)** A breach of confidentiality is a disclosure to a third party, without patient consent or court order, of private information that the physician has learned within the patient-physician relationship.

10. **A)** Euthanasia is the act of intentionally ending a life to provide relief from pain and/or suffering.

11. **B)** Physiatrists who will be giving expert testimony will be held to the Daubert standard. The information must be accepted by the medical community, published in the medical literature, have a scientific basis, and have a known error rate. If it does not meet these guidelines, then the testimony can be disqualified. The Comprehensive Employment Training Act of 1973 (CETA) provided training programs and public service jobs for individuals with disabilities. After 1982, this federally funded service was transferred to state level. Answer choice (C) refers to the Architectural Barriers Act of 1968, and choice (D) refers to the Education for All Handicapped Children Act of 1975.

12. **C)** The process of decision making involves the ability to make a choice either verbally or nonverbally, understand information regarding treatment options, utilize this information in a logical manner as it relates to their condition, and make a decision that is reliable and uniform with their values.

13. **D)** There are unique challenges that researchers face in conducting research in physical medicine and rehabilitation. Other concerns include overutilization of particular subjects in specialized populations, withholding standard of care practices in control groups, and the physician-patient relationship.

14. **A)** The AMA code of ethics suggests that gifts from patients can be accepted under the following conditions: (a) the physician is comfortable accepting the gift even if it becomes public knowledge; (b) the gift does not affect further medical care; (c) the gift does not present an emotional or financial hardship to the patient or the patient's family; (d) physicians may request the gift be in the form of a charitable donation. To avoid any perceived conflict of interest, it may be best to establish an office policy not to accept gifts above a certain value.

15. **C)** Beneficence is taking action that serves the best interest of the patient.

16. **D)** Informed consent is a process of communication between a patient and a physician that results in the patient's authorization or agreement to undergo a specific medical intervention.

17. **C)** Double effect is an action that produces two consequences, one positive and one negative. One example is giving morphine to a terminally ill patient. Morphine can have a positive effect in that it improves pain but it can negatively impact the respiratory system.

18. **B)** The ADA was passed in 1990 to protect the civil liberties of individuals with disabilities. It addressed issues in five key areas: state and federal services, employment, public transportation/accommodations, and telecommunications.

19. **B)** ACO consists of groups of physicians and hospitals that are held accountable for quality care provided to patients. This type of model system places a financial responsibility upon the health care provider to minimize unnecessary and duplicated expenditures. As a result, the providers will benefit from the savings realized by Medicare. The payment system is based on different programs including a shared savings program and advance payment initiative.

20. **D)** The Lystedt Law was passed in the state of Washington in 2009 and is named after a young athlete, Zachery Lystedt, who returned prematurely after sustaining a concussion during a middle school football game. As a result, he suffered from serious long-term consequences affecting his cognition and ability to function. Any athlete below the age of 18 years who is suspected of having a concussion cannot return to play unless given written permission by a health care professional trained specially in the diagnosis and treatment of concussion. The law also requires athletes and their parents to review and sign an educational form on concussions.

21. **A)** The patient in this scenario is a pregnant minor who has specific rights regarding confidentiality and treatment. Under law, a pregnant minor is not forced to disclose her condition to her parents for any reason. She may choose to get an abortion without parental consent. It is a violation of patient confidentiality for the caregiver to inform the parents of her diagnosis and/or pregnancy status. Ordering an x-ray on a pregnant patient is inappropriate here because it has potential to do harm to the fetus if the patient changes her mind about the abortion.

22. **B)** Autonomy is the right of an individual or patient to make his or her own informed decision.

23. **C)** NPI number is a unique 10-digit identification number issued to health care providers by CMS.

24. **C)** According to the American Medical Association (AMA), "a restrictive covenant is a contractual provision between a physician and his or her employer which prevents the physician from practicing in a specified geographic area for a given period of time if the physician's employment terminates."

25. **C)** The ADA establishes civil liberties for individuals with disabilities. Disabled individuals cannot be discriminated against in the workplace as long as they can perform their job under reasonable accommodations. Preemployment physicals are not allowed and can only be used after an individual has been hired. The list of acceptable diagnoses also includes conditions that can be perceived as disabilities (such as HIV).

26. **A)** The Social Security Act or Stark Law prohibits physicians from making referrals to health services (payable by Medicare) in which they receive financial compensation, including physical, occupational, and speech therapies, durable medical equipment, prosthetics, and orthotics among other services with a number of specific exceptions.

27. **D)** There are various ways in which a physiatrist and his or her team can promote cultural awareness. Over time, the inpatient units have had a greater representation of minority patients. Therefore, it is vital to improve communication and understanding and ultimately care. The following four approaches are suggested: (a) encourage education in cultural diversity, (b) create the best individualized program with consideration of one's values and belief and available resources in the community, (c) continue these practices on a consistent basis at administrative level, and (d) improve research and self-awareness.

28. **D)** Medicare pays for inpatient rehabilitation by using a PPS. A fixed amount of money is paid to the facility regardless of duration of hospitalization.

29. **D)** Compliance is the degree to which a patient follows medical advice.

30. **C)** Palliative care goals include comfort of the patient and improving quality of life.

31. **A)** The IDEA established guidelines for children (from birth to the age of 21 years) with disabilities to participate in a special education program and receive additional services to meet their needs. It creates an individualized curriculum that involves teachers as well as parents that will benefit the child as he or she develops. It applies to states that receive federal funding. There have been a number of amendments to the IDEA over the years. These services and devices are provided at no additional cost to their families.

32. **D)** Beginning in 2014, facilities will be required to report catheter-associated urinary tract infections (CAUTI) and new or worsening pressure injuries during the course of the hospitalization. Facilities that fail to comply will incur a 2% payment reduction.

33. **D)** The Privacy Rule outlines required guidelines to protect patient identifiable information. Designated organizations referred to as covered entities, including health care providers and health plans (eg, insurance company, Medicare/Medicaid), must follow these standards. Health information is allowed to be shared with those health care professionals directly involved in a patient's care, and it can be used to protect the public's health and reports to law enforcement. This information cannot be shared without authorization by the individual to family/friends, employers, or for marketing purposes. A patient has the right to see and receive a copy of his or her records. If any grievance occurs, the Office of Civil Rights works to ensure and enforce compliance of the Privacy Rule.

34. **D)** Medicare Part D primarily covers prescription drugs.

35. **A)** Abandonment is best described as ending a physician-patient relationship when a patient is in need of treatment, without making certain they have continuing care.

36. **B)** Health care proxy is an appointed agent who will make decisions if the primary person is unable to do so. The proxy should execute substituted judgement (ie, act in the manner that the patient would have wanted). It is best to discuss such decisions with the health care proxy before one becomes incapacitated.

37. **A)** The ADA was passed in 1990 to protect the civil liberties of individuals with disabilities. It addresses issues ranging from employment to public transportation/accommodations and telecommunications.

38. **D)** Under Medicare guidelines, a compliant diagnosis must be consistent with the following: bilateral joint replacement, or unilateral joint replacement with BMI of 50, or above the age of 85 years.

39. **C)** A conflict of interest occurs when a physician's self-interest challenges the patient's best interest. Therefore, he or she may potentially compromise clinical responsibilities and objectivity to benefit from a financial or other secondary gain.

40. **C)** Medicare Part A primarily covers the cost of inpatient hospitalization.

41. **B)** The Good Samaritan Law protects physicians from civil punishment when acting in an emergency situation. Emergency situations are defined differently by each respective state.

42. **C)** Living will conveys your preferences regarding medical care intended to sustain life. Examples are use of dialysis, artificial ventilation, tube feeding, and organ donation.

43. **C)** The treating physician may be asked for a letter of medical necessity to provide details of why recommended equipment is necessary to improve function. The letter should include appropriate documentation of the items listed in the question stem. The physician must show evidence that other lower cost options were considered, attempted, and unsuccessful, or not appropriate. The letter is not only needed for equipment such as wheelchairs, but may also be requested for the prescription of assistive technology.

44. **B)** As described in the Code of Federal Regulations (subpart B), IRFs can receive payment per discharge (prospective payment system) on the basis of distinct clinical characteristics as well as specific case- and facility-level adjustments. This minimal percentage, also known as the compliance threshold, was set at 75%. The Extension Act of 2007 lowered this percentage to 60% and is therefore referred to as the *60% rule*. It also established that comorbidities that met the criteria must be used to determine the total compliance threshold.

45. **B)** Nonmaleficence is one of the four core ethical principles. It means that the first objective is not to cause harm. In comparison, beneficence is the concept to "do good" first and foremost. Autonomy is the right of an individual to make an informed decision regarding his or her care. Beneficence is the idea of doing what is in the best interest of the patient. Justice is the act of being fair. Dignity, although important, is not one of the four core ethical principles.

46. **D)** Medicaid is jointly funded by the federal and state governments.

47. **B)** HIPAA stands for Health Insurance Portability and Accountability Act.

48. **A)** Advanced directives allow you to convey your decisions about end-of-life care ahead of time.

49. **D)** The Rehabilitation Act of 1973 not only became landmark legislation that established anti-discrimination for disabled persons, but also provided a variety of federally funded benefits. The National Housing Act Amendments removed obstacles for housing by creating the Office of Independent Living. The Urban Mass Transportation Act required mass transit to be accessible to disabled individuals.

50. **B)** The remaining choices are one of the 13 compliant Medicare diagnoses, which include (a) stroke; (b) spinal cord injury; (c) congenital deformity; (d) amputation; (e) major multiple trauma; (f) fracture of femur (long bones); (g) brain injury; (h) neurological disorders, including multiple sclerosis, motor neuron disease, polyneuropathy, muscular dystrophy, and Parkinson's disease; (i) burns; (j) active, polyarticular rheumatoid arthritis, psoriatic arthritis, and seronegative arthropathies resulting in functional impairment of activities of daily living (ADLs) or ambulation that has not improved from outpatient therapy, with the potential to improve with a more aggressive course; (k) systemic vasculitides with joint inflammation resulting in a significant functional impairment; (l) severe osteoarthritis involving two or more major weight-bearing joints (not a prosthesis) with deformity, atrophy, and loss of range of motion that led to a functional decline; and (m) bilateral joint replacement, unilateral joint replacement with body mass index (BMI) of 50 or above the age of 85 years.

51. **C)** Autonomy is one of the core principles of ethics. It is the right of an individual to make an informed decision regarding his or her care and treatment even if it is in contrast with the recommendations of his or her health care provider. An informed consent allows one to practice autonomy after considering the risks/benefits and alternatives. The remaining principles are also critical in the study of ethics. Nonmaleficence is the philosophy of "first, do no harm"; beneficence is the idea of doing what is in the best interest of the patient; and justice is the act of being fair.

52. **C)** Medicaid provides health coverage for low-income patients and individuals with disabilities.

53. **A)** Ethics is best defined as a branch of philosophy dealing with values pertaining to human conduct, considering the rightness and wrongness of actions, and the goodness or badness of the motives and ends of such actions.

54. **A)** Medicare is funded by the federal government. Medicaid is jointly funded by state and federal funds.

55. **D)** There are various rehabilitation settings including acute, subacute, day programs, outpatient, and home. The physiatrist must make the decision to determine the most appropriate disposition plan. When recommending an inpatient rehabilitation course, the following criteria must be evaluated: (a) Is the patient medically appropriate for admission? (b) Does the patient have attainable

rehabilitation goals with an appropriate rehab discharge plan? (c) Does the patient have rehabilitation potential in a reasonable time? (d) Does the patient require close medical management by a physician and nurse? (e) Does the patient require a comprehensive interdisciplinary team approach (physical therapy, occupational therapy, speech therapy, prosthetics, and orthotics)?

56. **A)** CARF is an international, nonprofit organization that establishes standards for health care organizations, including medical rehabilitation, employment and community services, child and youth services, behavioral health, aging services, and business and service management. It was founded in 1966 and has provided accreditation to various providers in 18 countries. Its mission focuses on maintaining the highest quality of care and performance for individuals living with a disability.

57. **D)** The designation of a proxy can vary from state to state, but the legally recognized proxy is the health care proxy assigned in advanced directives. The remaining choices are all examples of surrogate decision makers who could possibly be given that responsibility if one is not identified by the patient ahead of time.

58. **A)** Medicare provides health coverage for people older than 65 years.

59. **D)** The Stark Law governs physician self-referral for Medicare and Medicaid patients. It limits the conditions under which a physician can refer to an entity in which he or she has a financial interest.

60. **C)** The 60% rule (formerly the 75% rule) is a Medicare regulation stipulating that in order to be eligible for payments, 60% of an inpatient rehabilitation facility's patients must fall within a specific list of qualifying conditions. Knee replacement does not qualify as part of the 60% rule. In order for a joint replacement to qualify, they must have other comorbidities (obesity, bilateral joint replacement, or older than 85 years).

61. **C)** The Revenue Reconciliation Act of 1990 allows businesses to deduct a set amount of expenses used for making the workplace accessible for disabled individuals. The Targeted Jobs Tax Credit of 1978 allows a tax credit for companies that employ individuals with disabilities (for 1 year).

62. **D)** The K-level is based on the patient's expected potential and not on his or her current level of activity. It establishes reimbursement for various components so that individuals will receive prosthetics that correlate with their level of function. For example, an active individual would receive a more advanced device. The levels range from 0, where the individual cannot ambulate or transfer safely, to 4, where the individual participates in high-impact and energy activities.

63. **C)** In order for a patient to give his or her consent, he or she must have decision-making capacity. The individual obtaining the consent must fully disclose the risks and benefits and all treatment options, establishing an understanding on the behalf of the patient who is free from intimidation or force. The health care proxy is only called upon to give consent if the patient is not able to.

64. **D)** In this scenario, the patient should not have been examined extensively without receiving more information about the diagnosis from the referring physician. "First, do no harm," or nonmaleficence, was violated in this case because the physician may have delayed healing or caused further injury to the patient's hand. Autonomy is a patient's right to accept or refuse treatment. Justice describes a caregiver's responsibility to be fair when offering treatments and resources to patients. Informed consent is the act of explaining risks, benefits, and alternatives regarding specific treatments so that the patient can consent to treatment.

# 13

# *Pediatrics*

## QUESTIONS

1. Environmental factors that are implicated in the development of neural tube defects (NTDs) include:
   A) Maternal diabetes mellitus
   B) Folate deficiency
   C) Use of valproic acid
   D) Maternal hyperthermia
   E) All of the above

2. A Glasgow Coma Scale of 8 is suggestive of:
   A) Mild injury
   B) Moderate injury
   C) Severe injury

3. The most common site of spinal cord injury (SCI) in children is:
   A) Thoracic
   B) Lumbar
   C) Cervical
   D) Sacral

4. All of the following are anterior horn cell diseases affecting the motor neuron **except**:
   A) Spinal muscular atrophy
   B) Botulism
   C) Amyotrophic lateral sclerosis
   D) Poliomyelitis

5. An 8-year-old with a diagnosis of Duchenne muscular dystrophy (DMD) is referred for exercise. All of the following are allowed **except**:
   A) Swimming
   B) Daily walking
   C) Weight lifting
   D) Playing Wii

6. You are caring for a child with a known central nervous system (CNS) lesion. The child's lower extremities are characteristically kept in which position?
   A) Hip abduction, extension, and internal rotation, along with knee flexion, internal tibial rotation, and equinovarus foot posturing
   B) Hip adduction, extension, and internal rotation, along with knee extension, internal tibial rotation, and equinovarus foot posturing
   C) Hip adduction, flexion, and internal rotation, along with knee flexion, internal tibial rotation, and equinovarus foot posturing
   D) Hip adduction, extension, and external rotation, along with knee extension, external tibial rotation, and equinovarus foot posturing

ANSWERS TO THIS SECTION CAN BE FOUND ON PAGE 391    **371**

7. Each of the following is true of tibia vara (Blount's disease) **except**?
   A) Bowing of the proximal tibia is a result of abnormal function of the medial portion of the proximal tibial growth plate
   B) This disease is found most commonly in obese children who walk at 9 to 10 months
   C) It is more common in Whites than other racial groups
   D) Treatment is usually surgical, involving osteotomy of the proximal tibia and fibula

8. Arnold-Chiari malformation complicated by hydrocephalus occurs most commonly in which type of spina bifida?
   A) Spina bifida occulta
   B) Meningocele
   C) Myelomeningocele
   D) Myelocele

9. Which of the following is the major factor limiting ambulation in Duchenne muscular dystrophy (DMD)?
   A) Joint contracture
   B) Weakness
   C) Scoliosis
   D) Restrictive lung disease

10. Gastrointestinal symptoms in patients with cerebral palsy include all the following **except**:
    A) Gastroesophageal reflux
    B) Difficulty coordinating swallow or dysphagia
    C) Constipation
    D) Poor pancreatic enzyme secretion

11. Indications for botulinum toxin in children with cerebral palsy include all of the following **except**:
    A) Thumb-in-palm deformity
    B) Dynamic equinus during swing phase
    C) Fixed knee flexion contracture
    D) Focal dystonia

12. Which is/are the most common shunt complication(s) when treating hydrocephalus in an infant with myelomeningocele?
    A) Infection and obstruction
    B) Lower limb weakness
    C) Pain and swelling
    D) Incontinence of bowel and bladder

13. Of those patients with myelomeningocele (MMC) who complete high school, about what percentage go on to further education?
    A) Less than 10
    B) 20
    C) 40
    D) 50

14. Neural tube defects occur between _____ days of gestation:
    A) 7 and 18
    B) 18 and 30

C) 31 and 46

D) 47 and 65

15. Clinical features of peripheral vertigo include all of the following **except**:

A) Hearing loss

B) Past pointing and falling in the direction of disease

C) Vestibular and positional nystagmus

D) Cranial nerve dysfunction

16. The most common type of skull fracture after a head injury is:

A) Depressed

B) Linear

C) Comminuted

D) Open

17. Most children with spinal muscular atrophy (SMA) have:

A) Mental retardation

B) A single crease across their palm

C) Epilepsy

D) High cognitive function

18. A 4-year-old boy presents with a history of difficulty climbing stairs, falling, waddling gait, and large calf muscles. You suspect Duchenne muscular dystrophy (DMD). Of the following, the easiest and best confirmatory diagnosis test is:

A) Serum level of creatine kinase (CK)

B) Polymerase chain reaction (PCR) genetic test

C) Muscle biopsy

D) Family history

19. You are caring for a child with a known central nervous system (CNS) lesion. The child's upper extremities are characteristically kept in which position?

A) Shoulder adduction, flexion, and internal rotation with elbow flexion, wrist pronation and flexion, and finger and thumb flexion

B) Shoulder abduction, flexion, and external rotation with elbow flexion, wrist pronation and flexion, and finger and thumb flexion

C) Shoulder adduction, extension, and internal rotation with elbow flexion, wrist supination and flexion, and finger and thumb flexion

D) Shoulder abduction, flexion, and internal rotation with elbow extension, wrist pronation and flexion, and finger and thumb extension

20. What is the most common congenital lower limb deficiency?

A) Unilateral partial tibial deficiency

B) Fibular longitudinal deficiency

C) Partial proximal femoral deficiency

D) Bilateral partial tibial deficiency

21. In a child diagnosed with cerebral palsy (CP), independent sitting by what age is a good prognostic indicator for ambulation?

A) 6 months

B) 12 months

C) 24 months

D) 36 months

22. The occurrence of contractures in Duchenne muscular dystrophy (DMD) appears to be directly related to which of the following?
    A) Poor nutrition
    B) Obesity
    C) Prolonged static positioning of the limb
    D) Muscular atrophy

23. What percentage of cases of cerebral palsy are found to be due to complications of childbirth or birth asphyxia?
    A) 1% to 2%
    B) 5% to 10%
    C) 30% to 50%
    D) 50% to 75%

24. In patients with cerebral palsy, the use of augmentative communication:
    A) Enhances communication
    B) Creates difficulty in classroom activities
    C) Decreases parent interaction by speech
    D) Meets all the communication needs of the child

25. What percentage of myelomeningoceles (MMCs) are associated with hydrocephalus at birth?
    A) 5
    B) 15
    C) 25
    D) 50

26. Which best describes the sexual development of female patients with myelomeningocele (MMC)?
    A) Normal
    B) Markedly reduced
    C) Increased likelihood of late puberty
    D) Increased likelihood of precocious puberty

27. Ingestion of which of the following vitamins helps reduce the incidence of neural tube defects?
    A) Thiamine
    B) Pyridoxine
    C) Folic acid
    D) Vitamin $B_{12}$

28. Creatine kinase (CK) values in excess of 10,000 are usually seen in all of the following **except**:
    A) Duchenne muscular dystrophy
    B) Dermatomyositis
    C) Acute rhabdomyolysis
    D) Congenital myopathies

29. Retinal hemorrhages are pathognomonic of child abuse.
    A) True
    B) False

30. In which type of spinal muscular atrophy (SMA) can most of the patients sit but not walk?
    A) Type I
    B) Type II

C) Type III
D) Type IV

31. Duchenne muscular dystrophy (DMD) can affect all of the following **except**:
    A) Pulmonary system
    B) IQ
    C) Gastrointestinal (GI) system
    D) Cardiac system
    E) All of the above may be affected

32. A friend is telling you of his little girl who just celebrated her third birthday. Which of the following do you **not** expect her to be able to complete?
    A) Up and down stairs with hands on rail
    B) Jumps clearing ground and lands on feet together
    C) Walks down stairs alternating feet
    D) Pedals tricycle

33. Around what age should the first prosthetic fitting for a unilateral deficiency occur?
    A) 3 to 4 months
    B) 6 to 7 months
    C) When the child begins to walk
    D) When the child is able to navigate stairs

34. Which of the following is **not** a type of dyskinetic cerebral palsy (CP)?
    A) Dystonia
    B) Ataxia
    C) Athetosis
    D) Hemiballismus

35. A physiatrist evaluating patients in a muscular dystrophy clinic wants to start the boys with Duchenne muscular dystrophy (DMD) on an exercise program. Knowing that dystrophin-deficient muscle is very susceptible to exercise-induced muscle injury, the best way to begin the program would be:
    A) To allow the boys to play as hard and as long as they want, stopping only when they are too tired to play any more
    B) To have the boys exercise in a playful manner but with the supervision of a physical therapist
    C) To have the boys participate in the standard school physical program
    D) The exercise program is not a good idea, as it could make the disease progress faster

36. Risk factors for cerebral palsy include all the following **except**:
    A) Extreme or very low birth weight, or prematurity
    B) Multiple gestation pregnancy
    C) Chorioamnionitis
    D) First delivery for mother

37. When parental involvement in children with cerebral palsy is high:
    A) Children are more dependent
    B) Therapy is less important for function
    C) Compliance at home is improved
    D) Leisure time is reduced

38. Which of the following interventions was found to reduce the frequency of myelomeningocele (MMC)?
    A) Vitamin $B_{12}$
    B) Vitamin E
    C) Folic acid
    D) Ascorbic acid

39. Which of the following affects IQ scores of children with myelomeningocele (MMC)?
    A) Central nervous system infections
    B) Recurrent shunt revisions
    C) Ability to ambulate
    D) Pressure injury

40. Treatment of spasticity in cerebral palsy (CP) includes all of the following **except**:
    A) Botulinum toxin and phenol
    B) Oral or intrathecal baclofen
    C) Selective dorsal rhizotomy
    D) Hyperbaric oxygen therapy (HBOT)

41. Gower's sign is diagnostic of Duchenne muscular dystrophy.
    A) True
    B) False

42. All of the following can occur after moderate to severe head injury in children **except**?
    A) Executive function impairment
    B) Visuomotor integration impairment
    C) Memory impairment
    D) Accelerated closure of the epiphysis

43. The most common identifiable risk factor for childhood ischemic stroke is:
    A) Hematological disorders
    B) Congenital heart disease
    C) Central nervous system infection
    D) Vasculitis

44. Duchenne muscular dystrophy is a progressive hereditary disease with a predictable course. However, with corticosteroids and physical medicine and rehabilitation (PM&R) treatment, the disease course can be:
    A) Modified
    B) Cured
    C) Unaffected
    D) Halted

45. You observe a child who has been meeting developmental milestones. He or she is able to independently ambulate as well as come to stand independently. However, you note the child cannot go up and down stairs. Approximately how old would you expect this child to be?
    A) 12 months
    B) 15 months
    C) 18 months
    D) 24 months

46. What is the most common congenital limb deficiency?
    A) Left terminal transradial
    B) Left transhumeral
    C) Right terminal transradial
    D) Right transhumeral

47. Which is the most common type of cerebral palsy (CP)?
    A) Spastic quadriplegia
    B) Dyskinetic CP
    C) Spastic diplegia
    D) Mixed CP

48. A 12-year-old girl with limb-girdle muscular dystrophy is having trouble keeping up in school. She cannot ambulate fast enough to get to her next class on time. She is having difficulty writing her examination papers and finishing on time. The ultimate cause of the majority of her clinical problems is:
    A) Skeletal muscle weakness
    B) Spasticity
    C) Cardiomyopathy
    D) Joint contracture

49. Causes of cerebral palsy include all the following **except**:
    A) Toxoplasmosis, other agents, rubella, cytomegalovirus infection, herpes simplex (TORCH) infection during pregnancy
    B) Trauma to the child by age 2 years
    C) Infection of the brain and/or meninges by age 2 years
    D) Progressive lipid storage disease

50. Children with cerebral palsy should be referred to therapy:
    A) When they begin to show signs of walking
    B) When they display limitations in fine motor skills
    C) Only after the diagnosis is confirmed
    D) Even if the diagnosis is not established and abnormal muscle tone exists

51. What is the incidence of myelomeningocele (MMC) in the United States?
    A) 2 per 1,000 live births
    B) 20 per 1,000 live births
    C) 100 per 1,000 live births
    D) 10 per 1,000 live births

52. Which would best describe the ambulation potential for a patient with thoracic myelomeningocele (MMC)?
    A) Community ambulatory
    B) Household ambulatory
    C) Functional ambulatory
    D) Nonambulatory

53. All of the oral antispasticity medications are likely to cause sedation **except**:
    A) Baclofen
    B) Diazepam
    C) Dantrolene
    D) Tizanidine

54. Teenagers with complaints of difficulty climbing stairs, falls, decreased endurance, and episodic weakness are suggestive of:
    A) Neuropathic etiology
    B) Myopathic etiology
    C) Cerebral etiology
    D) Cerebellar etiology

55. Of the following types of brain injuries, which has the best prognosis for motor recovery?
    A) Diffuse axonal injury (DAI)
    B) Bilateral hematomas
    C) Focal contusion
    D) Diffuse hypoxia secondary to head injury

56. Phrenic nerve pacing may be required with spinal cord injury at which level?
    A) C3 to C5
    B) T3 to T5
    C) T7 to T8
    D) T12 to L4

57. Botulism is caused by:
    A) Gram-positive streptococci
    B) Gram-positive *Clostridium*
    C) Gram-negative *Escherichia coli*
    D) Gram-negative *Shigella*

58. You observe a child who is able to crawl on his or her hands and knees ("creeps"). At what age should this milestone be met?
    A) 6 months
    B) 9 months
    C) 10 months
    D) 12 months

59. An infant with features of intrauterine growth retardation (IUGR), small mouth, low-set abnormal ears, spasticity, and rocker-bottom feet is most consistent with which chromosomal syndrome?
    A) Trisomy 18 (Edwards' syndrome)
    B) 45, X (Turner syndrome)
    C) Trisomy 13 (Patau's syndrome)
    D) Trisomy 21 (Down syndrome)

60. The majority of cerebral palsy (CP) cases occur during which period?
    A) Prenatal
    B) Perinatal
    C) Infancy
    D) Childhood

61. Which of the following is consistent with myopathy?
    A) Brisk muscle stretch reflexes
    B) Weakness and atrophy
    C) Sensory loss
    D) Urinary retention

62. The incidence of cerebral palsy is:
    A) 1 to 2.3 per 1,000 live births
    B) 10 to 23 per 1,000 live births
    C) 8 per 1,000 live births
    D) 0.1 to 0.23 per 1,000 live births

63. In patients with cerebral palsy, precautions for therapeutic involvement:
    A) Are important for tracking severity
    B) Define safe limits of treatment
    C) Determine location of therapy
    D) Reduce parent interactions

64. What percentage of the population age 1 to 10 years has spina bifida occulta?
    A) 1
    B) 8
    C) 17
    D) 30

65. Which is the major cause of calcaneal deformity in myelomeningocele (MMC)?
    A) Unopposed contraction of foot dorsiflexors
    B) Unopposed contraction of plantar flexors
    C) Weakness of foot intrinsics
    D) Hip dislocation

66. Children with cerebral palsy (CP) are at risk for fractures and osteoporosis because of all of the following **except**:
    A) Malnutrition with calcium and vitamin D deficiency
    B) Immobility
    C) Antiepileptic medication
    D) Chronic respiratory infection

67. Common presentations of myopathy in infants and children include all of the following **except**:
    A) Hypotonia
    B) Delayed motor milestones
    C) Feeding problem
    D) Language problem
    E) Abnormality of gait

68. You are monitoring an 8-month-old (who was born preterm at 33 weeks) for developmental delays. You are suspicious of child abuse. One of the physical signs that may confirm your suspicion is:
    A) Bulging fontanels
    B) Enlarged head circumference
    C) Bruising in an unusual location such as the legs or the back
    D) Retinal hemorrhage
    E) All of the above

69. Spinal cord injuries are classified by which of the following scales?
    A) Glasgow Coma Scale
    B) American Spinal Injury Association/International Medical Society of Paraplegia (ASIA/IMSOP) spinal cord impairment scale

    C) The Wee Functional Independence Measure Scale
    D) Barthel index

70. All of the following are true in cases of myasthenia gravis (MG) **except**:
    A) It is an autoimmune disease
    B) It affects presynaptic receptors on the neuromuscular junction
    C) On repetitive nerve stimulation tests, there is a decremental response
    D) It can be diagnosed by edrophonium (Tensilon) test

71. A child should be able to pivot circles in prone by what age?
    A) 2 months
    B) 3 months
    C) 4 months
    D) 5 months

72. An infant with features of upward slant of palpebral fissures, low-set ears, prominent occiput, hypoplastic fingernails, and short sternum is most consistent with which chromosomal syndrome?
    A) Trisomy 18 (Edwards' syndrome)
    B) 45, X (Turner syndrome)
    C) Trisomy 13 (Patau's syndrome)
    D) Trisomy 21 (Down syndrome)

73. There are three different types of hemophilia. Which of the following is the hallmark of this disease?
    A) Hemarthrosis
    B) Spondylosis
    C) Retinal hemorrhages
    D) Hematuria

74. Which of the following muscular dystrophies is usually associated with a markedly reduced lifespan?
    A) Facioscapulohumeral dystrophy (FSHD)
    B) Becker's muscular dystrophy (BMD)
    C) Limb-girdle dystrophy
    D) Duchenne muscular dystrophy (DMD)

75. In a patient recently diagnosed with myotonic muscular dystrophy (MMD), all of the following are reasonable follow-up evaluations related to the diagnosis **except**:
    A) A check for insulin insensitivity and the presence of diabetes
    B) An electrocardiogram (ECG) evaluation for possible conduction abnormalities
    C) An ophthalmologic evaluation for cataracts
    D) An imaging study of the kidneys for stones

76. Which sport is **not** recommended for children with cerebral palsy?
    A) Swimming
    B) Adaptive horseback riding
    C) Weight lifting
    D) None of the above

77. When advising families with children with chronic illness and disability, practitioners should:
    A) Remain dogmatic on traditional therapies alone
    B) Allow for open discussion of benefits only

C) Allow for a risk-benefit discussion

D) Understand that families are angry and need to act out with defiance

78. What is the most common level of myelomeningocele (MMC)?
    A) Upper thoracic
    B) Cervical
    C) Lower thoracic
    D) Lumbar

79. The American Academy of Neurology suggests screening children with cerebral palsy (CP) for all of the following comorbidities **except**:
    A) Mental retardation
    B) Hearing and vision impairment
    C) Speech and language delay
    D) Oromotor dysfunction
    E) Seizures

80. Children with meningomyelocele (MMC) are likely to be nonambulatory at which spinal cord level?
    A) Thoracic
    B) Lumbar
    C) Sacral

81. Battle's sign in head trauma is suggestive of:
    A) Intracranial bleed
    B) Diffuse axonal injury
    C) Basilar skull fracture involving the temporal bone
    D) Basilar skull fracture involving the orbits

82. In infants, at what level does the spinal cord terminate?
    A) L2
    B) T12
    C) L4
    D) T10

83. A 9-year-old girl with a history of difficulty writing and frequent tripping is referred to your office for bracing. You notice stork legs, pes cavus, and hammer toes. The ankle tendon reflex is lost. Her mother had similar problems as a child. The above findings are suggestive of:
    A) Spinal muscular atrophy
    B) Charcot-Marie-Tooth disease (CMT)
    C) Friedreich's ataxia
    D) Congenital myopathy

84. A child should be able to maintain his or her head in the midline position by what age?
    A) 2 months
    B) 3 months
    C) 4 months
    D) 5 months

85. All of the following are proven teratogens **except**:
    A) Rubella virus
    B) Rubeolla virus
    C) Cytomegalovirus
    D) Toxoplasmosis

86. What is the most common connective tissue disease seen in children?
    A) Ankylosing spondylitis
    B) Juvenile rheumatoid arthritis (JRA)
    C) Reactive arthritis
    D) Systemic lupus erythematosus (SLE)

87. Which of the following complications is common in **both** Duchenne muscular dystrophy (DMD) and Becker's muscular dystrophy (BMD)?
    A) Cardiomyopathy
    B) Large bowel obstruction
    C) Ureteral reflux
    D) Obstructive respiratory disease

88. Clinically, what criterion can be used to differentiate between Duchenne muscular dystrophy (DMD) and Becker's muscular dystrophy (BMD)?
    A) Utilization of Gower's maneuver
    B) The ability to ambulate past the late teenage years
    C) Pseudohypertrophy of the calves
    D) Neck flexor weakness

89. A child with cerebral palsy who is likely to walk in the future should have at least what skill by age 2 years?
    A) Smiling
    B) Rolling
    C) Sitting
    D) Cruising

90. Adductor myotomies should:
    A) Be considered for the older child with a dislocated hip and pain
    B) Be considered early in severe spasticity to prevent dislocation
    C) Be delayed until 6 years
    D) None of the above

91. What is a frequent allergy in myelomeningocele (MMC)?
    A) Soap
    B) Poison ivy
    C) Latex
    D) Urine

92. Good prognostic indications for ambulation in children with cerebral palsy (CP) include all of the following **except**:
    A) Independent sitting by 2 years of age
    B) Fewer than three primitive reflexes by 18 months of age
    C) Hemiplegic CP
    D) Term birth

93. Which of the following is often seen in children with meningomyelocele (MMC)?
    A) Hydrocephalus
    B) Chiari malformation
    C) Neurogenic bladder
    D) Precocious puberty
    E) All of the above

94. A 9-year-old sustained C6 to C7 spinal cord injury. Three months after the injury, the parents report that his appetite is lacking and he has apathy, nausea, vomiting, and weakness. The most likely reason for these symptoms is:
    A) Hydrocephalus
    B) Hypercalcemia
    C) Decreased sodium
    D) Depression

95. A 16-year-old football player suffers a T10 fracture. He is paraparetic and has no pain or temperature sensation below T10. However, his proprioception, light touch, pinprick, and vibration are intact.
    These findings are suggestive of:
    A) Anterior spinal cord syndrome
    B) Posterior spinal cord syndrome
    C) Brown-Séquard syndrome
    D) Conus medullaris syndrome

96. The predominant type of neuropathy in Guillain-Barré syndrome (acute inflammatory demyelinating polyradiculoneuropathy) is:
    A) Motor
    B) Sensory
    C) Ataxia
    D) Autonomic

97. In the child's early years, all of the following are important parameters to monitor **except**:
    A) Head circumference
    B) Weight
    C) Height
    D) Body mass index

98. By what age should the palmar grasp reflex disappear?
    A) 2 months
    B) 4 months
    C) 6 months
    D) 12 months

99. What is the most common cause of limping and pain in the hip of children?
    A) Slipped capital femoral epiphysis (SCFE)
    B) Trochanteric bursitis
    C) Legg-Calvè-Perthes disease
    D) Transient toxic synovitis

100. The pathophysiology of Duchenne muscular dystrophy (DMD) involves:
    A) Merosin deficiency
    B) Abnormally low levels of dysferlin
    C) Absence of dystrophin
    D) Mutations of sarcoglycan

101. The laboratory serum creatine kinase level would most likely be highest in which of the following?
    A) A 5-year-old boy with Becker's muscular dystrophy (BMD)
    B) A 20-year-old man with BMD

C) A 5-year-old boy with Duchenne muscular dystrophy (DMD)

D) A 20-year-old man with DMD

102. The most common type of abuse in children with disabilities is:
   A) Verbal abuse
   B) Neglect
   C) Physical abuse
   D) Financial abuse

103. Intrathecal baclofen is a treatment that is recommended for:
   A) A child with mixed tone abnormalities who has failed to respond adequately to oral medications
   B) A child with mild spastic diplegia
   C) A child with mental retardation, seizure disorder, and orthopedic deformity
   D) A child with severe spasticity and parents with a known history of noncompliance

104. What percentage of those with myelomeningocele (MMC) will have normal urinary control?
   A) 50
   B) 25
   C) 10
   D) 1

105. The most likely cause of quadriplegic cerebral palsy (CP) is:
   A) Prematurity (less than 32 weeks)
   B) Perinatal stroke
   C) Hyperbilirubinemia
   D) Birth asphyxia

106. Children with meningomyelocele (MMC) have a higher incidence of:
   A) Environmental allergies
   B) Milk intolerance
   C) Latex allergy
   D) Medication allergies

107. During pediatric neurorehabilitation, all of the following are common focuses of rehabilitation **except**:
   A) Tone abnormalities and spasticity
   B) Preventing deep vein thrombosis
   C) Preventing heterotopic ossification
   D) Chronic subdural hematoma

108. Spinal cord injury without radiographic abnormalities (SCIWORA) is most common in:
   A) Infants and young children
   B) Adolescents
   C) Adults
   D) Old age geriatric population

109. In Erb's palsy, all of the following muscles are paralyzed **except**:
   A) Deltoid
   B) Bicep brachialis
   C) Supinator
   D) Intrinsic muscles of hand

110. You are providing rehabilitation to a 12-year-old spinal cord–injured boy. He has been complaining of intermittent headaches with nasal congestion and nausea. He perspires profusely on his face and neck. His blood pressure is elevated intermittently. The most likely level of his spinal cord injury is:
    A) T6
    B) T12
    C) L4

111. Which best describes the symmetric tonic neck reflex (STNR)?
    A) Flexion of the neck facilitates extension in the upper limbs and extension of the lower limbs. Extension of the neck facilitates flexion in the upper limbs and flexion of the lower limbs
    B) Flexion of the neck facilitates extension in the upper limbs and flexion of the lower limbs. Extension of the neck facilitates flexion in the upper limbs and extension of the lower limbs
    C) Flexion of the neck facilitates flexion in the upper limbs and flexion of the lower limbs. Extension of the neck facilitates extension in the upper limbs and extension of the lower limbs
    D) Flexion of the neck facilitates flexion in the upper limbs and extension of the lower limbs. Extension of the neck facilitates extension in the upper limbs and flexion of the lower limbs

112. A 5-year-old child is being lifted by the hand over a curb while crossing the street. Suddenly, the child experiences exquisite pain and refuses to move the affected arm. This child has most likely suffered a subluxation of which bone?
    A) Ulna
    B) Radius
    C) Humerus
    D) Scaphoid

113. A 12-year-old boy presents with waddling gait and difficulty in climbing stairs. On examination, he demonstrates significant weakness in his proximal lower extremity muscles, especially the quadriceps, and some calf hypertrophy. What is the genetic inheritance of this disorder?
    A) Autosomal dominant
    B) X-linked recessive
    C) Autosomal recessive
    D) There is no genetic linkage

114. Which gait characteristic is **least** likely to be associated with muscular dystrophy or myopathy?
    A) Toe walking in a child
    B) Ipsilateral foot drop
    C) Gluteus medius gait
    D) Increase in lumbar lordosis with standing or ambulation

115. Seizures occur in what percentage of children with cerebral palsy?
    A) 10
    B) 30
    C) 50
    D) 90

116. In patients with cerebral palsy, the ideal candidate for a selective posterior/dorsal rhizotomy is:
    A) An adolescent who is marginally ambulatory
    B) A child with mixed tone disorder
    C) A child with spasticity who has no orthopedic deformities
    D) A child with knee flexion contractures but severe spasticity

117. What are frequent signs and symptoms of spinal cord "tethering"?
    A) Infection
    B) Increased weakness
    C) Cognition loss
    D) Gastrointestinal upset

118. The key features of cerebral palsy include all of the following **except**:
    A) Abnormal movement and posture
    B) Onset in first 3 years of life
    C) Nonprogressive
    D) Mental retardation

119. Prenatal tests for neural tube defects performed at 16 to 18 weeks of gestation include all of the following **except**:
    A) Measure serum alpha-fetoprotein
    B) Acetylcholinesterase levels
    C) Ultrasound of abdomen
    D) Chromosomal assay

120. A 16-year-old sustains a head injury while playing football, and his amnesia resolves on day 5 of rehabilitation. You consider this amnesia to be:
    A) Mild
    B) Moderate
    C) Severe

121. All of the following conditions can predispose children to cervical spinal cord injury because of atlantoaxial dislocation **except**:
    A) Down syndrome
    B) Klippel-Feil syndrome
    C) Cerebral Palsy
    D) Morquio's syndrome

122. Lesions of the facial nerve distal to the nucleus (lower motor neuron involvement) result in:
    A) Paralysis of the lower facial muscles and the muscles of mastication
    B) Paralysis of the upper (forehead) and lower facial muscles
    C) Paralysis of the lower facial muscles with sparing of upper facial muscles (forehead)
    D) Paralysis of upper and lower facial muscles as well as the muscles of mastication

123. A 9-year-old suffered a traumatic brain injury (TBI). He is noted to be fidgety and have piano playing movements of the fingers, and has difficulty maintaining tongue protrusion. These symptoms are not seen when he is sleeping. This describes what type of movements?
    A) Chorea
    B) Tics
    C) Dystonia
    D) Tremors

124. With the asymmetric tonic neck reflex (ATNR), lateral rotation of the head on the trunk produces which of the following?
    A) Flexion in the upper and the lower limbs on the nasal side, and extension of both limbs on the occipital side
    B) Flexion in the upper and the lower limbs on the nasal side, and flexion of both limbs on the occipital side
    C) Extension in the upper and the lower limbs on the nasal side, and flexion of both limbs on the occipital side
    D) Extension in the upper and the lower limbs on the nasal side, and extension of both limbs on the occipital side

125. The most common cause of congenital torticollis is fibrosis of which muscle?
    A) Trapezius
    B) Levator scapulae
    C) Sternocleidomastoid (SCM)
    D) Scalenes

126. Which type of spinal muscular atrophy (SMA) is associated with good long-term survival?
    A) Type I (Werdnig-Hoffmann disease)
    B) Type II
    C) Type III (Kugelberg-Welander syndrome)
    D) Type IV

127. Restrictive lung disease is common in severe myopathies and is due primarily to:
    A) Recurrent pneumonia
    B) Obesity
    C) Respiratory muscle weakness
    D) Intrinsic lung damage

128. Which of the following statements is **not** true?
    A) Undernutrition is a goal in the management of cerebral palsy to enable parents to lift the children more easily
    B) Triceps skin fold helps determine nutritional status in cerebral palsy
    C) Poor nutritional intake is associated with decreased community participation
    D) Poor swallow, reflux, and constipation contribute to poor nutrition in cerebral palsy

129. Comparing phenol with botulinum toxin in the treatment of spasticity for children with cerebral palsy, which of the following is true?
    A) Phenol is quicker and has fewer side effects
    B) Phenol is a less expensive option but more difficult technically to perform
    C) Botulinum toxin is longer lasting but less predictable
    D) Botulinum toxin has been subjected to fewer studies than phenol has

130. What is a leading cause of death in infants with myelomeningocele (MMC)?
    A) Symptomatic Chiari II malformation
    B) Infection
    C) Hydrocephalus
    D) Renal failure

131. Each of the following conditions arises from overuse **except**:
    A) Nursemaid's elbow
    B) Little leaguer's elbow

C) Golfer's elbow

D) Medial epicondylitis

132. At what age can a child achieve fine pincer grasp?
   A) 1 year old
   B) 2 years old
   C) 3 years old
   D) 4 years old

133. At what age should a child achieve scissor grasp?
   A) 6 months
   B) 8 months
   C) 9 months
   D) 12 months

134. Which type of grasp should a 6-month-old child have?
   A) Palmar grasp
   B) Pincer grasp
   C) Fine pincer grasp
   D) Scissor grasp

135. At what age does a child demonstrate disappearance of head lag when pulled to sit?
   A) 3 weeks
   B) 2 months
   C) 4 months
   D) 6 months

136. In Erb's palsy one may see:
   A) Benediction sign
   B) Claw hand
   C) Waiter's tip
   D) Ape hand

137. Children with cerebral palsy often have which of the following visual impairments:
   A) Strabismus
   B) Exotropia
   C) Esotropia
   D) All of the above

138. What condition is characterized by infants with "wide" or "short" heads?
   A) Dolichocephaly
   B) Scaphocephaly
   C) Brachycephaly
   D) Mesaticephaly

139. The WeeFIM (pediatric functional independence measure) functional assessment in the pediatric population may be measured beginning at what age?
   A) Birth
   B) 6 months
   C) 12 months
   D) 24 months

140. Which of the following syndromes is associated with Wilms' tumor?
    A) Denys-Drash syndrome
    B) Aniridia, genitourinary abnormalities, and mental retardation
    C) Beckwith-Wiedemann syndrome
    D) All of the above

141. What does IEP stand for?
    A) Early intervention program
    B) Individualized education program
    C) Internal external programming
    D) Institution for early programming

142. A child with which condition should be monitored for the need for speech therapy?
    A) Cerebral palsy
    B) Bulbar palsy
    C) Intracranial hemorrhage
    D) All of the above

143. Motor development may be delayed due to which of the following causes:
    A) Myopathy
    B) Basal ganglia infarct
    C) Cognitive impairment
    D) All of the above

144. Feeble or eventually lost fetal movements may be the earliest sign of a motor disability.
    A) True
    B) False

145. Which of the following is an electromyogram (EMG) finding characteristic of a congenital myopathy?
    A) End-plate potentials
    B) Miniature end-plate potentials
    C) Short-duration small-amplitude polyphasic potentials
    D) Long-duration large-amplitude polyphasic potentials

146. What must accompany rehabilitation in those with myelomeningocele (MMC) as they move to adulthood?
    A) Anticipation and prevention of life-threatening events
    B) Rechecks as needed
    C) Avoidance of activity
    D) Insistence on employment

# *Pediatrics*

## ANSWERS

1. **E)** In addition to the environmental factors listed, maternal obesity, use of carbamazepine, antihistamines, and sulfonamide medication increase the risk of NTD in women of child-bearing age.

2. **C)** The Glasgow Coma Scale examines three variables: eye opening, verbal response, and motor abilities. Scores can range from 3 to 15. A score of 8 or less indicates a severe injury, 9 to 12 a moderate injury, and 13 to 15 a mild injury.

3. **C)** The most mobile portion of the spinal column is the cervical region (hence the most vulnerable). Approximately 55% of SCI in children involve the cervical spine, 30% involve the thoracic spine, and 15% the lumbar spine.

4. **B)** Botulism is due to toxins produced by *Clostridium botulinum*. These toxins block the release of acetylcholine at the neuromuscular junction.

5. **C)** Children with DMD should avoid high-resistance exercises such as weight lifting. Keeping an active life with sustained nonresistive activities, such as swimming, is best.

6. **B)** Extensor patterns are usually seen in the lower extremity of children with CNS lesions. The extension posture of the lower limb includes hip adduction, extension, and internal rotation, along with knee extension, internal tibial rotation, and equinovarus foot posturing. Flexor patterns are seen in the upper extremities. This includes shoulder adduction, flexion, and internal rotation with elbow flexion, wrist pronation and flexion, and finger and thumb flexion.

7. **C)** Blount's disease, or tibia vara, is most common in African American children. As such, it should be expected in all children in this population who suffer from persistent tibial bowing past the age of 2 years.

8. **C)** This malformation is seen in more than 90% of the cases with myelomeningocele. The protruding sac contains meninges, spinal cord, and spinal fluid. Spina bifida occulta results when there is failure of fusion of the posterior elements of the vertebrae. Meningocele is characterized by a protruding sac, which contains meninges and spinal fluid, whereas myelocele is the presence of a cystic cavity in front of the anterior wall of the spinal cord.

9. **B)** Weakness has been shown to be the most significant contributing factor to loss of ambulation in neuromuscular disease. Prior randomized trials have shown no benefit to early surgical treatment of contractures in DMD. Weakness was noted to be the major cause of loss of ambulation in DMD, and not contracture formation. Contracture formation might actually assist with ambulation.

10. **D)** Motor function of the swallowing muscles and the bowel is affected by cerebral palsy. Pancreatic enzyme secretion is affected in children with cystic fibrosis.

11. **C)** A fixed contracture is not an indication for treatment with botulinum toxin A. All of the other choices relate to increased or abnormal muscle tone and may be relieved (at least partially) by botulinum toxin.

12. **A)** The two most common shunt complications are infection and obstruction. Signs and symptoms vary with the age of the child.

13. **D)** About one-half of those who finish high school go on to further education.

14. **B)** The nervous system is derived from ectoderm. The anterior neuropore closes around 23rd day of intrauterine life. The posterior neuropore closes at 26 and 27 days of intrauterine life.

15. **D)** Cranial nerve dysfunction, intact hearing, and loss of consciousness are suggestive of central vertigo.

16. **B)** Linear fracture is most common after a head injury and usually does not require neurosurgical intervention. If the fracture crosses the suture line in infants, leptomeningeal cyst can occur later in life.

17. **D)** SMA is a disease affecting the anterior horn cells (motor neurons) that causes neurogenic atrophy of muscles. The brain is not affected. They have high cognitive abilities. Therefore, providing them with tools for ambulation and mobility are important. Patients with Down syndrome usually have a single crease across their palms instead of two creases.

18. **B)** CK may be increased by 10,000 times, but not diagnostic of DMD. A muscle biopsy is diagnostic, but invasive. The PCR genetic test is a simple blood test that is confirmatory.

19. **A)** Full flexor pattern is commonly seen in the upper extremity of children with CNS lesions. Upper extremity flexor patterns include shoulder adduction, flexion, and internal rotation with elbow flexion, wrist pronation and flexion, and finger and thumb flexion. Extensor patterns are typically seen in the lower extremities.

20. **B)** Fibula hemimelia is the most common congenital lower limb deficiency. One-fourth of the time, this deficiency occurs bilaterally.

21. **C)** As described by Molnar, if independent sitting occurs by age 2 years, prognosis for ambulation is good. "Will my child walk?" is usually the most frequent question asked by the parent of a newly diagnosed child with CP.

22. **C)** Transition to a wheelchair, because it leads to prolonged static positioning of the limbs, is the largest contributor to the formation of joint contractures in DMD. Although poor nutrition and obesity might lead to wheelchair use sooner, they are not primary causes of joint contractures. Muscular atrophy is not directly related to contractures, although the pseudohypertrophy seen in the calf muscles of boys with DMD is associated with tightness in the heel cord and ankle plantar flexion contractures.

23. **B)** About 5% to 10% of cases of cerebral palsy are due to complications of childbirth or birth asphyxia.

24. **A)** Augmentative communication is important in patients with cerebral palsy who have difficulty communicating. This has been shown to improve all communication efforts and has not been shown to create difficulty in the classroom or decrease parent interaction. It may not, however, meet all of the communication needs of the child.

25. **B)** Approximately 15% of these babies have severe hydrocephalus and require immediate shunting.

26. **D)** Between 12% and 15% of girls with MMC show precocious puberty; 95% have menses.

27. **C)** Folic acid is given to pregnant women to decrease the risk of neural tube defects.

28. **D)** Dystrophic and inflammatory myopathies cause highly elevated CK levels. Congenital myopathies cause mild to moderate elevations of CK.

29. **B)** Retinal hemorrhages can occur after hypoxic or ischemic injury, vaginal birth, side impact car accidents, or child abuse. The sequelae can be visual impairment.

30. **B)** SMA type I (Werdnig-Hoffmann disease) has its onset before 6 months of age. Most patients cannot sit, and the condition has a mortality rate of more than 90% by 3 months of age.
SMA type II has an onset between 6 and 18 months of age. Most patients can sit but not walk. Life expectancy in these patients is to the second decade.
SMA type III (Kugelberg-Welander syndrome) usually presents at about 18 months of age. Most patients can walk and have a normal life expectancy.

31. **E)** DMD is a multisystem disease affecting:
    1. Musculoskeletal system causing weakness and scoliosis
    2. Pulmonary system affecting respiratory function and sleep problem (due to weakness of intercostal and diaphragmatic muscles)
    3. Cardiac system causing cardiomyopathy
    4. IQ and causing mental retardation
    5. GI system causing problems with megacolon and malabsorption

32. **C)** She would be able to complete all of the following with the exception of walking down stairs alternating feet. This is typically accomplished by the age of 4.

33. **B)** At 6 to 7 months, a normally developing child should achieve sitting balance. It is at this time they should undergo the first fitting for a unilateral device. A device with a more sophisticated terminal device is provided at 11 to 13 months when the child begins to walk.

34. **D)** Each is a characteristic type of CP except hemiballismus. Dystonia is characterized by slow rhythmic movements with tone changes generally found in the trunk and extremities, whereas the ataxic-type involves uncoordinated movements associated with nystagmus, dysmetria, and a wide-based gait. Slow writhing involuntary movements, particularly in the distal extremities, describe athetosis.

35. **B)** Intervention with submaximal exercise training in neuromuscular disease has been shown to improve physical performance and increase muscle efficiency while reducing fatigue and improving quality of life. However, in children, the exercise program must be worked into an enjoyable, playful setting. Supervision is necessary to make sure that the children do not play to exhaustion, which could produce muscle damage and overwork weakness.

36. **D)** Obstetric care has improved, but other causes of cerebral palsy have increased, such as prematurity and the incidence of multiple gestation pregnancy. Chorioamnionitis is now recognized as a risk factor for cerebral palsy.

37. **C)** When parents are involved in the care of children with cerebral palsy, the compliance for medications and exercise in the home is improved.

38. **C)** Folic acid supplementation was first shown to decrease the rate of neural tube deficits in the early 1980s in Wales.

39. **A)** IQ scores are adversely affected by central nervous system infections but not by recurrent shunt revisions.

40. **D)** HBOT is considered an alternative therapy in patients with CP. Its primary use is in wound care.

41. **B)** Gower's sign is suggestive of proximal muscle weakness, which can occur in any myopathic process.

42. **D)** Following moderate to severe brain injuries, all of the options listed, except for accelerated closure of the epiphysis, have been reported in various studies. Language impairment has also been reported.

43. **B)** All of the risk factors are causes of stroke in children, but congenital heart disease is the most common.

44. **A)** Corticosteroids and PM&R can help prolong independence by several years, hence modifying the disease course. No definitive cure is available yet.

45. **C)** This child is 18 months old. At this point, it is unlikely he or she would be able to navigate steps.

46. **A)** The most common congenital limb deficiency is a left terminal transradial deficiency.

47. **C)** Spastic diplegia is the most common type of CP. Approximately 75% of those with CP is of this type. There is greater involvement of the lower extremities in comparison with the upper extremities of those with spastic diplegia. Dyskinetic and mixed CP, which exhibits patterns of both spastic and dyskinetic CP, make up approximately 25% of those with CP.

48. **A)** The vast majority of clinical problems encountered in neuromuscular disease can be directly linked to skeletal muscle weakness. Despite other comorbid conditions, studies have indicated that what causes most of the functional problems and impairs quality of life for people with neuromuscular disease is muscle weakness.

49. **D)** Cerebral palsy is by definition due to a nonprogressive brain insult.

50. **D)** Early identification of abnormal tone and motor development may precede diagnosis, but early intervention treatment should be instituted.

51. **A)** Rates have varied in the United States from 2.34 per 1,000 live births to as low as 0.51 per 1,000 live births. The declining rate could be related to awareness of the need for dietary supplements during pregnancy, especially folic acid.

52. **C)** Most patients with lumbar lesions will have some level of ambulation, but those with thoracic MMC can be functional ambulators.

53. **C)** All of the other medications exact their effect through the central nervous system (CNS) **except** for dantrolene, which works at the skeletal muscle level. Dantrolene inhibits the release of calcium from the sarcoplasmic reticulum during excitation-contraction coupling and suppresses the uncontrolled calcium release.

54. **B)** All of the symptoms described are common in muscle diseases.

55. **C)** In general, focal deficits recover better than diffuse deficits. Younger age also predicts a better recovery.

56. **A)** The phrenic nerve is formed from nerve roots C3-5 and supplies the diaphragm. Patients who require permanent ventilatory support can be candidates for phrenic nerve pacing.

57. **B)** Botulism affects the presynaptic neuromuscular junction. The condition is caused by gram-positive *Clostridium botulinum* toxins. The toxins affect the release of acetylcholine, resulting in cranial nerve and muscle weakness.

58. **B)** A child usually "creeps" at 9 months. They can usually pull to stand through half-kneel at 10 months, while independently ambulating at 1 year of age. Sitting with a straight back occurs at 6 months.

59. **A)** The listed clinical features all describe someone with Edwards' syndrome or trisomy 18. Turner syndrome is characterized by being a female of short stature with a webbed neck, a broad "shield" chest, and wide-set nipples. In trisomy 21, the infant presents with the following features: upward slant of palpebral fissures, low-set auricles, prominent occiput, hypoplastic fingernails, and short sternum. Patau's syndrome, trisomy 13, is characterized by intrauterine growth retardation, coloboma (a gap in part of the structure) of the iris, cleft lip and palate, and urinary tract abnormalities.

60. **A)** Approximately 70% to 80% of cerebral palsy cases occur during the prenatal period. Some of the risk factors for CP include prenatal intracranial hemorrhage, placental complications, gestational toxins, or teratogenic agents.

61. **B)** Although the various forms of myopathy are clinically dissimilar, they all involve loss of muscle strength, causing loss of reflexes rather than hyperreflexia, along with weakness and atrophy. Sensation remains intact, as only muscle fibers are affected. Urinary retention is not part of these diseases.

62. **A)** With improvements in obstetric care and the increased survival of premature infants, the incidence of cerebral palsy has remained the same over the past several decades (about 1–2.3 per 1,000 live births).

63. **B)** The American Academy of Pediatrics policy statement on prescribing therapies states that safety limits should be defined.

64. **C)** Studies show a 17% incidence of spina bifida occulta in normal individuals age 1 to 10 years, with no neurologic involvement and incomplete closure of the posterior elements of the spine.

65. **A)** Calcaneal deformities result from unopposed contraction of foot dorsiflexors and can be present at birth or develop later.

66. **D)** In children with cerebral palsy, immobility, malnutrition secondary to oromotor dysfunction, and antiepileptic medications (particularly older generation medications) are associated with decreased bone mineral density.

67. **D)** Speech may be affected in patients with myopathy if the facial muscles are involved, but language is not affected.

68. **E)** Infants with nonaccidental trauma (shaken baby syndrome) may have all of the signs, which should make you suspicious. CT of the head usually reveals subdural hematomas of varying chronicity. Contusions and intracerebral hemorrhage can be seen.

69. **B)** ASIA/IMSOP utilizes documentation of motor, sensory, and sphincter functions. Ten key muscles are graded using the Medical Research Council (MRC) scale, and sensation is assessed over 28 dermatomes.
The Glasgow Coma Scale is used in traumatic brain injury.
The Wee functional independence score measures self-care, mobility, cognition, and communication in children.
The Barthel index is used to measure performance in activities of daily living following conditions such as stroke.

70. **B)** MG affects postsynaptic receptors of the myoneural junction. Transmission of acetylcholine is blocked. Predominant clinical findings include fatigability of ocular, bulbar, and skeletal muscles. This can result in ptosis, diplopia, slurred speech, difficulty with chewing, respiratory problems, and weakness (proximal more than distal).

71. **D)** A child should be able to pivot circles while prone at 5 months of age. They can maintain their heads in the midline position at 2 months of age. By 3 months, they should be able to prone prop on extended elbows. At 4 months, they can roll prone to supine.

72. **D)** The clinical features listed all describe someone with Down syndrome or trisomy 21. Turner syndrome is characterized by being a female of short stature with a webbed neck, a broad "shield" chest, and wide-set nipples. In trisomy 18, the infant suffers from intrauterine growth retardation (IUGR), small mouth, and rocker-bottom feet. Patau's syndrome, trisomy 13, is characterized by IUGR, coloboma (a gap in part of the structure) of the iris, cleft lip and palate, and urinary tract abnormalities.

73. **A)** Hemarthrosis is the hallmark of hemophilia. There are three different types of hemophilia (A, B, C), which are deficiencies of factor VIII, factor IX, and factor XI, respectively. Hemarthrosis is defined as bleeding into the joints causing pain, swelling, and limited joint movement.

74. **D)** Although facioscapulohumeral dystrophy can be quite heterogeneous in its clinical presentation and course, it is typically only slowly progressive. The same is true of BMD and limb-girdle dystrophy. Only DMD is usually associated with a markedly shortened life expectancy. DMD is a progressive myopathy that is universally fatal, with death usually occurring from respiratory or cardiac complications.

75. **D)** Myotonic muscular dystrophy affects skeletal muscle, smooth muscle, myocardium, brain, and ocular structures. Associated findings include frontal pattern baldness, gonadal atrophy (in males), cataracts, insulin insensitivity, and cardiac dysrhythmias.

76. **D)** Sports are a key component of a healthy lifestyle for children, including those with cerebral palsy. Damiano's study refuted that weightlifting is contraindicated in cerebral palsy.

77. **C)** According to the American Academy of Pediatrics policy statement on complementary and alternative medicine, families that request complementary treatments should engage in an open, risk-benefit discussion.

78. **D)** The majority of children with MMC have lumbar lesions, with one-fourth having midlumbar lesions. Very few have cervical and upper thoracic levels.

79. **E)** Children with cerebral palsy (CP) have an increased incidence of seizures, sleep problems, and hydrocephalus, but screening for these conditions is not recommended.

80. **A)** Generally, children with sacral level MMC are able to ambulate with or without crutches or canes. Involvement of peroneal and foot muscles in patients with lumbar lesions will result in limited but some ambulation with an assistive device (depending on quadriceps, hamstrings, and hip flexors involvement). Thoracic MMC lesions may cause total paralysis of the lower limbs.

81. **C)** Battle's sign is retroauricular ecchymosis. In addition, hemotympanum and otorrhea are suggestive of temporal bone fracture. Raccoon eyes are periorbital ecchymoses and suggest an anterior skull base fracture.

82. **A)** The spinal cord terminates at L1 in adults and L2 in infants.

83. **B)** Hereditary sensory-motor neuropathy (HSMN) type I and II are also known as CMT. It is a progressive motor and sensory demyelinating neuropathy (mainly autosomal dominant). The distal muscles of the lower extremity are affected more than the upper extremities. Spinal muscular atrophy and Friedreich's ataxia are autosomal recessive conditions.

84. **A)** A child should be able to maintain his or her head in the midline position at 2 months of age. By 3 months, children should be able to prone prop on extended elbows. At 4 months, they can roll prone to supine, while at 5 months, they should be able to roll supine to prone.

85. **B)** Exposure to potential teratogens increases the chances of malformations in the fetus. Of those listed, the only one not proven to be teratogenic is Rubeolla virus.

86. **B)** JRA is the most common connective tissue disease in children. A diagnosis of JRA is made in the presence of arthritis lasting 6 weeks or longer with an onset earlier than 16 years of age. The incidence is 13.9 per 100,000 per year, and the etiology remains unknown.

87. **A)** Significant cardiac involvement occurs in both DMD and BMD. Dystrophin has been localized to the membrane surface of cardiac Purkinje fibers, and defective dystrophin expression probably contributes to the cardiac conduction disturbances seen in DMD and BMD. Death has been attributed to congestive heart failure in as many as 40% of patients with DMD. The other choices are not seen in this setting. Restrictive (not obstructive) lung disease is common in DMD (and to a lesser extent in BMD) and is due to weakness of the diaphragm, chest wall, and abdominal musculature. The ureter and the large bowel, having smooth muscle, are not primarily involved in DMD or BMD.

88. **B)** The most useful clinical criterion to distinguish BMD from DMD is the continued ability of the patient to walk into the late teenage years. Those with BMD will typically remain ambulatory beyond 16 years of age, whereas even the outlier DMD patients generally stop ambulating between 13 and 16 years of age. Gower's maneuver, pseudohypertrophy of the calves, and neck flexor weakness can be seen in both BMD and DMD and are not useful in distinguishing the two diagnoses.

89. **C)** Patients with cerebral palsy who are able to sit by age 2 years have a good prognosis for future ambulation.

90. **B)** Patients with severe spasticity are at risk for hip dislocation. Adductor myotomies have been shown to decrease that risk if performed early enough.

91. **C)** Although the prevalence of latex allergy in the general population is estimated to be less than 1% to 2%, its prevalence in children with MMC ranges from 20% to 65% because of the repeated exposure.

92. **D)** Term birth does not signify any specific insult or abnormality of movement or posture and therefore does not help to prognosticate the ability to ambulate in children with CP.

93. **E)** Hydrocephalus can be seen with MMC or after closure of the defect. Leakage of cerebrospinal fluid stops and therefore requires shunting. Chiari malformation is a caudal displacement of brain stem and ventricles, which can cause apnea, stridor, nystagmus, opisthotonus, and dysphagia. Neurogenic bladder is commonly seen in patients with MMC. Precocious puberty occurs more commonly in girls secondary to activation of the hypothalamic-pituitary axis, probably due to hydrocephalus.

94. **B)** Hypercalcemia occurs in 25% of such patients 1 to 12 weeks after the injury and is due to bone resorption. Calcium levels above 12 mg/dL can cause the symptoms listed. Although depression can cause apathy and loss of appetite, this combination of symptoms including nausea and vomiting is most consistent with hypercalcemia.

95. **A)** In anterior spinal cord syndrome, there is paresis and analgesia below the lesion, but vibration and position sense are preserved as these are mediated by the posterior columns. In Brown-Séquard syndrome, there is ipsilateral motor paralysis, loss of touch as well as proprioception, and contralateral loss of pain and temperature below the level of the lesion.

96. **A)** Although all of the answer choices can be seen, motor involvement predominates. *Campylobacter jejuni*, *Mycoplasma pneumoniae*, cytomegalovirus, and Epstein-Barr virus are common known causes.

97. **D)** Head circumference, height, and weight are all important parameters that must be closely monitored in a child's early years. BMI is not routinely monitored.

98. **C)** The palmar grasp reflex is seen when an object is placed in the infant's hand and strokes their palm. The fingers will close and they will grasp it. It is seen initially at birth and should disappear by 6 months of age.

99. **D)** Transient toxic synovitis is the most common cause of limping and hip pain in children. SCFE is commonly seen in preadolescent-adolescent obese boys and is a separation of the proximal femoral epiphysis through the growth plate. Trochanteric bursitis is not commonly seen in children. In Legg–Calvè–Perthes disease, there is avascular necrosis at the femoral head. It is seen in children age 4 to 10 years who have pain in the groin that radiates to the anterior/medial thigh toward the knee.

100. **C)** The absence of dystrophin is the basis of the pathophysiology of DMD. Most of the genes in the affected area of the X chromosome encode for components of the dystrophin-glycoprotein complex.

101. **C)** A normal serum creatine kinase value essentially helps to exclude either BMD or DMD. Higher creatine kinase values are noted in the early disease stages and tend to decrease over time with loss of muscle fibers. DMD children can present with a significantly elevated creatine kinase value, typically in the range of 20,000 international units/liter or greater, and is usually higher than in BMD.

102. **B)** Although any type of abuse can occur, neglect is the most common type of abuse in children with disabilities.

103. **A)** Intrathecal baclofen should be considered for a child with significant spasticity or dystonia interfering with function and who has had an adequate trial of oral medications.

104. **C)** Fewer than 10% of children with MMC have normal urinary control. Continence is an important issue and must be addressed.

105. **D)** Prematurity usually causes diplegic cerebral palsy (CP), as white matter adjacent to the ventricles is affected. Stroke and congenital malformations more frequently cause hemiplegic CP. Hyperbilirubinemia causes athetoid or dystonic CP. Severe anoxia causes diffuse brain injury and hence quadriplegic CP.

106. **C)** Compared with the general population, children with MMC have a 20% or higher rate of latex allergy.

107. **D)** Chronic subdural hematomas and hydrocephalus can develop during the rehabilitation phase, but are not focuses of therapy.

108. **A)** SCIWORA is most common in children below 8 years of age. The vertebral column in this population has more elasticity, hence fracture and dislocation are less common. However, myelopathy or central cord injury can occur. MRI of the spine is more sensitive than CT or radiography to reveal SCIWORA injuries.

109. **D)** Erb's palsy involves injury to the upper trunk of the brachial plexus. Intrinsic muscles of the hand are supplied by the ulnar nerve, which is supplied by C8-T1. In Erb's palsy, the arm is held in adduction and internal rotation at the shoulder, extension at the elbow, pronation of the forearm, and flexion at the wrist.

110. **A)** This patient has an acute and potentially life-threatening syndrome called autonomic dysreflexia. This can occur with complete spinal cord injuries at the T6 level or above and is due to imbalanced sympathetic discharges of the splanchnic outflow.

111. **D)** The STNR describes the effects of flexing and extending the head. On flexion of the neck, flexion in the upper limbs and extension of the lower limbs is observed. On extension of the neck, the opposite pattern will be seen.

112. **B)** In this situation described, the child is most at risk for subluxation of the radial head and neck distal to the annular ligament. This is referred to as nursemaid's elbow.

113. **B)** The abnormal gene for Duchenne muscular dystrophy (DMD) and Becker's muscular dystrophy (BMD) is on the short arm of the X chromosome at position Xp21. Both DMD and BMD are inherited X-linked recessive diseases affecting primarily skeletal muscle and myocardium. Mutations in the dystrophin gene that result in a complete loss of dystrophin lead to the DMD phenotype. Mutations that cause the production of a reduced amount of dystrophin, or the production of a truncated, dysfunctional form of dystrophin, produce the BMD phenotype. Both DMD and BMD are progressive myopathies, although DMD is much more severe and is universally fatal. BMD shows a similar pattern of muscle weakness to that of DMD but with later onset and much slower rate of progression.

114. **B)** The gait characteristic least likely to be associated with a myopathic process is an ipsilateral foot drop. In general, muscular dystrophy and the myopathic process typically affect the proximal more than the distal muscles. Because of hip abduction weakness, gluteus medius gait or a Trendelenburg gait can be noted with myopathic disorders. A child presenting with toe walking

should be carefully evaluated for a neuromuscular disorder. In muscular dystrophy with hip extensor weakness, the stability of the hip can be maintained by lumbar lordosis, which places the center of gravity line posterior to the hip joint.

115. **B)** Seizures occur in about 30% of children with cerebral palsy.

116. **C)** Patients with spasticity but no orthopedic deformities have the best outcome after selective posterior/dorsal rhizotomy.

117. **B)** Cord tethering may result in increasing weakness, scoliosis, pain, urologic dysfunction, or orthopedic deformities.

118. **D)** Cerebral palsy is a disorder of movement and posture that occurs in the first 2 to 3 years of life, usually from a single event that is nonprogressive. Mental retardation can occur as a result of insult to the brain, but is not a key feature.

119. **D)** Chromosomal assay is not specific for the diagnosis of neural tube defects.

120. **B)** Posttraumatic amnesia is considered mild if it persists less than 24 hours after the injury. It is considered moderate if it persists between 1 and 7 days and severe if it lasts 8 days or longer.

121. **C)** The odontoid process helps to prevent dislocation of C1 onto C2. Aplasia of the odontoid process can occur in mucopolysaccharidosis (Morquio's syndrome) or Klippel-Feil syndrome. In Down syndrome, congenital hypoplasia of the articulation of C1 and C2 can occur.

122. **B)** When forehead muscles are involved in facial nerve palsy, it is indicative of a lower motor neuron lesion distal to the nucleus. The muscles of mastication are supplied by cranial nerve V. Lower facial muscles are involved in both upper and lower motor neuron facial palsies. Bilateral upper motor neuron innervation of the upper facial muscles leads to sparing of these muscles in an upper motor neuron lesion.

123. **A)** Chorea describes brief, random, repetitive, rapid, purposeless movements. Dystonia is a repetitive, sustained abnormal posture that typically has a twisting quality. Tics are stereotyped, repetitive nonrhythmic movements that mainly involve the head and upper body. Tremor is a rhythmic oscillation.

124. **C)** This is the classical fencer's posture of extension in the upper and the lower limbs on the nasal side, and flexion of both limbs on the occipital side.

125. **C)** The most common cause of congenital torticollis is fibrosis of the SCM.

126. **C)** SMA Type III, or Kugelberg-Welander syndrome, is associated with good long-term survival but dependent on respiratory function. It is an autosomal recessive disorder characterized by proximal weakness predominantly of the legs. Fasciculations are common, and scoliosis is frequent.

127. **C)** Respiratory impairment in the setting of a myopathy is due to weakness of the diaphragm, chest, and abdominal musculature. The other listed factors have not been shown to play a significant role in restrictive lung disease.

128. **A)** Appropriate nutrition is needed in children with cerebral palsy to maximize brain, muscle, and bone development. Undernourished children are at risk for multiple health problems, which may result in poor community participation.

129. **B)** Although phenol injections may last longer than botulinum toxin injections, they are more difficult injections to perform and are associated with more side effects.

130. **A)** Symptomatic Chiari II malformation remains the leading cause of death for infants with MMC.

131. **A)** Nursemaid's elbow is subluxation of the radial head from sudden traction in an extended and pronated arm. Medial epicondylitis is sometimes called golfer's elbow or little leaguer's elbow. Little leaguer's elbow occurs in a skeletally immature individual, which furthermore involves inflammation of the medial epicondylar apophysis. Throwing leads to repeated valgus stress on the growth plate, which causes pain with resisted wrist flexion and pronation.

132. **A)** Fine pincer grasp involves using the DIP of the index finger and thumb, compared to pincer grasp which incorporates the PIP of the index finger and sides of the thumb as well to grasp the object.

133. **B)** Scissor grasp involves using all four fingers and the side of one's thumb. This is achieved at 8 months.

134. **A)** Palmar grasp involves picking up an object with the whole hand. Scissor grasp is achieved at 8 months and uses all four fingers and the side of the thumb. Pincer grasp uses the thumb and index finger. Fine pincer grasp is achieved at 12 months and uses the thumb and DIP of the index finger.

135. **C)** A child can support his or her head to at least 45° when pulled to sit at this age. A child should be able to sit unsupported by 6 months of age. Children with low tone who are unable to achieve this milestone may be described as "floppy."

136. **C)** Erb's palsy affects the upper roots C5-6 and may present with a waiter's tip hand. Klumpke's palsy is a brachial plexus injury involving the lower roots, primarily C8-T1. It presents with a claw hand from injury to ulnar innervated hand intrinsic muscles, as well as flexor carpi ulnaris and half of the flexor digitorum profundus. The Benediction sign appears the same as a claw hand; however, it occurs as a result of median nerve injury to the lateral two lumbricals, in which one is unable to fully make a fist. Claw hand causes inability to fully open a fist with paralysis of the medial two lumbricals. Ape hand also occurs from an injury to the median nerve, specifically affecting the abductor pollicis and opponens pollicis muscles and leaving the adductor pollicis intact, and therefore usually results from injury distal to the brachial plexus.

137. **D)** Exotropia and esotropia are types of strabismus, or misalignment of the eyes. Exotropia involves one eye turning horizontally outward compared to the other, and esotropia involves one eye turning inward.

138. **C)** Brachycephaly occurs when the width becomes more than 80% of the length. In normocephalic or mesaticephalic children, the width is 75% to 80% of the length. Patients become dolichocephalic when the width becomes less than 75% of the length. Dolicocephaly is another name for scaphocephaly. It is characterized by a long head, in which the occipitofrontal diameter (OFD) is disproportionately longer than the width (biparietal diameter [BPD]) and often appears in premature infants.

139. **B)** The WeeFIM functional independence measure is designed to measure functional assessment beginning at 6 months up to 7 years of age. Children aged 0 to 6 months use a 0 to 3 module questionnaire to measure precursors to function. Children above age 7 years use the adult FIM

assessment construct unless their functional level is equivalent to a child younger than 7 years, in which case they may also use the WeeFIM. The three constructs measured are cognition, self-care, and mobility.

140. **D)** Patients with Wilms' tumor may have associated findings such as hemihypertrophy of the limb or aniridia. They have nephroblastomas and may have associated gonadoblastomas along the gastrourinary (GU) tract. Patients with Denys-Drash syndrome have pseudohermaphroditism in addition to kidney disease, and patients with Beckwith-Wiedemann syndrome have macroglossia.

141. **B)** An individualized education program is a system implemented during the school-age years that includes modifying the curriculum and/or environment to maximize learning potential aside from providing therapeutic services. Early intervention is a government sponsored program involving therapy and other services prior to the school-age years, from infancy or onset of need until age 3 years.

142. **D)** Children with cerebral palsy may have oromotor dysfunction in speech production, or cognitive dysfunction in receptive or expressive language pathways from involved areas of the brain. All patients referred for speech therapy first need to rule out hearing loss, which may present as early as 6 to 8 months, when parents may notice decrease in spontaneous babbling vocalizations.

143. **D)** Motor development may be compromised peripherally by myopathy or centrally by cognitive impairment. A child who has motor deficits but compensates well leads the differential of etiologic diagnosis toward myopathy rather than cognitive impairment.

144. **A)** Decreased or ceased fetal movements prior to birth may be the earliest presentation of a motor disability such as congenital myopathy. In the postnatal period, deterioration due to a progressive neuromuscular disease may be masked by the relatively fast pace of early motor development.

145. **C)** Short-duration small-amplitude (SDSA) polyphasic potentials are often seen in children presenting with congenital myopathies or other neuromuscular disorders. Congenital myopathy should be in the differential of any infant presenting with hypotonia referred for EMG. Myotubular (centronuclear) myopathy is an example of a congenital myopathy most consistently presenting with abnormal spontaneous action potential activity at rest. SDSA are also present in dystrophic myopathies and polymyositis/dermatomyositis; however, muscular dystrophy can rarely present with low-density lipoprotein from fiber splitting in chronic disease. SDSA polyphasic potentials are action potentials with a dropout of muscle fibers, and are associated with myopathic diseases. Less commonly they are associated with neuromuscular junction disorders or severe neuropathic diseases. Miniature end-plate potentials represent a monophasic, single quantum version of a biphasic end-plate action potential of summated quanta, both of which can be found in either children or adults.

146. **A)** MMC presents lifelong challenges to affected patients, their families, and clinicians. Surveillance and education are required to prevent life-threatening events related to ventriculoperitoneal shunt malfunction, Chiari II malformation, renal failure, infection, and latex allergy—all in conjunction with maximizing function.

# 14

# *Industrial Rehabilitation*

## QUESTIONS

1. All of the following are true regarding workers' compensation **except**:
   A) The injured worker does not need to prove that the employer is at fault for her or his injury
   B) Lost income is generally only partially replaced by workers' compensation income, and does not cover 100% of lost wages
   C) Workers' compensation varies little from state to state because it is governed by federal law
   D) Workers' compensation provides both medical payments and supplemental lost wages while the injured worker recovers

2. An impairment is:
   A) The loss or abnormality of body structure or of a physiological or psychological function
   B) The nature and extent of functioning at the level of the person
   C) The nature and extent of a person's involvement in life situations in relation to activities, health conditions, and contextual factors, and may be restricted in nature, duration, and quality
   D) Invariably associated with a disability and a correlated handicap

3. The Valpar Component Work Sample Series is an example of the work sample approach to vocational testing, which measures:
   A) Motor responses
   B) General intelligence and academic performance
   C) Occupational interests
   D) None of the above

4. The FABER test evaluates for:
   A) Possible pathology in the knee
   B) Possible pathology in the sacroiliac joint and hip
   C) Cervical stenosis
   D) Evidence of radiculopathy

5. Heel walking tests motor strength of the ankle dorsiflexors and involves the following nerve root(s):
   A) S1
   B) L4-5
   C) L3-4
   D) L1-2

6. Maximal medical improvement is achieved once a condition:
   A) Yields normal laboratory and radiological findings
   B) Has used up all allowable workers' compensation funding
   C) Requires no further diagnostic testing or intervention
   D) Has been diagnosed for 6 months

ANSWERS TO THIS SECTION CAN BE FOUND ON PAGE 413

7. The risk of using an acute care model for a patient presenting with a chronic problem includes all of the following **except**:
   A) Potentially overlooking psychosocial issues that may be contributing
   B) Providing unnecessary expectations that there will be a "quick fix"
   C) Empowering patients and addressing multiple dimensions of care issues
   D) Not necessarily considering occupational and lifestyle issues

8. Under the current U.S. workers' compensation system:
   A) The injured worker can sue a third party involved in the injury
   B) The injured worker needs to pay his or her own medical bills
   C) The injured worker is not paid for time off
   D) The injured worker must sue his employer to regain lost earnings

9. In the medicolegal workers' compensation context, an aggravation refers to:
   A) A permanent worsening of a prior condition by a particular event
   B) Signs or symptoms of a prior illness or injury occurring in the absence of a new provocative event
   C) A temporary worsening of a prior condition by an injury
   D) An injury causing a latent disease process to appear

10. Vocational testing assesses all of the following **except**:
   A) General intelligence
   B) Aptitudes, interests, and work skills
   C) Aptitude for specific occupations, as listed in the Dictionary of Occupational Titles
   D) Ability to speak

11. Musculoskeletal injuries generally resolve and can be considered chronic by:
   A) 1 month
   B) 3 months
   C) 6 months
   D) 1 year

12. If fingertips are more than 10 cm from the floor with testing maximum trunk flexion, the following reasons should be considered **except**:
   A) Symptom amplification
   B) Nerve root compression
   C) Tightness of the quadriceps
   D) Paraspinal muscle spasm

13. What is the definition of the term "symptom magnification"?
   A) Perceived (subconscious) concern with body integrity and body function
   B) Conscious attempt to deceive for social rewards
   C) Conscious or subconscious, self-destructive, socially reinforced behavioral response pattern
   D) Anger related to a specific job-related injury

14. Indications for spine surgery include all of the following **except**:
   A) Cauda equina syndrome
   B) History and examination findings that are not consistent with imaging results and/or electrodiagnosis (EMG)
   C) Progressive neurologic deficits
   D) Certain types of fractures, tumors, and infections

15. All the following are true **except**:
    A) Many treatments such as splinting, surgery, and ointments date back 5,000 years
    B) The Code of Hammurabi specified physician fees and monetary damages for those who harm others
    C) The United States developed workers' compensation laws before the European nations
    D) The 18th century physician and author Bernardino Ramazzini is considered the father of occupational medicine

16. A reasonable degree of medical certainty indicates:
    A) Less likely than not
    B) Greater than or equal to 51% certain
    C) Greater than or equal to 95% certain
    D) Within the realm of possibility

17. Vocational rehabilitation principles include all of the following **except**:
    A) Placing the individual back with a previous employer if a position is available
    B) Vocational testing regardless of the previous employment
    C) Assessing the premorbid skills of a client to see if a suitable position exists
    D) Vocational testing if the patient cannot return to previous employment

18. What is the most common cause of disability in workers below the age of 45 years:
    A) Neck pain
    B) Shoulder pain
    C) Low-back pain
    D) Knee pain

19. Initial care in a patient with acute onset of nonspecific low back pain (with no serious conditions noted on initial assessment) includes:
    A) Nonsteroidal anti-inflammatory drugs (NSAIDs), if not contraindicated
    B) Use of narcotic medication for primary pain control
    C) Valium to control muscle spasm
    D) Bed rest for 2 weeks

20. All of the following are goals of a causality examination **except**:
    A) Confirming the original diagnosis was correct and due to injury, event, or exposure
    B) Confirming a person's current complaints and findings has not been confounded by sickness behavior (conscious or unconscious)
    C) Identifying the most appropriate form of treatment intervention
    D) Verifying current symptoms and physical examination findings is consistent with a diagnosis and are not indicative of an unrelated new diagnosis

21. Which of the following is true concerning lumbar epidural steroid injections?
    A) Provide permanent relief from persistent lumbar radiculopathy
    B) Markedly reduce functional impairment
    C) Primarily indicated for axial back pain
    D) Provide temporary relief for patients presenting with lumbar radiculopathy

22. Which of the following statements is true for an injured worker?
    A) The direct costs of medical care exceed the indirect costs
    B) Low-back pain is not a significant source of disability in young workers

C) The indirect costs of medical care exceed the direct costs

D) The National Academy of Sciences found that musculoskeletal injuries are a trivial cause of health care costs

23. The following are all true statements about occupational rehabilitation **except**:
   A) Job matching can help select a particular job for a worker with specific abilities
   B) Functional capacity evaluations can help assess validity and functional ability to clarify appropriate work restrictions
   C) Work conditioning may improve the worker's strength and cardiovascular fitness after a period of prolonged inactivity
   D) Positive Waddell's signs on examination indicates a musculoskeletal nidus for pain

24. Funding for state vocational rehabilitation agencies is primarily supplied by:
   A) The federal government
   B) The state government
   C) Both the state and federal governments equally
   D) Charitable organizations

25. General principles of disability prevention include all of the following **except**:
   A) Primary prevention efforts designed to prevent worsening of an impairment
   B) Secondary prevention efforts to identify and treat a pathologic condition and reduce the risk factors for further disablement
   C) Tertiary prevention efforts to limit the restriction of a person's participation in an area, such as employment, by actively facilitating such or by removing a barrier
   D) Ensuring that disabled individuals retire as soon as possible

26. Regarding the straight leg raise test:
   A) The test is positive if the patient complains of axial pain
   B) The test is positive if there is pain below the knee with greater than 70° of straight leg raising
   C) The test is positive if pain is relieved by dorsiflexing the ankle
   D) The test is positive if pain in the affected leg occurs with straight leg raising the patient's unaffected extremity

27. Which position causes the highest lumbar intradiskal pressure?
   A) Standing
   B) Walking
   C) Lying supine
   D) Sitting

28. Ways to improve functional outcomes in occupational injuries include all the following **except**:
   A) Early intervention correlates with early resolution
   B) Evaluations and treatment should ideally occur in more than one location
   C) The worker should remain at work as much as possible
   D) Initial and subsequent visits should be brief and problem focused

29. The maximum that should be lifted on an occasional basis during light duty is:
   A) 10 lb
   B) 20 lb
   C) 50 lb
   D) 100 lb

**30.** The Rehabilitation Act of 1973:
  A) Extended civil rights protection to persons with disabilities
  B) Included antidiscrimination and affirmative action in employment
  C) Was broadened by the Rehabilitation Act Amendments of 1978 to include independent living programs, under the responsibility of the Rehabilitation Services Administration
  D) All of the above

**31.** The expenses that a business might incur to comply with the provisions of the Americans with Disabilities Act in hiring a disabled worker can be partially mitigated by:
  A) An "access" tax credit for eligible expenses against income taxes
  B) The Targeted Jobs Tax Credit (TJTC)
  C) Only hiring the person part-time so that the employer does not have to provide health care
  D) The Full Employment Act

**32.** When evaluating a patient with an acute onset of low-back pain, identifiable "red flags" requiring further workup include all of the following **except**:
  A) Night pain that interrupts sleep
  B) Pain that is relieved by rest
  C) History of trauma
  D) Unexplained weight loss

**33.** *Cumulative trauma disorders* is a term that primarily refers to which of the following conditions?
  A) Carpal tunnel syndrome
  B) Recurrent low-back pain
  C) Patella tendinitis
  D) Plantar fasciitis

**34.** Once injured workers agree to receive Workers' Compensation benefits:
  A) They can sue their employer for negligence
  B) They cannot sue third parties who are involved
  C) They can sue their employer and third parties
  D) They forgo their right to sue their employer

**35.** Which of the following is **not** true of independent medical examinations (IMEs)?
  A) The physician performing the IME bills the company requesting the examination and not the patient
  B) Because the examination is performed by a physician, a doctor-patient relationship is started at that time
  C) The report will often need to address issues of causation, impairment, and functional ability
  D) The IME doctor should not order treatment for the examinee

**36.** Vocational rehabilitation is an example of:
  A) An ameliorative program
  B) A corrective program
  C) Both
  D) Neither

**37.** Which of the following sources of income is included in the benefit cap for Social Security Disability payments (ie, counts against the beneficiary's payments)?
  A) Veterans' payments
  B) Disability pensions from government jobs

C) Workers' compensation benefits

D) All the above

38. Waddell's nonorganic signs include:
    A) Point tenderness with palpation
    B) Loss of sensation representing the distribution of a specific nerve root or peripheral nerve
    C) No complaints of low-back pain with axial simulation
    D) Negative-seated straight leg raise test while the patient is distracted and findings of increased pain with formal supine straight leg raise testing

39. Clinical symptoms of cauda equina syndrome include all of the following **except**:
    A) Radicular pain and numbness involving both legs
    B) Loss of perineal sensation/saddle anesthesia
    C) Unaffected gait pattern
    D) Urinary frequency, urinary retention or incontinence

40. Which of the following statements is true according to a National Academy of Sciences study?
    A) A large percentage of injured workers account for a small percentage of costs
    B) A small percentage of injured workers account for a small percentage of costs
    C) A small percentage of injured workers account for a large percentage of costs
    D) A large percentage of injured workers account for a large percentage of costs

41. The maximum weight that should be lifted on an occasional basis during medium duty is:
    A) 10 lb
    B) 20 lb
    C) 50 lb
    D) 100 lb

42. Direct expenditures related to disability include all of the following **except**:
    A) Loss of income
    B) Medical and personal care
    C) Assistive technology
    D) Income support

43. Disincentives for vocational rehabilitation include all of the following **except**:
    A) There are no disincentives for vocational rehabilitation
    B) Fear on the part of disabled individuals that their cash and medical benefits will be jeopardized if they demonstrate that they can work, even on a part-time basis
    C) Stereotypes that characterize the disabled as inevitably unproductive members of society
    D) Employers' attitudes toward the disabled

44. Low-back pain and back injuries occurring in the work force:
    A) Are uncommon in workers between ages 30 and 60 years
    B) Become chronic and last more than 90 days in most cases
    C) Are a primary cause of absenteeism from work
    D) Do not require a complete medical history and physical examination

45. Spurling's test is used to help evaluate for:
    A) Cervical disk herniations
    B) Lumbar spondylosis
    C) Injury to the brachial plexus
    D) Lumbar disk herniations

**46.** Which of the following is the lowest risk factor for occupational injury claims?
  A) Job dissatisfaction
  B) Low educational status
  C) Smoking
  D) Low income

**47.** Which of the following is true regarding employment evaluations?
  A) Preemployment evaluations should be done before interviewing a potential employee
  B) Preplacement evaluations have been determined to be illegal under current federal law
  C) Ergonomists can help evaluate worksite modifications
  D) Job site analyses rely solely on job descriptions for their recommendations

**48.** Which condition is associated with the highest risk, for a given individual, of having a significant disability?
  A) Rheumatoid arthritis
  B) Multiple sclerosis
  C) Cerebrovascular disease
  D) Emphysema

**49.** The presence of a job coach is a unique feature of which type of employment program?
  A) Transitional employment
  B) Projects with industry
  C) Supported employment
  D) Sheltered workshops

**50.** Functional capacity evaluations (FCEs):
  A) Evaluate a worker's ability to perform a particular type of job
  B) Do not evaluate a worker's tolerance for performing selected job tasks
  C) Usually take less than 30 minutes to complete
  D) Do not require specially trained therapists

**51.** Work hardening focuses on improving all of the following **except**:
  A) Strength and flexibility
  B) Conditioning
  C) Functional ability for a specific job
  D) General cardiovascular fitness

**52.** A 38-year-old woman "clocked out" at work and was getting into her car in the parking lot when she slipped, twisting her ankle. Should this injury be covered under workers' compensation?
  A) Yes, because it arose out of the course of her employment
  B) Yes, because it was her own fault that she slipped
  C) No, because she already clocked out
  D) No, because the minor injury will probably heal on its own

**53.** Which of the following is **not** a known physical risk factor for occupational injury claims?
  A) Contact stress
  B) Inadequate sleep
  C) Whole body vibration
  D) Forceful movement

54. The condition associated with the highest prevalence of individuals with activity limitations is:
    A) Mental retardation
    B) Diabetes mellitus
    C) Heart disease
    D) Visual disorders

55. Which of the following programs has been clearly superior in returning disabled individuals to gainful, nonsheltered employment?
    A) Sheltered workshops
    B) Day programs
    C) Home-based programs
    D) None of the above

56. Permanent worsening of a previous condition by a particular event is called:
    A) Aggravation
    B) Precipitation
    C) Exacerbation
    D) Recurrence

57. Which of the following is **not** a known risk factor for occupational injury claims?
    A) Smoking
    B) Job dissatisfaction
    C) High educational level
    D) Deconditioning

58. Which workers' compensation act was enacted in 1970/1971?
    A) The Employers' Liability Law
    B) The Occupational Safety and Health Act (OSHA)
    C) The Code of Hammurabi
    D) No-fault insurance

59. All of the following are true, **except**:
    A) An injury refers to a specific event that occurred
    B) An occupational illness may arise gradually, and not necessarily after a particular event
    C) Cumulative trauma disorder refers to a specific medical diagnosis and helps clarify the pathoanatomic event
    D) Carpal tunnel syndrome is a type of cumulative trauma disorder

60. Estimates of the percentage of disabled individuals in the United States range from:
    A) 3% to 5%
    B) 5% to 10%
    C) 15% to 20%
    D) 25% to 30%

61. On-the-job training programs:
    A) Can include tax incentives for potential employers
    B) Mandate that employers retain employees after the program has been completed
    C) Guarantee that the counselor will place the newly trained individual if the employer does not retain him or her
    D) Are illegal in most states, due to liability issues

62. All of the following are true about neck pain **except**:
    A) Most people with neck pain experience complete resolution of symptoms
    B) Between 50% and 85% of the population who experience neck pain at some initial point will report neck pain again within 1 to 5 years
    C) Findings are similar in the general population, workers, and patients following motor vehicle accidents
    D) A normal neurologic exam is common

63. Testing extensor hallucis longus (EHL) strength provides information about which of the following nerve roots:
    A) L1
    B) L2
    C) L3
    D) L5

64. Establishing a diagnosis for a patient with complaints of low-back pain on whom you are considering a referral for spine surgery is based on:
    A) MRI findings primarily
    B) Subjective history primarily
    C) Objective findings on examination only
    D) Diagnostic testing should not be performed for nonspecific low-back pain

65. A patient with low-back pain is sent to a physician for an independent medical exam. The physician is looking for evidence of symptom magnification. Which of the following tests are **not** performed when checking for Waddell's signs?
    A) Tenderness
    B) Distraction
    C) Slump test
    D) Regional weakness

66. A 52-year-old male underwent surgery for an open midshaft femur fracture and has been unable to work due to the injury for 8 months. What type of disability is he considered to have?
    A) Temporary
    B) Permanent
    C) Partial
    D) Total

67. A 45-year-old female with low-back pain due to a herniated disk is unable to stand for longer than 15 minutes at a time. Her standing limitation is defined as a/an _____.
    A) Impairment
    B) Handicap
    C) Disability
    D) Flaw

68. An employee is required to perform a certain duty for 7 hours out of a 9-hour work day. Which of the following physical requirement durations fits this description?
    A) Occasionally
    B) Frequently
    C) Often
    D) Constantly

69. A 35-year-old male veterinarian is required to lift 25- to 40-lb dogs daily for up to one-third of his regular work day. His job fits into which of the following strength ratings?
    A) Sedentary work
    B) Light work
    C) Medium work
    D) Heavy work
    E) Very heavy work

70. Principles of managing patients with neck pain include:
    A) Electrodiagnostic testing performed within the first week of symptoms
    B) Imaging tests done as soon as possible
    C) Use of appropriately selected nonsteroidal anti-inflammatory drugs (NSAIDs) or nonpre-scription medication as a first-line treatment for pain
    D) Strict bed rest

71. Illness behaviors are most often seen in which phase of injury?
    A) Acute
    B) Subacute
    C) Chronic
    D) Same in all phases

72. Workplace factors associated with an increased risk of neck pain include:
    A) Use of chairs with armrests
    B) Low levels of psychological job strain
    C) Using telephone headsets
    D) Working with the cervical spine in flexion for prolonged periods

# *Industrial Rehabilitation*

1. **C)** While the Occupational Safety and Health Act (OSHA) provides national guidelines for workers' compensation policy, each state has an administrative agency that governs employee safety, workers' benefits, employers' behaviors, and procedures for appeal. For this reason, there are state-to-state variations in compensation rate, coverage, and duration of benefits.

2. **A)** An impairment is the loss or abnormality of body structure, and can be physiological or psychological. Answer choice (B) is the definition of activity, and (C) the definition of participation, both of which can represent a dimension of disablement in the biopsychosocial model of the World Health Organization paradigm. Impairment is not invariably associated with a disability or handicap.

3. **A)** Motor responses are measured in this very practical testing, which includes a series of tasks such as drill press operation, circuit board assembly, or bench assembly. Aptitudes and intelligence are not the focus of this testing.

4. **B)** FABER is an acronym for **f**lexion, **ab**duction, **e**xternal **r**otation. This is also known as Patrick's test. It is also sometimes referred to as FABERE (indicating extension after the flexion, abduction, and external rotation to elicit pain). It is a stress maneuver to detect hip and sacroiliac pathology. It is performed by placing the affected hip in flexion, abduction, and external rotation with the foot placed on the opposite knee. The pelvis is stabilized with the examiner's hands on the contralateral anterior superior iliac spine. The test is positive if there is pain in the ipsilateral hip or sacroiliac region.

5. **B)** Heel walking and toe walking are utilized to evaluate muscle strength and spinal innervation. Heel walking is a quick screen for L4-5 aggravation, and toe walking is a screen for S1 innervation.

6. **C)** Maximal medical improvement (MMI) occurs once the medical condition has resolved or has become stable with no further changes expected. Further diagnostic testing intervention is not recommended. The injured worker is not expected to significantly change in the near term with regard to pain level or functional ability. An impairment rating might be appropriate once MMI has been obtained.

7. **C)** Using an acute care model for chronic illness provides patients with expectations that a medication, injection, or surgery will cure the problem. The risk is that psychosocial, occupational, and lifestyle issues, and the importance of utilizing a multidimensional biopsychosocial approach will be overlooked.

8. **A)** Employees can sue a third party if they believe that party is somehow responsible for their injury. In turn, that third party may sue the employer if it believes the employer is legally liable for the accident. If this occurs, the employer's liability coverage would pay any damages awarded by the court to the third party to compensate for the bodily injury to the employee.

9. **A)** In the medicolegal arena, an exacerbation is a temporary worsening. To establish aggravation of a condition, the physician must document that an actual permanent worsening of the condition has occurred. Occasionally, this applies if the employee has a medical condition unrelated to work that is aggravated by a work injury.

10. **D)** Vocational testing assesses general intelligence, aptitude, and interest of various occupations.

11. **B)** Musculoskeletal injuries generally resolve within 12 weeks. A condition is considered chronic if it persists beyond the expected normal healing time.

12. **C)** Evaluation of normal lumbar flexion should reveal fingertips no greater than 10 cm from the floor. Reasons for limited lumbar flexion include nerve root irritation from possible disk herniation, tight hamstrings, and spasm of the paraspinal muscles. Symptom amplification should also be considered, and in these situations, it is prudent to retest several times to determine whether there is significant variability.

13. **C)** Dr Leonard Matheson defined symptom magnification as "a conscious or unconscious self-destructive socially reinforced behavioral response pattern consisting of reports or displays of symptoms which function to control the life circumstances of the sufferer."

14. **B)** Cauda equina syndrome, progressive neurologic deficits, certain types of fractures, infections, and tumors are all indications for spinal surgery. Surgery **may** also be indicated for patients with consistent history, examination findings, and diagnostic imaging. Patients with documented leg and back pain secondary to a herniated disk, stenosis, or spondylolisthesis with poor response to conservative treatment (typically lasting at least 3 months) **may** also be surgical candidates. Surgical intervention for patients presenting with purely axial back pain has not been demonstrated.

15. **C)** The United States lagged behind Europe in adopting policies to protect workers injured on the job. In fact, Chancellor Otto von Bismarck of Germany was the first to adopt a system of compensation for injured workers in 1884. In the late 1800s, the industrial revolution had created unsafe work conditions in factories throughout the United States. Both adults and children were being maimed and killed on the job, and employers routinely dodged liability for workers' accidents. Injured workers had little recourse but to sue employers for compensation, and few employees could afford to do this. Employers had powerful defenses against employee lawsuits, assumption of risk, comparative negligence, and fellow employee negligence. In 1908, the U.S. Federal Employers' Liability Act was passed. Applying to railroad workers, it removed contributory negligence and the voluntary assumption of risk by workers as an employer's defense. In 1917, the U.S. Supreme Court affirmed that workers' compensation laws were constitutional, and by 1920, 42 states had adopted such laws.

16. **B)** The phrase reasonable degree of medical certainty is a medicolegal term meaning "more likely than not." In other words, if there is a preponderance of evidence supporting a conclusion, the phrase "reasonable degree of medical certainty" can be applied.

17. **B)** If the client was employed prior to the onset of the disability, resuming employment with a previous employer always holds the most potential. If the patient can return to his or her previous employment, usually vocational testing is not indicated.

18. **C)** In workers younger than 45 years, low-back pain is the most common cause of disability. Low-back pain affects 2% to 4% of the working population annually. Eighty percent of the working population will likely have an episode of low-back pain on at least one occasion.

19. **A)** The patient should be assured that rapid recovery can be expected if the initial assessment reveals no evidence of a serious condition. Nonprescription analgesics will provide sufficient pain relief for most patients with acute back pain. Most patients will not require bed rest. Bed rest greater than 4 days has the potential to cause debilitating effects.

20. **C)** The causality exam consists of review of records, interview, physical examination, test results, and conclusions. Objective findings on examination should carry a greater weight of evidence than subjective findings in supporting the diagnosis. Goals of the causality examination do not include identifying the most appropriate form of treatment intervention.

21. **D)** Lumbar epidural steroid injections provide temporary pain relief for patients from persistent lumbar radiculopathy. The injections have no proven effect on functional impairment, need for surgery, or pain relief lasting more than 3 months. Epidural steroid injections are not indicated for patients presenting with axial (nonradicular) back pain only.

22. **C)** The cost of medical care (direct costs) for the injured worker is far less than the cost of lost productivity and wages, not to mention the administrative costs associated with Workers' Compensation claims (indirect costs).

23. **D)** The Waddell's signs are nonorganic findings often discovered in the evaluation of low-back pain. The presence of three of the five signs is clinically significant, although not necessarily for malingering. When a patient exhibits such findings, it indicates that disturbances other than physical pathology might be contributing to the patient's condition.

24. **A)** The federal government supplies approximately 80% of the funding for vocational rehabilitation agencies. The states supply the remaining 20%.

25. **D)** Insuring retirement as soon as possible is not part of disability prevention.

26. **D)** Crossover pain (pain when the contralateral limb is raised) is a stronger indication of nerve root compression than pain elicited from raising the ipsilateral (affected) limb. Straight leg raising is positive if there is pain below the knee with more than 30° and less than 70° straight leg raising. When straight leg raising is positive, the pain is increased by dorsiflexing the ankle and relieved by plantar flexing the ankle.

27. **D)** Research has shown that sitting increases intradiskal pressure more than any other sedentary position. Provision of a chair with a supported backrest, armrests, and back support may reduce intradiskal pressure.

28. **B)** Ideally, care should be rendered in one location.

29. **B)** Workers on light duty can lift up to 20 lb on an occasional basis and up to 10 lb on a frequent basis.

30. **D)** All of the answers are true.

31. **A)** The access tax credit was created to ease the burden of compliance with the Americans With Disabilities Act on small businesses. The TJTC is an incentive for employers to hire the "hardcore" unemployed, those on supplementary security income (SSI).

32. **B)** Red flags are indicative of potentially serious conditions. These include (but are not limited to) major trauma from a motor vehicle accident or fall from a height; minor trauma or strenuous lifting in older patients; history of cancer; history of fevers, chills, or unexplained weight loss; urinary retention; urinary frequency or overflow incontinence; saddle anesthesia; and severe progressive neurologic deficits in the lower extremity.

33. **A)** Cumulative trauma disorders primarily refer to carpal tunnel syndrome, but may also include lateral epicondylitis, cubital tunnel syndrome, de Quervain's tenosynovitis, myofascial pain, and rotator cuff tendinitis. These disorders are the result of a repetitive movement that results in tissue damage.

34. **D)** Workers' compensation laws are by definition "no fault." In exchange for the employer's assumption of responsibility, the worker surrenders the privilege to litigate against the employer as a result of the injury.

35. **B)** Physicians who perform an IME are providing a service to an insurer, employer, or attorney by evaluating the claimant and medical records and then rendering specific opinions related to diagnosis, causation, medical tests and treatment, fitness for duty, maximal medical improvement, and permanent partial impairment. There is no physician-patient treating relationship when an IME is performed. The physician completing the IME does not assume the role of the treating physician and does not provide any treatment recommendations directly to the patient.

36. **B)** Vocational rehabilitation is an example of a corrective program. Corrective programs are designed to facilitate the individual's ability to return to work and to reduce or remove the disablement. An ameliorative program provides payment for income support and medical care directly.

37. **C)** Workers' compensation benefits count against the individual's payments. The other sources of income listed in the question stem do not.

38. **D)** Dr Waddell described nonorganic signs of low-back pain. If two or more of the tests, including subjective evaluation, are positive, the examiner should be concerned about issues other than peripheral nociception (organic pain) creating the pain behavior. Four tests comprising Waddell's signs include nonorganic tenderness with light superficial palpation, axial simulation by applying light downward pressure on the patient's head, distraction while performing seated straight leg raising, and regional sensory loss with sensory examination testing. Behavioral signs can also be revealed with muscle testing. Muscles may give way after briefly exerting normal strength, and strength exerted may be variable if testing rapid alternating strength.

39. **C)** Cauda equina typically involves radicular pain and numbness involving both legs, although symptoms may be more severe in one extremity. Leg weakness may present with foot drop, stumbling gait, or difficulty getting up from a chair. Pain in the lower extremities may diminish as the paralysis progresses. There may be difficulty voiding or loss of urinary or anal sphincter control. Saddle anesthesia/loss of perineal sensation is typical.

40. **C)** This is the correct answer, as it illustrates the importance of a small yet costly group. It has been estimated that 25% of the cases of work-related back injuries account for around 90% (87%–93%) of the costs.

41. **C)** A person with the functional ability to do medium work can lift 50 lb on an occasional basis.

42. **A)** Disability frequently results in the impoverishment of the individual, and income support programs remain a huge expense for society. Indirect costs of disability are the loss of income or homemaker potential experienced by the individual.

43. **A)** Until they are assured that they would be able to feasibly support themselves, many individuals remain leery of demonstrating that they can work at all. Stereotypes and prejudice still abound and further limit the disabled in obtaining employment.

44. **C)** Low-back pain affects about 80% of adults at some time in their lives. Low-back pain and back injuries commonly occur in workers from ages 30 to 60 years. Back injuries are a primary cause of absenteeism from work. Most individuals with low-back pain experience near-complete resolution of symptoms within 30 days.

45. **A)** Spurling's test is used to help diagnose cervical disk herniations or cervical spondylosis. This test should be performed cautiously. While in the seated position, the patient is asked to rotate and laterally flex the head to the unaffected side first, followed by the affected side. The examiner uses one hand to lightly compress downward on the head to axially load the cervical spine. If this is tolerated well, then include extension of the neck, which narrows the neural foramen and reproduces radicular arm pain that can be associated with a cervical disk herniation or cervical spondylosis (foraminal stenosis).

46. **D)** Job dissatisfaction, smoking, and low education are all factors influencing the reporting of low-back pain. Low income can be a risk factor as well, but it is less so than the others.

47. **C)** The field of ergonomics endeavors to enhance the interaction between a person and his or her work environment. An ergonomic evaluation can help identify specific job-related position and equipment needs and may lead to worksite modifications to improve the worker's productivity and reduce the risk of workplace injury. An offer of employment can be contingent on successfully completing a preemployment evaluation.

48. **B)** Multiple sclerosis, although not as common as the other conditions listed, carries a far greater risk of causing an individual to have a significant disability.

49. **C)** Supported employment is a very intensive approach to returning the most severely disabled individuals to work. A job coach accompanies the client for as long as 6 months, at least on a part-time basis, assisting with job modifications, relationships with coworkers, and even performance on the job, as needed. Supported employment has succeeded in returning individuals with severe disabilities to productive employment.

50. **A)** The purpose of an FCE is to estimate a worker's capability to perform a job task. FCEs emphasize validity and consistency and identify poor effort by using a set of objective task-based measurements. There is much debate about the value of FCE testing, but there is agreement that FCE tests a worker's tolerance to perform selected job tasks.

51. **D)** Work hardening prepares a worker for a specific job by improving strength, conditioning, flexibility, and overall functional ability. This differs from work conditioning, which is typically needed after a prolonged period of reduced activity to improve an injured worker's strength and cardiovascular fitness. Work conditioning is not tailored to a specific job.

52. **A)** Injuries or illnesses are typically covered under workers' compensation laws when they "arise out of and in the course of employment." Many state workers' compensation systems exclude coverage for injuries sustained while an employee is commuting to and from work. There are many exceptions to this rule, such as where the scope of the employee's duties includes travel.

53. **B)** Although inadequate sleep has received much attention lately for its association with medical error, it is not known to be a physical risk factor for occupational injury claims.

54. **C)** Heart disease, because of the prevalence of the condition itself and the chance that it will cause a disability, results in the highest prevalence of individuals with activity limitations.

55. **D)** Sheltered workshops are certified by the U.S. Department of Labor to pay "subminimum" wages to disabled individuals with diminished earning capacity. An example of this type of public, nonprofit organization is "Goodwill." Day programs primarily provide supervised day activities and are not designed to lead to productive employment. Home-based programs help to set the disabled individual up with employment such as telephone soliciting that can be done at home. None of these programs have resulted in significant reintegration of their disabled clients into competitive community employment.

56. **A)** Aggravation is a permanent worsening of a previous condition by a particular event. Exacerbation is a temporary worsening of previous condition by injury. Recurrence is defined as signs and symptoms of a previous illness or injury occurring in the absence of a new provocative event.

57. **C)** Risk factors for occupational injuries include smoking, low educational level, job dissatisfaction, lower socioeconomic status, deconditioning, and previous history of injuries or disabilities.

58. **B)** OSHA was passed in 1970 in part to provide consistency and regulation of states' workers' compensation systems. The Code of Hammurabi is one of the earliest recorded legal codes; it regulated the society of ancient Babylon, including specifying compensation for employment and services rendered.

59. **C)** The term *cumulative trauma disorder* actually applies to many clinical entities affecting diverse tissues. A cumulative trauma disorder is generally caused by repetitive stresses applied at sufficient force or frequency to result in tissue damage. Cumulative trauma disorders are more common in the upper limbs. At-risk jobs are those that require rapid speed or high force of movement, use of poorly designed tools, static or overhead work positions, and vibration.

60. **C)** Multiple sources, including the U.S. Census Bureau and the International Center for the Disabled, have conducted surveys that indicate that 15% to 20% of the population have at least some level of disability. Most frequently, this disability required the use of a gait aid for ambulation, or help with activities of daily living.

61. **A)** Tax incentives are frequently offered to provide an incentive to potential employers. Participating employers frequently retain the employees they have trained, but are not mandated to do so. Similarly, no guarantees are made that other positions will be found, but the success rate of these programs is substantial.

62. **A)** Most people with neck pain do not experience a complete resolution of symptoms. Between 50% and 85% of people experiencing neck pain at some initial point will report neck pain again 1 to 5 years later. The numbers in the general population appear to be similar compared with workers and with patients following motor vehicle crashes.

63. **D)** EHL strength correlates with the L5 nerve root. Gastroc-soleus strength correlates with S1 nerve root. Quadriceps strength relates to the L3-4 nerve root. Hip flexor strength reflects to the L1-2 nerve root.

64. **D)** It is essential to match a patient's subjective complaints, objective findings on examination, and diagnostic testing before considering a referral for spine surgery. A diagnosis based on MRI, in the absence of objective clinical findings, may not be the cause of a patient's pain. This could potentially lead to an attempt at operative correction with resulting chronic low-back pain and disability. Diagnostic testing should not be done routinely for nonspecific low back pain.

65. **C)** Waddell's signs are used to confirm or deny symptom magnification and to predict poor prognosis. Symptom magnification is a disproportionate behavior to a physical impairment. The presence of more than three of the five Waddell's signs is highly suggestive of symptom magnification. The five signs are diffuse tenderness, stimulation tests (axial loading or simulated rotation), distraction, regional sensory change/weakness, and overreaction. Diffuse tenderness is discomfort with light palpation of the skin. Stimulation tests are maneuvers that are typically nonpainful, such as pressing on top of the head or rotation of the pelvis and shoulders in the same direction at the same time. A stimulation test is positive if patient experiences pain. Distraction is when pain is produced with a straight leg raise, but not with straightening of the leg in a seated position. Regional changes include an inconsistent sensory loss or weakness in an entire region, such as an extremity or side of the body. Overreaction is an inconsistent painful response to a stimulus. This test is positive when the same stimulus is repeated later without the same painful reaction. The slump test is not part of Waddell's signs, but it is performed to confirm or rule-out radicular symptoms potentially caused by a lumbar disk problem.

66. **A)** A disability is considered to be temporary when there is a possibility of curing the injury or illness and when the disability is present for 12 months or less. Permanent disability is considered by most to be a disability that is present for more than 12 months. Partial and total disability pertains to the rating of a disability by a jurisdiction, such as Workers' Compensation or Veterans Affairs. Partial disability is any percentage of disability less than 100% and total disability is when a person is considered to have 100% disability.

67. **C)** An impairment is described as the physical abnormality of structure or function referring to anatomical, physiological, or psychological conditions. In this question the impairment would be the herniated disk. A disability is considered an inability to perform a task normally as compared to the average population because of an associated impairment. In this question, the standing limitation is considered a disability because of the impairment of her herniated disk. A handicap is related to societal and environmental roles and being unable to fulfill them because of an associated impairment. For example, if the female mentioned in this question was unable to apply for a job because she could not stand greater than 15 minutes, this would be considered a handicap.

68. **D)** There are three words that are used to describe how often a task is performed throughout a work day. Occasionally is defined by up to one-third of the work day, however no more. Frequently is performing a task from one-third up to two-thirds of the work day. Constantly is performing a task two-thirds of the time or more. "Often" is not a word that is used to describe how often a task is performed.

69. **C)** **Sedentary**—Work involves mostly sitting and occasional periods of standing and walking. Less than 10 lb of force may be required for a maximal lift and carry. Lifting, carrying, pushing/pulling, should be less than 5 lb for occasional work, (occasional meaning up to one-third of the work day).
**Light work**—Requirements: Walking or standing required a significant amount of time (or) sitting with pushing/pulling arm or leg controls (or) working at constant pace with pushing/pulling of items whose weight is negligible; 10 to 20 lb of force required occasionally and/or 10 lb required frequently (one-third to two-thirds of the time).
**Medium work**—Physical demands required more so than those mentioned for light work; 20 to 50 lb of force required occasionally and/or 10 to 25 lb required frequently.
**Heavy work**—50 to 100 lb of force required occasionally and/or 25 to 50 lb of force required frequently and/or 10 to 20 lb of force constantly (two-thirds of the work day or more).
**Very heavy work**—More than 100 lb of force required occasionally and/or more than 50 lb of force frequently, and/or more than 20 lb of force constantly.

70. **C)** The American College of Occupational and Environmental Medicine recommends that the initial assessment of patients with cervical spine problems focuses on identifying the presence of "red flags" such as fever, serious neurologic involvement, or major trauma. In the absence of red flags, imaging and other tests are not recommended in the first 4 to 6 weeks of neck pain, as it almost never results in a meaningful change in clinical management. Electrodiagnostic testing should not be performed until 3 weeks after injury—tests are usually negative within the first 3 weeks. Nonprescription medication or an appropriately selected nonsteroidal anti-inflammatory medication, appropriate adjustment of physical activity (if necessary), and the use of thermal modalities such as heat and/or ice can be used to relieve discomfort.

71. **C)** Illness behaviors are often seen in patients with a chronic pain syndrome. Symptoms become the central focus of the patient's life. Behaviors include grimacing, loud sighing, inconsistency on examination, slow movements, and overly involved family members.

72. **D)** Workplace factors associated with increased neck pain include repetitive and precision work, prolonged sedentary work positions, working with the cervical spine in flexion for prolonged periods of time, keyboard poorly positioned too close to the desktop edge, mouse position requiring flexion of shoulders of more than 25°, use of chairs without armrests, using telephone shoulder rests, using a computer monitor requiring poor head posture (eg, a head tilt of more than 3°), high levels of psychological job strain, low coworker social support, and job insecurity.

# 15

# *Pain*

## QUESTIONS

1. Which of the following is **not** recommended as a first-line medication for low-back pain?
   A) Acetaminophen
   B) Naproxen
   C) Tramadol
   D) Meloxicam

2. 6-monoacetylmorphine is a unique metabolite of which substance?
   A) OxyContin
   B) Codeine
   C) Heroin
   D) Cocaine

3. When referring to the "scotty dog," which of the following part of the dog correctly pairs with its associated anatomy?
   A) Transverse process = nose
   B) Pedicle = nose
   C) Lamina = neck
   D) Inferior articular process = ear

4. A 72-year-old male presents to your outpatient office for increasing low-back pain (over the last 4 weeks) with radiation into bilateral lower extremities. Symptoms worsen with standing and walking. Symptoms are improved with sitting and the patient states that he feels extremely comfortable when pushing a shopping cart. He denies weakness, changes in sensation, or bowel/bladder incontinence. He has not yet tried any medications or physical therapy. According to his history, which of the following is least likely to recommended at this time?
   A) Nonsteroidal anti-inflammatory drugs (NSAIDs)
   B) Lumbar stabilization program with focus on flexion-based exercises (Williams exercises)
   C) Interlaminar, caudal, or transforaminal epidural steroid injections under fluoroscopic guidance
   D) Decompression of spinal canal and neural foramina

5. Which of the following medications alleviates pain by inhibiting prostaglandin synthesis, is somewhat selective for cyclooxygenase-2, and has analgesic, antipyretic, and anti-inflammatory actions?
   A) Meloxicam (Mobic)
   B) Ketorolac (Toradol)
   C) Diclofenac (Voltaren)
   D) Acetaminophen (Tylenol)

ANSWERS TO THIS SECTION CAN BE FOUND ON PAGE 439

6. Which of the following is **incorrect** regarding complex regional pain syndrome (CRPS) I?
   A) There is a preceding noxious event with an obvious nerve lesion
   B) Spontaneous pain or hyperalgesia-hyperesthesia is not limited to a single nerve territory and disproportionate to the inciting incident
   C) Edema, skin blood flow (temperature), or sudomotor abnormalities, motor symptoms, or trophic changes are present on the affected limb, in particular at distal sites
   D) Other diagnoses are excluded

7. Which of the following exercises involves the least amount of force on the low back and are therefore used in the early stages of lumbar rehabilitation?
   A) Sit-ups
   B) Leg raises
   C) Curl-ups
   D) Lying prone and extending the spine while extending arms and legs

8. The first line of treatment for bothersome phantom limb sensation, phantom limb pain, and residual limb pain is:
   A) Desensitization techniques
   B) Pharmacologic techniques
   C) Biofeedback techniques
   D) Use of transcutaneous electrical nerve stimulation (TENS) unit

9. Pain caused by a stimulus that does not normally provoke pain is known as:
   A) Anesthesia
   B) Allodynia
   C) Hyperesthesia
   D) Hyperalgesia

10. Which is **not** an indication for a spinal cord stimulator (SCS) implantation?
    A) Complex regional pain syndrome (CRPS)
    B) Peripheral vascular disease (PVD)
    C) Nonischemic nociceptive pain
    D) Failed back surgery syndrome (FBSS)

11. Which of the following statements is **not** true regarding facet joint–mediated pain?
    A) Rehabilitation should be focused on exercises with neutral or flexion posture to reduce stress on facet joints
    B) Diagnostic use of facet joint–nerve blocks and therapeutic radiofrequency ablation are treatment options
    C) To minimize the false-positive response that occurs with one injection, two separate blocks using different-duration anesthetics are recommended
    D) Facet joint–mediated pain is likely elicited on flexion or repetitive end-range flexion

12. Mirtazapine, venlafaxine, and duloxetine are _____ and are used to treat depression and chronic pain.
    A) Tricyclic antidepressants
    B) Benzodiazepines
    C) Selective serotonin reuptake inhibitors (SSRIs)
    D) Serotonin-norepinephrine reuptake inhibitors (SNRIs)

13. TENS is often used for pain control and is an acronym for:
    A) Tension stimulator
    B) Transcutaneous electrical nerve stimulation
    C) Toxic epidermal necrolysis syndrome
    D) Ten stimulation modes

14. Which type of nerve fibers transmit the first sensation of pain?
    A) A delta fibers
    B) C fibers
    C) A beta fibers
    D) B fibers

15. Functional instability, leading to low-back pain, is thought to be the result of:
    A) Tissue damage
    B) Poor muscular balance
    C) Poor muscular control
    D) All of the above

16. Phantom pain is a type of:
    A) Neuropathic pain
    B) Nociceptive pain
    C) Psychogenic pain
    D) Somatoform pain

17. A patient asks what side effects can be expected after undergoing a lumbar L5-S1 interlaminar epidural steroid injection. Which of the following is not a potential complication of this particular injection?
    A) Headache
    B) Epidural abscess
    C) Epidural hematoma
    D) Tetraplegia

18. The WHO recommends a three-step "ladder" for cancer pain relief. In which order should pain medication be administered?
    A) Mild opioids, non-opioids, strong opioids
    B) Strong opioids, mild opioids, non-opioids
    C) Non-opioids, mild opioids, then strong opioids until the patient is free of pain
    D) Mild opioids, strong opioids, surgical intervention

19. Complex regional pain syndrome (CRPS) type I is:
    A) Sympathetic-mediated pain limited to a peripheral nerve distribution
    B) Reported in 25% of tetraplegic stroke patients
    C) Also known as *causalgia*
    D) Also known as *reflex sympathetic dystrophy*

20. Which of the following statements is **not** true regarding central poststroke pain (CPSP)?
    A) CPSP develops in 8% of stroke patients
    B) Functional MRI (fMRI) is required for the diagnosis of CPSP
    C) Pain is characterized most often as a burn
    D) There is no intervention proven to alter the development of CPSP

21. Occipital neuralgia refers to pain in the distribution of the:
    A) Temporal nerve
    B) Lingual nerve
    C) Greater and lesser occipital nerves
    D) Facial nerve

22. Which of the following is true regarding discogenic lumbar pain?
    A) There is strong familial predisposition to discogenic lumbar pain
    B) Intradiscal pressures increase when one changes his or her position from sitting to standing
    C) There is a strong association between discogenic lumbar pain and alcoholism
    D) For nonradicular low-back pain with degenerative disk disease, fusion appears to have a superior outcome when compared with standard nonsurgical therapy, and also is better than intensive interdisciplinary rehabilitation

23. When treating a patient with new onset/acute temporomandibular disorder (TMD), which of the following choices have been found to be effective?
    A) Oral rest, nonsteroidal anti-inflammatory drugs (NSAIDs), antidepressants, and narcotics
    B) Oral rest, NSAIDs, antidepressants, and behavioral modifications
    C) Narcotics, behavioral modifications, oral splinting, and NSAIDs
    D) Heat, NSAIDs, antidepressants, and long-term use of benzodiazepines

24. Spondylolysis, a common cause of low-back pain, is thought to arise secondary to:
    A) Repetitive hyperflexion of the lumbar spine
    B) Repetitive hyperextension of the lumbar spine
    C) Repetitive side bending of the lumbar spine
    D) Repetitive rotation of the lumbar spine

25. Which of the following is a rehabilitation treatment option commonly used for phantom limb pain?
    A) Transcutaneous electrical nerve stimulation
    B) Sensory discrimination training
    C) Mirror therapy
    D) All of the above

26. Opioid receptors belong to the _____ family.
    A) G-protein–coupled receptor
    B) N-methyl-D-aspartate (NMDA) receptor
    C) alpha-amino-3-hydroxy-5-methyl-4-isoxazolepropionic acid (AMPA) receptor
    D) gamma-aminobutyric acid (GABA) receptor

27. A 55-year-old man who works in construction presents with pain over his upper back. He states that he bent over to lift a heavy object and felt a sharp pain midline. On examination, he has obvious spasm with tenderness to palpation over his paravertebral muscles in the region of T7-T9. Neurological examination is within normal limits. You make the diagnosis of:
    A) Discitis
    B) Thoracic radiculopathy
    C) Vertebral fracture
    D) Thoracic sprain/strain

28. Which is true regarding BOTOX® and its use for patients with chronic migraines?
    A) Considered a preventative (prophylactic), rather than an acute treatment option
    B) Indicated in chronic migraine patients who have 10 or more headache days each month

C) Indicated for headache lasting 2 or more hours each day

D) An option for patients under 18 years of age

29. Which painful disorder is characterized by the presence of distinct sensitive spots in a palpable taut band of skeletal muscle fibers that produce local and referred pain?

A) Myofascial pain syndrome (MPS)

B) Fibromyalgia

C) Trochanteric bursitis

D) Somatoform pain disorders

30. A 24-year-old man presents to you with right forearm pain. He states that the pain began 6 months ago, after an elevator door closed on his right forearm. On exam, the right forearm has shiny skin, with decreased hair growth, and the area is very tender to touch. You make a presumptive diagnosis of:

A) Cellulitis

B) Scleroderma

C) Complex regional pain syndrome (CRPS)

D) Synovitis

31. Which of the following medications is **not** effective in treating chronic low-back pain?

A) Tramadol

B) Tricyclic antidepressants

C) Nonsteroidal anti-inflammatory drugs

D) Systemic steroids

32. A 60-year-old obese woman presents to you for initial evaluation of left lower extremity pain, associated with numbness and tingling. She states that the pain is located in the posterior thigh and radiates down to the calf. The patient is having a difficult time with toe walking. On the basis of her description, you expect which of the following nerve roots to be involved?

A) L4

B) L5

C) S1

D) S2

33. Nociceptors are:

A) Pacinian corpuscles

B) Meissner corpuscles

C) Merkel's disks

D) Free nerve endings

34. A 30-year-old man presents to you for initial evaluation of intermittent headaches. The headache is unilateral and is associated with lacrimation and ptosis. The most likely diagnosis is:

A) Classic migraine

B) Cluster headache

C) Tension headache

D) Shingles

35. Neuropathic pain, itchiness, and impaired sensation can occur as a result of burn injury involving nerve endings in which of the following layers?

A) Epidermal

B) Dermal

    C) Subcutaneous fat

    D) Deep fascia

36. Which of the following opioid analgesics has the longest half-life, producing longer periods of pain relief?

    A) Morphine

    B) Codeine

    C) Oxycodone

    D) Oxymorphone

37. A "sharp," "burning," "electric-like," or "skin-sensitive" pain at the end of a residual limb is called:

    A) Phantom pain

    B) Stump pain

    C) Neuroma

    D) Causalgia

38. A 32-year-old male presents to your office with complaints of persistent right sacroiliac (SI) joint pain after right sacral fracture 9 months prior. He underwent no surgical intervention for this injury. What has the greatest diagnostic value in validating his diagnosis of sacroiliitis?

    A) X-ray of the right hip

    B) MRI of the right hip

    C) Fluoroscopic SI joint injection

    D) Bone scan

39. A patient presents with numbness and pain in a well-circumscribed distribution on the anterolateral thigh. These symptoms are exacerbated by walking or extending of the hip. No weakness of the lower limb is noted. You make the diagnosis of:

    A) Peripheral neuropathy

    B) Peroneal nerve entrapment

    C) Lateral femoral cutaneous neuropathy

    D) Sciatic neuropathy

40. This therapeutic technique uses many forms of both auditory and visual physiologic monitoring in an attempt to educate patients to alter physiologic functions that are usually not under conscious control. This technique has been used in chronic pain conditions, including headaches, low-back pain, and fibromyalgia.

    A) Pilates

    B) Yoga

    C) Biofeedback

    D) Tai chi

41. The most common location for an interdigital (Morton's) neuroma is between which of the following metatarsal heads?

    A) 1st and 2nd

    B) 2nd and 3rd

    C) 3rd and 4th

    D) 4th and 5th

42. Which of the following is considered a nonparticulate steroid preparation?

    A) Dexamethasone (Decadron)

    B) Triamcinolone (Kenalog)

C) Methylprednisolone (Depo-Medrol)
D) Betamethasone (Celestone)

43. Pregabalin (Lyrica) and gabapentin (Neurontin) work by blocking specific _____ channels on neurons and are preferred first-line medications for diabetic neuropathy.
    A) Sodium
    B) Calcium
    C) Potassium
    D) Magnesium

44. Allodynia is:
    A) Pain resulting from a stimulus that does not normally produce pain
    B) An increased painful sensation in response to additional noxious stimuli
    C) A decreased sensitivity to painful stimuli
    D) The absence of the sense of pain while remaining conscious

45. Which of the following cervical facet joints has a referral pattern of pain into below the spine of the scapula?
    A) C4-C5
    B) C5-C6
    C) C6-C7
    D) C7-T1

46. Which of the following is **not** an application based on the gate control theory?
    A) Spinal cord stimulation
    B) Massage
    C) Transcutaneous electrical nerve stimulation (TENS)
    D) Medial branch block

47. C fibers are:
    A) Small myelinated fibers responding to high-intensity mechanical stimulation
    B) Large myelinated fibers that transmit temperature sensation
    C) Small unmyelinated fibers that transmit burning pain
    D) Large unmyelinated fibers that transmit noxious information from a variety of modalities

48. Ten liters of 100% oxygen at the onset of headache has been shown to be effective in treating:
    A) Classic migraine
    B) Cluster headache
    C) Tension headache
    D) Shingles

49. A 75-year-old man presents to you 3 months after sustaining a stroke, with resulting right-sided weakness. He complains of pain over his right shoulder and decreased range of motion. Scarf sign is positive. The patient is noted to have decreased range of motion in all planes. The most likely diagnosis is:
    A) Rotator cuff syndrome
    B) Adhesive capsulitis
    C) Shoulder dislocation
    D) Glenohumeral subluxation

50. Which of the following cervical facet joints has a referral pattern of pain into the occiput?
    A) C2-C3
    B) C3-C4
    C) C4-C5
    D) C5-C6

51. Which of the following structures lacks innervation and therefore cannot transmit pain?
    A) Anterior vertebral body
    B) Posterior longitudinal ligament
    C) Anterior longitudinal ligament
    D) Internal annulus fibrosus

52. Which of these neuropathic pain agents works by potentially binding to μ-opioid receptors and inhibits norepinephrine reuptake, producing analgesia?
    A) Amitriptyline (Elavil)
    B) Gabapentin (Neurontin)
    C) Pregabalin (Lyrica)
    D) Tapentadol (Nucynta)

53. Spinal cord stimulation (SCS) is indicated for the treatment of the following:
    A) Failed back syndrome, complex regional pain syndrome, arachnoiditis, phantom limb pain
    B) Failed back syndrome, complex regional pain syndrome, epidural fibrosis, phantom limb pain
    C) Radicular pain syndrome or radiculopathies, complex regional pain syndrome, epidural fibrosis, phantom limb pain
    D) All of the above

54. Which of the following nonsteroidal anti-inflammatory drugs (NSAIDs) does not inhibit platelet aggregation?
    A) Celecoxib (CeleBREX)
    B) Ketorolac (Toradol)
    C) Diclofenac (Voltaren)
    D) Aspirin

55. A 75-year-old female with a recent left middle cerebral artery cerebrovascular accident (CVA) presents to your outpatient office with complaints of right shoulder pain. On evaluation, her right upper extremity is flaccid. Her right shoulder is exquisitely painful to light touch, is edematous, and warm. Special tests including Neer's, Hawkin's, and Yergason's tests are negative. Her pain is most likely caused by:
    A) Shoulder subluxation
    B) Complex regional pain syndrome (CRPS)
    C) Bicipital tendonitis
    D) Impingement syndrome

56. A 20-year-old man presents to you for initial evaluation of low-back pain and morning stiffness. He denies trauma to the area. On physical examination, there is decreased spinal mobility and decreased chest expansion. You make a diagnosis of:
    A) Spinal stenosis
    B) Reactive arthritis
    C) Ankylosing spondylitis
    D) Psoriatic arthritis

57. Symptoms associated with temporomandibular disorder (TMD) can include all of the following **except**:
    A) Changes to vision
    B) Unilateral pain in muscles of mastication, radiating to temples, side of face, or ear
    C) Tinnitus or other ear symptoms
    D) Nocturnal clenching or bruxism

58. The phenomenon when an initial dose of a substance loses its effectiveness over time, requiring a higher dose to achieve that same effect is known as:
    A) Dependence
    B) Addiction
    C) Tolerance
    D) Withdrawal

59. A 45-year-old man with diabetes mellitus presents to you complaining of severe pain over his right thigh, difficulty ambulating, and leg weakness. He states that the pain started suddenly around his inguinal area. At first, pain was dull and aching, but then intensified within 2 hours, and became severe and debilitating. He does not recall any trauma to the area. He also complains of associated numbness over the right anterior thigh and medial leg. You make a diagnosis of:
    A) Lumbar radiculopathy
    B) Polymyalgia rheumatica
    C) Avascular necrosis of femoral head
    D) Diabetic amyotrophy

60. Temporomandibular disorder (TMD) can be caused by:
    A) Myofascial pain dysfunction
    B) Internal derangement of the joint space
    C) Degenerative joint disorders
    D) All of the above

61. A 45-year-old woman presents to your outpatient office with severe pain on gentle touching of the left wrist. You also note loss of hair over the painful area, swelling, and decreased range of motion at the left wrist. Five months ago, the patient suffered a left proximal ulnar fracture after a fall. Which of the following terms best describes this phenomenon?
    A) Hyperesthesia
    B) Hyperalgesia
    C) Hyperpathia
    D) Allodynia

62. The gold standard diagnosis of sympathetically mediated complex regional pain syndrome (CRPS) type I is by:
    A) X-ray
    B) Triple-phase bone scan
    C) Electromyogram (EMG)/nerve conduction studies (NCS)
    D) Sympathetic blockade of the stellate ganglion with local anesthetic

63. The most common level of cervical facet joint–mediated pain is:
    A) C1-C2
    B) C2-C3
    C) C3-C4
    D) C4-C5

64. A patient presents to you with low-back pain, which she attributes to her being diagnosed with osteoporosis. Osteoporosis is usually not visible on conventional radiographs until at least ____% of bone mineral has been lost.
    A) 10 to 15
    B) 15 to 20
    C) 25 to 30
    D) 35 to 40

65. A 70-year-old man presents to you 1 year after a stroke with complaint of severe, persistent, paroxysmal, often intolerable pain on the hemiplegic side, which is not responsive to any analgesic treatment. Before looking at his old imaging studies, you suspect that the patient's stroke affected which of the following areas of his brain:
    A) Medulla
    B) Substantia nigra
    C) Thalamus
    D) Globus pallidus

66. A 34-year-old woman with multiple sclerosis presents to your office with facial pain. The pain is described as stabbing, electric pain, is unilateral over the jaw, and is intermittent. What is the most likely diagnosis?
    A) Occipital neuralgia
    B) Trigeminal neuralgia
    C) Osteonecrosis of jaw
    D) Osteomyelitis

67. Amitriptyline (Elavil) is a _____ and is used to treat depression and neuropathic pain.
    A) Tricyclic antidepressant (TCA)
    B) Benzodiazepine
    C) Selective serotonin reuptake inhibitor (SSRI)
    D) Serotonin-norepinephrine reuptake inhibitor (SNRI)

68. _____ is an oral analogue of lidocaine used in the treatment of neuropathic pain.
    A) Mexiletine
    B) Ketamine
    C) Pregabalin
    D) Amitriptyline

69. Which of the following drugs has the highest morphine milligrams equivalent factor?
    A) Fentanyl transdermal patch
    B) Fentanyl oral spray
    C) Fentanyl nasal spray
    D) Fentanyl oral lozenge

70. Which statement is **not** true regarding migraine?
    A) Analgesic overuse is associated with an increased risk of chronic pain
    B) Migraine can be induced by sildenafil
    C) The severity and frequency of attacks tend to increase with increasing age
    D) Migraine is associated with an increased risk of developing myocardial infarction in men

71. A patient presents with pain over the lateral aspect of his elbow. The examiner fully extends the patient's elbow, pronates the forearm, and asks the patient to make a fist. He then resists the patient's attempt to extend and radially deviate the wrist, eliciting pain over the lateral elbow. This test is known as:
    A) Hawkin's test
    B) Watson's test
    C) Cozen's test
    D) Yergason's test

72. The cell bodies of first-order, or primary, thoracic visceral pain fibers are found in:
    A) Dorsal root ganglion
    B) Trigeminal ganglion
    C) Mesenteric ganglion
    D) Inferior cervical ganglion

73. What is the pain wind-up phenomenon?
    A) Increased pain intensity by repeated stimulation
    B) Recruitment of silent nociceptors after tissue injury causing increased pain intensity
    C) Increased muscle tone caused by severe pain
    D) Central sensitization caused by repeated stimulation of nociceptive C fibers

74. Which nerve innervates the L4-L5 facet joint?
    A) L2 and L3 medial branches
    B) L3 and L4 medial branches
    C) L4 and L5 medial branches
    D) L4 dorsal ramus

75. A 45-year-old female complains of widespread pain over the upper back, lower back, neck, right hip, chest, abdomen, left shoulder, and left arm for the past 4 months. She also complains of severe generalized fatigue and difficulty falling asleep during this same time period. The intensity level of pain has been similar throughout this time period. What is the most likely diagnosis?
    A) Rheumatoid arthritis
    B) Fibromyalgia (FM)
    C) Myofascial pain syndrome
    D) Entrapment neuropathy

76. A patient presents with pain and paresthesias in the first three fingers of the hand and the skin over the thenar eminence. The pain does not awaken the patient at night. Pain can be provoked by resisted elbow flexion and pronation, as well as by resisted finger flexion. You make the diagnosis of:
    A) Carpal tunnel syndrome (CTS)
    B) Pronator syndrome
    C) C5 radiculopathy
    D) C8 radiculopathy

77. The majority of burns result from:
    A) Fire/flame injuries
    B) Scald injuries
    C) Electrical injuries
    D) Chemical injuries

78. Which of the following side effects has been seen with long-term use of high-dose opioids?
    A) Increased lactation
    B) Decreased libido
    C) Increased cortisol response to stress
    D) Hostility and anxiety

79. Which nerve innervates the C5-C6 facet joint?
    A) C4 and C5 medial branches
    B) C5 and C6 medial branches
    C) C6 and C7 medial branches
    D) C4 and C7 medial branches

80. Which sympathetic block can be performed for pelvic visceral pain?
    A) Stellate-ganglion block
    B) Celiac plexus block
    C) Hypogastric plexus block
    D) Lumbar sympathetic block

81. A 65-year-old woman presents to your outpatient office secondary to diffuse pain throughout her body for the past 9 months. She states she has pain throughout her spine and on physical exam is positive for tenderness in 13 of 18 paired tender points. She also complains of sleep difficulty during this same time period. What is the best treatment at this point?
    A) No treatment is necessary if there are no signs of neurologic deficits.
    B) Recommend holding off on any cardiovascular exercise at this time, as it may worsen her symptoms.
    C) Consider trial of pregabalin (Lyrica)
    D) Consider trial of opioids

82. Which of the following medications alleviates pain by inhibiting cyclooxygenase in the central nervous system and has analgesic and antipyretic, but **not** anti-inflammatory actions?
    A) Meloxicam (Mobic)
    B) Ketorolac (Toradol)
    C) Diclofenac (Voltaren)
    D) Acetaminophen (Tylenol)

83. What is the goal of chronic pain management?
    A) Decrease the use of medications
    B) Enable people with pain to function better and enjoy daily activities
    C) Eliminate pain
    D) Help people with pain return to their previous work

84. A 72-year-old male with history of diabetes mellitus, peripheral vascular disease, and lumbar spinal stenosis presents to your outpatient office with complaints of pain status post left below the knee amputation (BKA or transtibial) 3 weeks ago that has continued to worsen. He describes an electrical and burning pain in the distribution of his amputated distal left lower extremity. He denies any low-back pain or the pain worsening with standing, walking long distances, or lying down. This can be described as:
    A) Phantom sensation status post BKA
    B) Phantom pain status post BKA
    C) Stump pain
    D) Lumbar stenosis

85. Modalities such as paraffin baths, cold packs, and cryotherapy work to alleviate pain through:
    A) Conduction
    B) Convection
    C) Conversion
    D) Evaporation

86. The most common needle used for image-guided lumbar epidural injection is:
    A) 18-gauge
    B) 22-gauge
    C) 25-gauge
    D) 27-gauge

87. Which of the following is **incorrect** regarding migraine headaches?
    A) There is a family history associated with migraine headaches
    B) Prodrome is not present in migraine
    C) Migraines generally occur more commonly in women than in men
    D) Peak prevalence occurs during midlife

88. All of the following are goals of chronic pain management **except**:
    A) Elimination of all pain
    B) Return to work
    C) Maximize activity and function
    D) Restoration of a normal sleep cycle

89. An unpleasant abnormal sensation, whether spontaneous or evoked, is known as:
    A) Anesthesia
    B) Allodynia
    C) Dysesthesia
    D) Hyperalgesia

90. Patients with chronic pain can display:
    A) Sleep fragmentation
    B) Difficulty falling asleep
    C) Decreased quality of sleep
    D) All of the above

91. The most common level affected in a degenerative spondylolisthesis is:
    A) L2-L3
    B) L3-L4
    C) L4-L5
    D) L5-S1

92. Which intervention may be used for diagnosis of facet joint–mediated pain?
    A) Fluoroscopically guided facet joint injection
    B) Interlaminal epidural injection
    C) Fluoroscopically guided medial branch ablation
    D) Transforaminal epidural injection

93. Which of the following medications alleviates pain by inhibiting prostaglandin synthesis and release and inhibits platelet aggregation, and its therapeutic response may take 2 weeks for arthritis treatment?
    A) Meloxicam (Mobic)
    B) Ketorolac (Toradol)

C) Diclofenac (Voltaren)

D) Aspirin

94. Methadone hydrochloride works as:
   A) An *N*-methyl-D-aspartate (NMDA) receptor antagonist
   B) A gamma-aminobutyric acid (GABA) agonist
   C) An acetylcholine receptor blocker
   D) A blocker of release of calcium from the sarcoplasmic reticulum

95. An increased response to a stimulus that is normally painful is known as:
   A) Anesthesia
   B) Allodynia
   C) Hyperesthesia
   D) Hyperalgesia

96. What type of exercise should be avoided in patients with osteoporotic compression fractures?
   A) Walking for 40 minutes, three times a week
   B) Spinal flexion exercises
   C) Progressive resistive back extension exercises
   D) Swimming

97. Which pharmacologic intervention is most appropriate for the treatment of neuropathic pain in a T6 American Spinal Injury Association (ASIA) classification A paraplegic with insomnia and urinary leakage between catheterizations?
   A) Amitriptyline (Elavil)
   B) Fluoxetine (Prozac)
   C) Gabapentin (Neurontin)
   D) Trazodone (Desyrel)

98. Hyperalgesia is considered:
   A) Pain due to a stimulus that does not normally provoke pain
   B) Increased response to a stimulus that is normally painful
   C) Increased sensitivity to stimulation
   D) An unpleasant abnormal sensation, whether spontaneous or evoked

99. The anticonvulsants carbamazepine (Tegretol) and oxcarbazepine (Trileptal) are especially effective in trigeminal neuralgia. The actions of these two drugs are mediated principally through _____ channels.
   A) Sodium
   B) Calcium
   C) Potassium
   D) Magnesium

100. A college football player presents for initial evaluation of left anterior thigh pain. He states that he was hit by a blunt force on his anterior thigh earlier in the day. On exam, you note that his thigh is warm to touch and is swollen, and the patient has difficulty flexing his knee. He had an x-ray of the area that only showed soft tissue swelling. You make the diagnosis of:
   A) Quadriceps muscle contusion
   B) Compartment syndrome
   C) Fracture of the femur
   D) Hamstrings tear

101. Modalities such as ultrasound work to alleviate pain through:
    A) Conduction
    B) Convection
    C) Conversion
    D) Evaporation

102. Which of the following opioid analgesics has the longest half-life, producing longer periods of pain relief?
    A) Morphine
    B) Codeine
    C) Methadone
    D) Oxymorphone

103. Modalities such as whirlpool baths and fluidotherapy work to alleviate pain through:
    A) Conduction
    B) Convection
    C) Conversion
    D) Evaporation

104. Which of the following is associated with sacroiliitis?
    A) Bowel and/or bladder dysfunction
    B) Positive Patrick's test
    C) Paresthesia of the lateral thigh
    D) Weakness of extension of the great toe

105. The initial gate control theory by Melzack and Wall proposed that stimulation of _____ fibers modulates the dorsal horn "gate" and therefore reduces the nociceptive input from the periphery.
    A) A beta
    B) B
    C) C
    D) A delta

106. A patient calls to complain of an extremely painful persistent bifrontal headache and nausea that began shortly after receiving an L4-L5 epidural steroid injection 2 days prior. He states that the headaches have been worsening. What is the best treatment option for this patient at this time?
    A) Second L4-L5 epidural steroid injection
    B) Occipital nerve block
    C) Epidural blood patch
    D) Fluid and oral analgesics

107. A 61-year-old male patient with metastatic colon cancer is being seen in your pain clinic. He is managed on OxyContin 20 mg twice a day, oxycodone 10 mg every 4 hours, and Dilaudid 2 mg every 6 hours for pain. What morphine equivalent dosing is this patient receiving?
    A) 176 morphine milligram equivalent
    B) 182 morphine milligram equivalent
    C) 188 morphine milligram equivalent
    D) 196 morphine milligram equivalent

108. Which of the following drugs has the lowest morphine milligrams equivalent factor?
    A) Codeine
    B) Hydrocodone

C) Hydromorphone
D) Tapentadol

109. A 63-year-old female slipped, fell, and broke her hip. She was managed surgically with open reduction internal fixation (ORIF) and sent to acute in-patient rehabilitation. On arrival, she is taking Dilaudid IV 2 mg every 4 hours. You decide to switch her to oral (PO) pain medications. Which of the following regimens has the closest morphine milligram equivalent?
    A) Oxycodone 5 mg every 3 hours
    B) Oxycodone 5 mg every 4 hours
    C) Oxycodone 10 mg every 3 hours
    D) Oxycodone 10 mg every 4 hours

110. Which of the following drugs has the lowest morphine milligrams equivalent factor?
    A) Methadone
    B) Hydrocodone
    C) Morphine
    D) Tramadol

111. Which of the following dosages of medication will achieve a morphine equivalence of 60 morphine milligrams?
    A) Dilaudid 2 mg every 6 hours
    B) Oxycodone 10 mg every 6 hours
    C) Morphine 15 mg every 8 hours
    D) Tramadol 50 mg every 4 hours

112. Which of the following medications has the greatest per milligram potency?
    A) Morphine
    B) Oxycodone
    C) Codeine
    D) Methadone

113. A patient in your clinic had begun a regimen of oxycodone 20 mg every 6 hours for low-back pain 6 months ago, as he has been refractory to other methods of treatment. Today he presents to clinic and states that for the past month he has only been taking oxycodone 10 mg every 6 hours due to adequate pain relief. What reduction in morphine equivalents does this change represent?
    A) 20 morphine milligram equivalent
    B) 40 morphine milligram equivalent
    C) 60 morphine milligram equivalent
    D) 80 morphine milligram equivalent

114. Which of the following is the correct morphine milligram equivalent conversion factor for methadone 40 mg/day?
    A) 4 morphine milligram equivalent
    B) 8 morphine milligram equivalent
    C) 12 morphine milligram equivalent
    D) 16 morphine milligram equivalent

115. Which of the following analgesic regimens will have the highest morphine milligram equivalence?
    A) Tramadol 100 mg every 4 hours
    B) Oxycodone 10 mg every 6 hours

C)  Dilaudid 4 mg every 8 hours

D)  OxyContin 30 mg every 12 hours

116. A 44-year-old female is in the surgical ICU (SICU) following a cholecystectomy. She is given tapentadol 50 mg every 4 hours for postsurgical pain. Her pain is well controlled. What equivalent morphine dosage is she receiving?

A)  100 morphine milligram equivalent

B)  120 morphine milligram equivalent

C)  140 morphine milligram equivalent

D)  160 morphine milligram equivalent

117. A 32-year-old male heroin user is being treated for drug addiction and is being given methadone 20 mg/day for detox therapy. How much morphine equivalence is this patient currently receiving?

A)  60 morphine milligram equivalent

B)  80 morphine milligram equivalent

C)  100 morphine milligram equivalent

D)  120 morphine milligram equivalent

118. Which of the following opioid medication regimens will have the lowest morphine milligram equivalence?

A)  OxyContin (extended release) 20 mg every 12 hours

B)  Oxycodone 5 mg every 4 hours

C)  Morphine 30 mg every 12 hours

D)  Tramadol 50 mg every 6 hours

119. Which of the following morphine milligram equivalents corresponds to a regimen of Dilaudid 2 mg every 8 hours?

A)  16 morphine milligram equivalents

B)  20 morphine milligram equivalents

C)  24 morphine milligram equivalents

D)  28 morphine milligram equivalents

120. A 67-year-old male is taking 5 mg hydrocodone every 6 hours for pain as he tries to pass a kidney stone. What morphine equivalent dose is he consuming per day?

A)  20 morphine milligram equivalent

B)  40 morphine milligram equivalent

C)  60 morphine milligram equivalent

D)  80 morphine milligram equivalent

121. A 16-year-old female gymnast suffered a major fall resulting in femur fracture; she is seen by orthopedics for open reduction, internal fixation (ORIF) and is started on 60 mg codeine every 6 hours to manage pain. What morphine equivalent is being delivered to this patient per day?

A)  20 morphine milligram equivalent

B)  24 morphine milligram equivalent

C)  30 morphine milligram equivalent

D)  36 morphine milligram equivalent

122. Which dosing adjustment should be employed to reduce a patient's total morphine milligram equivalence by 20?

A)  Change OxyContin 30 mg every 12 hours to OxyContin 20 mg every 12 hours

B)  Change tramadol 100 mg every 4 hours to tramadol 100 mg every 6 hours

    C) Change Dilaudid 6 mg every 6 hours to Dilaudid 4 mg every 6 hours

    D) Change morphine 30 mg every 4 hours to morphine 30 mg every 8 hours

123. Which of the following drugs has the highest morphine milligrams equivalent factor?
    A) Hydrocodone
    B) Morphine
    C) Codeine
    D) Oxycodone

124. A 54-year-old construction worker who is well known to your clinic presents for management of his low-back pain. He is currently taking oxycodone 10 mg every 8 hours and ibuprofen 400 mg every 6 hours as needed for pain. Assuming full compliance to current regimen, what daily morphine equivalence is this patient currently receiving?
    A) 30 morphine milligram equivalent
    B) 45 morphine milligram equivalent
    C) 60 morphine milligram equivalent
    D) 75 morphine milligram equivalent

125. Which pair of medications has the same morphine milligram equivalence?
    A) Tramadol 50 mg every 6 hours, and Dilaudid 4 mg every 12 hours
    B) Oxycodone 10 mg every 4 hours and methadone 10 mg every 6 hours
    C) Hydrocodone 10 mg every 4 hours and oxycodone 15 mg every 6 hours
    D) Hydrocodone 60 mg once a day, morphine 20 mg three times daily

126. A 74-year-old male has recently undergone lumbar laminectomy. Following his surgery, he is given oxycodone 10 mg every 6 hours for pain. His pain is well controlled but he complains of nausea and attributes it to his current pain management regimen. You decide to switch the patient to tramadol. Which of the following regimens have the same morphine equivalence dosing as the patient's current pain regimen?
    A) Tramadol 100 mg every 6 hours
    B) Tramadol 50 mg every 4 hours
    C) Tramadol 100 mg every 4 hours
    D) Tramadol 50 mg every 6 hours

# *Pain*

## ANSWERS

1. **C)** For most patients with low-back pain, regardless of the duration of symptoms, acetaminophen and nonsteroidal anti-inflammatory drugs (NSAIDs) are first-line options for pain relief.

2. **C)** There are three active metabolites of heroin (diacetylmorphine): 6-monoacetylmorphine (6-MAM), morphine, and the much less active 3-monoacetylmorphine (3-MAM). 6-MAM is then either metabolized into morphine or excreted in the urine. Since 6-MAM is a unique metabolite of heroin, its presence in the urine confirms that heroin was used by the patient.

3. **A)** Transverse Process = Nose
   The outline of the "scotty dog" can be seen on an oblique view of the lumbar spine. The parts of the dog include:
   Transverse process = nose
   Pedicle = eye
   Pars interarticularis = neck
   Superior articular process = ear
   Inferior articular process = front leg

4. **D)** The patient here most likely is presenting with pain secondary to lumbar spinal stenosis. Of the following options, surgery would be least likely indicated for this patient at this time. His symptoms are acute/subacute. He has not yet tried conservative treatment and is currently without neurological symptoms. Therefore, he is not a surgical candidate at this time.

5. **A)** Meloxicam (Mobic). Alleviates pain by inhibiting prostaglandin synthesis, is somewhat selective for cyclooxygenase-2, and has analgesic, antipyretic, and anti-inflammatory actions.

6. **A)** In CRPS II there is the presence of nerve injury, unlike **no** nerve injury found in CRPS I. The International Association for the Study of Pain established the following criteria that must be present for a clinical diagnosis for CRPS to be made:
   - Preceding noxious event without obvious nerve lesion (CRPS I) or with obvious nerve lesion (CRPS II)
   - Spontaneous pain or hyperalgesia-hyperesthesia not limited to a single nerve territory and disproportionate to the inciting incident
   - Edema, skin blood flow (temperature) or sudomotor abnormalities, motor symptoms, or trophic changes are present on the affected limb, in particular at distal sites
   - Other diagnoses are excluded

7. **C)** Sit-ups cause more than 3,000 N of compressive loads on the spine because of psoas activity. Leg raises also cause relatively high compressive forces. Lying prone and extending the spine while extending the arms and legs cause more than 6,000 N of compression to the spine. Curl-ups cause lower forces on the spine, so they are a better choice for anterior abdominal strengthening in the early stages of rehabilitation, or in those who have increased pain and cannot tolerate increased spinal loading exercises.

8. **A)** Desensitization techniques such as tapping, slapping, wrapping, and massaging the residual limb have been shown to reduce phantom limb pain and abnormal sensations. Many patients find that wearing a prosthesis diminishes their phantom pain.

9. **B)** Allodynia is pain from a stimulus that ordinarily will not provoke pain. Anesthesia is a loss of sensation. Hyperesthesia is an increased sensation or sensitivity. Hyperalgesia is increased pain response from a normally painful stimulus (the degree of pain is disproportionate to the stimulus).

10. **C)** Indications for SCS include CRPS, inoperable ischemic limb pain, PVD, FBSS, and angina pectoris.

11. **D)** Rehabilitation exercises are performed primarily with the spine in a neutral posture or in flexion to reduce stress on facet joints. Spine stabilization, core stabilization exercises, posture correction, and a strengthening program to restore functional movements should be initiated. Facet joint–mediated pain is often elicited on extension or with rotation-extension combined movements. Point tenderness may occur in the paravertebral regions. Diagnostic facet joint–nerve blocks and therapeutic radiofrequency ablation are also treatment options, if indicated.

12. **D)** Serotonin-norepinephrine reuptake inhibitors (SNRIs). SNRIs are used to treat depression and chronic pain.

13. **B)** TENS stands for transcutaneous electrical nerve stimulation. The TENS unit is a portable device that utilizes electrical stimulation for pain control. It is presumed to decrease pain via the gate controlled theory of pain.

14. **A)** A delta fibers (group III fibers) are 2 mm to 5 mm in diameter, are myelinated, have a fast conduction speed (5 m/s–40 m/s), and are the first fibers to transmit the sensation of pain.

15. **D)** Tissue damage, poor muscular balance, and poor muscular control are thought to lead to functional instability of the low back. These cause the joints to become lax and alter the anatomy of the lumbar spine, leading to a feeling of instability.

16. **A)** Phantom pain is pain from a part of the body that has been lost, or from which the brain no longer receives signals. It is a type of neuropathic pain. Phantom limb pain is a common pain experience of amputees. Whereas phantom sensation is common, phantom pain is not and needs to be treated aggressively. It is often described as shooting, crushing, burning, or cramping.

17. **D)** This question asks for potential complications of a lower lumbar interlaminar epidural steroid injection. Tetraplegia may occur after cervical epidural steroid injection secondary to direct trauma to the spinal cord. This has occurred specifically in heavily sedated patients. Caution should be used especially in the cervical region, as there may be catastrophic consequences. Dural puncture with subsequent postdural puncture headache, epidural abscess, and epidural hematoma can occur with any level (cervical, thoracic, lumbar) interlaminar epidural injection.

18. **C)** Non-opioids, mild opioids, then strong opioids should be the progression until the patient is free of pain.

19. **D)** CRPS type I is also known as reflex sympathetic dystrophy (RSD) or shoulder-hand syndrome. It is the most common subtype of RSD in stroke patients (reported in about 12%–25% of hemiplegic stroke patients). CRPS type II, also known as causalgia, is a sympathetic-mediated pain limited to a peripheral nerve distribution.

20. **B)** CPSP (formerly known as thalamic pain or Dejerine-Roussy syndrome) is a central neuropathic pain syndrome that can occur after cerebrovascular accident. It develops in 8% of stroke patients. Elimination of other causes of pain after stroke must occur before diagnosing CPSP, since CPSP is a diagnosis of exclusion. Pain is characterized most often as a burn; however, aching, pricking, lacerating, shooting, squeezing, throbbing, and heaviness are all possible qualitative descriptors.

21. **C)** Occipital neuralgia is usually caused by an entrapped nerve root at the neck, usually C2 level, supplying the greater and lesser occipital nerves. At times, the nerve can be entrapped more cephalad, as the nerve courses through muscles in the neck or the posterior scalp. Patients will present with shooting pain and/or scalp hypersensitivity to light touch.

22. **A)** There is strong familial predisposition to discogenic lumbar pain. Discogenic pain is also associated with advanced age, male sex, and smoking. Intradiscal pressure is higher in the sitting position than in the standing position. For nonradicular low-back pain with degenerative disk disease, fusion does not appear to be better than intensive interdisciplinary rehabilitation.

23. **B)** When treating new onset/acute TMD, the treatments below have been found to be applicable:
    - Heat: A heating pad, hot towel, or water bottle to the involved side of the face can decrease muscle spasms.
    - Oral rest: Downgrade diet to mechanically soft for 2 weeks, avoid yawning and laughing with mouth open. Restrict repetitive jaw motions such as chewing gum and/or biting fingernails.
    - Medications:
      - NSAIDs (ibuprofen, naproxen, indomethacin) are commonly prescribed for use for a 2-week period.
      - Antidepressants are often indicated secondary to the strong link between TMD and psychological factors. Tricyclic antidepressants are most widely used.
      - Benzodiazepines can be used and help with sleep; however, they should be limited to 2 weeks because of dependency risk.
      - Narcotic use should be avoided.
    - Oral splinting: Can improve the temporomandibular joint (TMJ) and the masticatory motor system to reduce abnormal muscle function and protect teeth from attrition and abnormal occlusal loading. As a result, masticatory muscle pain decreases.
    - Behavioral modification: Relaxation techniques, conditioning, and biofeedback have been useful.
    - Rehabilitation therapy: Exercise programs are designed to improve muscular coordination, relax tense muscles, and increase range of motion and strength. Manual therapy, muscle stretching and strengthening exercises are the most useful techniques for reeducation and rehabilitation of the masticatory muscles. Use of splints in combination with therapy has been found to drastically decrease pain, compared to therapy or splints alone. Shortwave diathermy, ultrasound, laser, and transcutaneous electrical nerve stimulation (TENS) are used to reduce inflammation, and increase muscular relaxation and blood flow by changing capillary permeability.
    - Acupuncture: The mechanism is unclear, but acupuncture may relieve pain by stimulating the production of endorphins, serotonin, and acetylcholine within the central nervous system.

24. **B)** Spondylolysis refers to a defect of the pars interarticularis. If a child, adolescent, or young adult presents with low-back pain, spondylolysis should be high on the differential diagnosis. It is thought to arise from repetitive hyperextension of an immature spine. Sports such as football and gymnastics increase the risk of developing spondylolysis.

25. **D)** Phantom pain refers to a painful sensation perceived in a body part that is no longer present following surgical or traumatic removal. This pain most commonly occurs after amputation of a limb (phantom limb pain). Transcutaneous electrical nerve stimulation has been considered beneficial to help treat phantom limb pain and can be started early in the postoperative period without any side effects. Sensory discrimination training, or tactile stimulation, has also been proven to decrease phantom limb pain because of reversal of cortical reorganization. Virtual reality and mirror treatment with a "mirror box" has been used to provide pain relief for these patients. Other treatment options can include use of compression stockings, stump shrinkers, heat/cold, manipulation, vibration, acupuncture, and massage.

26. **A)** There are three distinct opioid receptors—mu, delta, and kappa. All of these receptors belong to the G-protein–coupled receptor family, with cyclic adenosine monophosphate (cAMP) acting as an intracellular second messenger.

27. **D)** Thoracic sprain/strain usually occurs with heavy lifting or excessive repetitive motion. Sprain refers to injury to ligaments, whereas strain refers to injury to muscle. Sprain/strain commonly presents with pain and muscle spasm. The neurological examination should be normal.

28. **A)** BOTOX is the first and only preventive treatment approved by the U.S. Food and Drug Administration (FDA) for adults (18 years and older) with chronic migraine (15 or more headache days a month, each lasting 4 hours or more). BOTOX therapy is not approved for adults with migraine who have 14 or fewer headache days a month. Thirty-one BOTOX injections should be administered into seven specific head and neck sites. When labeled doses are injected in recommended areas, it may produce results lasting up to 3 months. Initial migraine treatment options should include lifestyle modifications such as regular exercise, adequate sleep, avoidance of caffeine and alcohol intake. Nonpharmacologic treatment may include biofeedback-assisted relaxation. Abortive therapies include use of nonsteroidal anti-inflammatory drugs with or without caffeine, ergots, and triptans. Other prophylactic therapy may include use of beta-blockers (propranolol), calcium channel antagonists, tricyclic antidepressants such as amitriptyline, sodium valproate, and serotonin reuptake inhibitors.

29. **A)** MPS is defined as a painful disorder characterized by the presence of distinct sensitive spots in a palpable taut band of skeletal muscle fibers that produce local and referred pain. This disorder can also be accompanied by anxiety and depression. Symptoms can be reproduced by digital pressure over the tender areas of the muscle where the patient's usual pain occurs.

30. **C)** CRPS is a pain syndrome, usually preceded by an inciting event, either trauma or a period of immobilization. It is associated with a hyperactive sympathetic nervous system. It is characterized by intense pain and sensitivity to light touch, with both nociceptive and neuropathic features. Swelling and excessive or lack of hair growth when compared with the other extremity is usually noted.

31. **D)** Multiple studies have found systemic steroids not to be effective for chronic low-back pain.

32. **C)** S1 affects sensation in the posterior thigh and calf. Toe walking is affected because the gastroc soleus muscle is affected.

33. **D)** Nociceptors are free nerve endings that transmit the sensation of pain. There are thermal, chemical, and mechanical nociceptors for various stimuli.

34. **B)** Cluster headaches usually present as a sharp unilateral headache, are localized to the orbital area, and are far more common in men than in women. To diagnose cluster headaches, one of the following autonomic signs must be present during the headache on the same side as the headache: lacrimation, ptosis, miosis, rhinorrhea, or conjunctival injection (red eye).

35. **B)** Nerve endings in the dermal layer are responsible for transmitting sensation and pain back to the central nervous system.

36. **D)** Morphine, codeine, and oxycodone have a half-life of 2.5 to 3.5 hours. Oxymorphone has a half-life of 7 to 9 hours.

37. **B)** Amputation residual limb pain is a "sharp," "burning," "electric-like," or "skin-sensitive" pain at the end of an amputated residual limb. Unlike phantom pain, it occurs in the actual existing body part. Residual limb pain is due to a damaged nerve in the residual limb region, sometimes with neuroma formation. A neuroma can cause pain and skin sensitivity. Causalgia should present with other sympathetic-mediated symptoms, such as swelling, hyperthermia or hypothermia, or sweating in the acute stage.

38. **C)** SI joint dysfunction, or sacroiliitis, causes back, buttock, leg, or groin pain with tenderness over the SI joint. This joint is an L-shaped articulation of the sacrum and the ilium. Pain in the SI joint can be caused by hypermobile or hypomobile joint patterns, spondyloarthropathy, pyogenic or crystal arthropathy, and fracture of the sacrum and pelvis. There are many tests that can be utilized to assist in the diagnosis of sacroiliitis. Clinical tests include Patrick's (flexion, abduction, external rotation, and extension [FABERE]) test, Gaenslen's test, and iliac compression test. Nonprovocative tests include Yeoman's test, Gillet's test, and seated flexion test. Imaging can help aid in the diagnosis, including x-ray, bone scan, CT, or MRI. However, these are most useful to rule out other disease etiologies. Fluoroscopic SI joint injections using an anesthetic and steroid have the most diagnostic value of these answer choices. It can be both diagnostic and therapeutic.

39. **C)** Lateral femoral cutaneous neuropathy (also known as *meralgia paresthetica*) refers to entrapment of the lateral femoral cutaneous nerve. Patients will present with anterior lateral thigh numbness and pain. It is a purely sensory nerve entrapment, so there should be no muscle weakness.

40. **C)** A commonly used form of biofeedback in chronic pain is electromyogram (EMG) biofeedback, but there are other types.

41. **C)** 3rd and 4th. The most common location for an interdigital (Morton's) neuroma is between the 3rd and 4th metatarsal heads.

42. **A)** Attention should be paid to which steroid preparation is given during a transforaminal epidural steroid injection. The nonparticulate, soluble synthetic glucocorticoid—dexamethasone sodium phosphate—has been favored over particulate steroid preparations because of fear that the larger particles might be more likely to cause spinal cord infarction or stroke, if accidentally injected into the vertebral artery (clearly seen in experimental animal studies). Of the answer choices, dexamethasone (Decadron) is the only nonparticulate steroid preparation, while the others are not.

43. **B)** Medications such as pregabalin and gabapentin work by blocking calcium channels and have been shown to decrease neuropathic pain.

44. **A)** Allodynia is pain resulting from a stimulus that does not normally produce pain. Hyperalgesia is an increased painful sensation in response to additional noxious stimuli. Analgesia is defined as the absence of the sense of pain without losing consciousness and other sensations. Hypoalgesia or hypalgesia is a decreased sensitivity to painful stimuli.

45. **C)** C6-C7. C6-C7 has a referral pattern of pain into below the spine of the scapula.

46. **D)** The gate control theory was proposed by Melzack and Wall in the mid-1960s. The concept of the gate control theory is that nonpainful input can override painful input by "closing the gate of control," which results in suppression of pain. In medial branch block, the peripheral pain signal input is simply blocked with injected anesthetic medication.

47. **C)** A sharp, pricking, stinging pain sensation caused by a needle, pin prick, or a skin cut is transmitted by the A delta fibers. Burning pain caused by inflammation or burned skin is transmitted by C fibers.

48. **B)** Cluster headache. Ten liters of 100% oxygen at the onset of a headache has been shown to be effective in treating cluster headaches.

49. **B)** Adhesive capsulitis occurs when the connective tissue around the glenohumeral joint becomes inflamed. This leads to pain, stiffness, and decreased range of motion. People with a history of a stroke, diabetes, or lung or heart disease are at a higher risk for developing adhesive capsulitis.

50. **A)** Pain referral patterns from the cervical zygapophyseal joints has been described by Dwyer and Bogduk. Pain from the C2-C3 segmental level can radiate to the upper cervical level and extend at least onto the occiput.
    Pain referral patterns from the cervical zygapophyseal joints have been described by Dwyer and Bogduk. Pain from the C6-C7 segmental level can radiate over a more or less quadrangular area covering the supraspinous and infraspinous fossa. C6-C7 pain is distinguished from C5-C6 by its extension below the spine of the scapula.

51. **D)** The sinuvertebral nerve innervates the anterior vertebral body, the external annulus, and the posterior longitudinal ligament. The anterior longitudinal ligament is innervated by the gray rami communicans, which branch off the lumbar sympathetic chain. The internal annulus fibrosus and nucleus pulposus do not have innervations.

52. **D)** Nucynta is a newer opioid agonist indicated for the management of:
    1. Moderate to severe chronic pain in adults.
    2. Neuropathic pain associated with diabetic peripheral neuropathy (DPN) in adults.
    This is the only opioid agonist that also offers some potential neuropathic pain relief. It works by potentially binding to mu-opioid receptors and inhibits norepinephrine reuptake, producing analgesia. All other answer choices can be used for neuropathic pain, but have a different mechanism of action.

53. **D)** SCS relieves pain by applying electrical stimulation resulting in paresthesias covering or overlapping areas where pain may occur. However, this is done without discomfort or changes to motor function. The most common indication for SCS use in the United States is failed back syndrome (FBS). However, it may be also used for:

- Radicular pain syndrome or radiculopathies resulting in pain secondary to FBS or herniated disk
- Postlaminectomy pain
- Multiple back operations
- Unsuccessful disk surgery
- Degenerative disk disease (DDD)/herniated disk pain refractory to conservative and surgical interventions
- Peripheral causalgia
- Epidural fibrosis
- Arachnoiditis or lumbar adhesive arachnoiditis
- Complex regional pain syndrome (CRPS), reflex sympathetic dystrophy (RSD), or causalgia

54. **A)** Studies have shown that celecoxib, a selective COX-2 inhibitor, does not inhibit platelet aggregation.

55. **B)** The International Association for the Study of Pain established the following criteria that must be present for a clinical diagnosis for CRPS:
- Preceding noxious event without obvious nerve lesion (CRPS I) or with obvious nerve lesion (CRPS II)
- Spontaneous pain or hyperalgesia-hyperesthesia not limited to a single nerve territory and disproportionate to the inciting incident
- Edema, skin blood flow (temperature) or sudomotor abnormalities, motor symptoms, or trophic changes are present on the affected limb, in particular at distal sites
- Other diagnoses are excluded

This patient has poststroke shoulder pain and shows signs of allodynia, edema, and warmth. This patient most likely is in stage 1 of CRPS. Neer's and Hawkin's tests are negative making it less likely that impingement syndrome is the cause of her pain. Yergason's test is negative making the diagnosis of bicipital tendonitis less likely. Other causes for shoulder pain in a hemiplegic patient include shoulder subluxation and brachial plexus/peripheral nerve injury.

56. **C)** Ankylosing spondylitis is three times more common in men than in women, usually presents in the late teens, and is associated with morning stiffness and aching pain in the lower back (at times affecting the buttocks). On physical examination, one can find tenderness to palpation over the sacroiliac joints and decreased spinal mobility.

57. **A)** It is often difficult to separate physical, behavioral, habitual, traumatic, and psychophysiologic factors in patients with temporomandibular disorder (TMD). A thorough history is important. Symptoms can include:
- Diffuse jaw pain
- Unilateral pain in muscles of mastication, radiating to temples, side of face, or ear
- Joint clicking
- Limited mouth opening with/without lateral deviation of jaw
- Tinnitus or other ear symptoms
- Nocturnal clenching or bruxism
- Spasticity of muscles of mastication with prolonged chewing
- Recent alteration in bite
- Psychological stress causing nocturnal teeth grinding

- Facial trauma
- Chronic/heavy computer use
- Dental work

58. **C)** Addiction is the continued use of medication (or engagement in rewarding stimuli) despite adverse consequences. Addiction has a physical and psychological component. Dependence is the body's physical reliance on a drug or medication in order to prevent withdrawal. Withdrawal is an abnormal physical and psychologic condition brought on by a cessation of a medication (typically an opioid).

59. **D)** Diabetic amyotrophy is the most common cause of focal femoral neuropathy. The onset is sudden, pain is debilitating, and patients often exhibit difficulty with ambulation.

60. **D)** TMD can be caused by:
    - Myofascial pain dysfunction involving the temporalis, masseter, lateral, and medial pterygoid
    - Internal derangement of the joint space involving trauma, muscle hyperactivity, condylar restriction, disc perforation, or displacement
    - Degenerative joint disorders, including rheumatoid arthritis, psoriasis, pseudogout, ankylosing spondylitis, and lupus erythematosus
    - Fractures
    - Infections
    - Tumors
    - Psychophysiologic factors including stress, tension, depression, habitual clenching and grinding of the teeth, and fingernail biting
    - Malalignment of the jaws or internal components of the joint space

61. **D)** This patient's clinical presentation is consistent with complex regional pain syndrome. Allodynia is pain due to a stimulus that does not normally provoke pain (such as gentle touching in this case). Hyperalgesia is an increased response to a stimulus that is normally painful. Hyperesthesia is an increased sensitivity to stimulation. Hyperpathia is exaggerated response to a painful stimulus.

62. **D)** Alleviation of pain with sympathetic blockade is the gold standard in diagnosing sympathetically mediated CRPS type I. Although CRPS is primarily a clinical diagnosis, several diagnostic studies may be helpful to rule out other pathologies, including doppler flowmeter, infrared thermography, quantitative sudomotor axon reflex testing, and vital capillaroscopy. Imaging may also be used to exclude other diagnoses, such as use of plain films (demineralization can occur), MRI (marrow edema, soft tissue swelling, joint effusion can be seen), and bone scintigraphy (increased periarticular activity in the affected limb). The sensitivity and specificity is variable in triple-phase bone scans. Therefore, the gold standard in diagnosis of CRPS is with sympathetic blockade of the stellate ganglion with local anesthetic.

63. **B)** The most common symptomatic level of cervical facet (zygapophyseal) joint pain determined by controlled diagnostic block is C2-C3. The prevalence of C2-C3 facet joint pain has been estimated to be 50% to 53% in patients whose chief complaint is posterior headache after whiplash injury.

64. **C)** For this reason, x-ray is generally not useful for the diagnosis of osteoporosis. Bone mineral density is used in the diagnosis and is measured using dual energy x-ray absorptiometry (DEXA).

65. **C)** Central pain syndrome (CPS; also called thalamic pain syndrome or Dejerine-Roussy syndrome) is most commonly preceded by numbness on the affected side, which is later replaced by a burning and tingling sensation. CPS can be severe and debilitating, presenting at times with hypersensitivity to touch. Less commonly, some patients develop severe ongoing pain with little or no stimuli. The thalamus is thought to play a major role in relaying sensory/pain information between a variety of subcortical areas and the cerebral cortex.

66. **B)** The trigeminal nerve supplies sensation over the jaw through the mandibular division. Trigeminal neuralgia causes neuropathic pain, is more common in women and multiple sclerosis patients, and is described as a sharp, electric pain. It is usually unilateral and intermittent.

67. **A)** Tricyclic antidepressant (TCA). Amitriptyline (Elavil) is a tricyclic antidepressant and is used to treat depression and neuropathic pain.

68. **A)** Mexiletine is an orally active local anesthetic, antiarrhythmic agent, that is structurally similar to lidocaine and is considered an oral analogue of lidocaine for neuropathic pain treatment. Ketamine is the most commonly used *N*-methyl-D-aspartate (NMDA) antagonist for neuropathic pain. Pregabalin (Lyrica), similar to gabapentin (Neurontin), binds to the alpha-a2delta subunit of the voltage-dependent calcium channel in the central nervous system. It decreases the release of neurotransmitters, such as glutamate, noradrenaline, and gamma-aminobutyric acid. Amitriptyline (Elavil) is a tricyclic antidepressant (TCA) used for neuropathic pain.

69. **A)** Fentanyl has a relatively short plasma half-life, thus most formulations will have a short duration of its action. Fentanyl patch is unique; since it stays in place for 72 hours the effective time the drug remains in the system is increased. As a result, the morphine milligram equivalence factor is increased with Fentanyl patch relative to oral and spray formulations. The morphine milligram equivalence factor for Fentanyl patch is 7.2, for Fentanyl oral spray is 0.18, for Fentanyl nasal spray is 0.15, and for Fentanyl oral lozenge is 0.13.

70. **C)** The severity and frequency of migraine attacks tend to decrease with increasing age. The other answers are all true.

71. **C)** Cozen's test. Cozen's test is used to diagnose lateral epicondylitis. The patient radially deviates and extends the wrist against resistance. A positive test is pain over the lateral epicondyle. This test can also be performed with resisted 3rd finger extension.

72. **A)** The cell bodies of first-order, or primary, pain fibers are located in either the dorsal root ganglia or the trigeminal ganglia. The trigeminal ganglia are specialized nerves for the face, whereas the dorsal root ganglia provide sensory innervation for the rest of the body.

73. **D)** Pain wind-up is a phenomenon caused by repeated stimulation of peripheral nerve fibers, leading to progressively increasing electrical response in the second-order neurons. The process is also termed as *central sensitization*, which leads to hyperalgesia, allodynia, and spontaneous pain.

74. **B)** Each lumbar and thoracic facet joint (except L5-S1 facet joint) is innervated by the medial branches of the dorsal rami exiting at the same level and one level above. The L4-L5 facet joint is innervated by the L3 and L4 medial branches.

75. **B)** Fibromyalgia (FM).
FM is a syndrome defined by chronic widespread pain for at least 3 months' duration. The majority of patients are women and prevalence increases with age.
According to the 1990 American College of Rheumatology (ACR) criteria:
A patient must have pain in the axial skeleton, pain above and below the waist, and pain in palpation in at least 11 of 18 paired tender points throughout the body.
However, the ACR revised their FM criteria in 2010, as the tender point exam has been controversial and is difficult to perform. Tender points have a questionable specificity, and an alternative to the tender point exam for FM was developed and therefore accepted.
According to the 2010 ACR FM Diagnostic Criteria, a patient is diagnosed with FM if:
1. Widespread pain index (WPI) is at least 7 and symptom severity (SS) scale is at least 5. Or the WPI score is 3 to 6 and the SS scale is at least 9.
2. The symptom has been present at a similar level for least 3 months.
3. The patient does not have another disorder that would otherwise explain his or her pain.

*WPI quantifies the extent of bodily pain with questioning patients having pain in 19 different body regions. Each body region scores 1 point. The patient in this question scores a WPI of 8, based on her eight different regions of pain. The SS scale quantifies symptom severity by scoring problems with fatigue, cognitive dysfunction, and loss of sleep over the past week. This is done with a 0 to 3 scale for each, 0 representing no problem and 3 representing severe problem. The patient in this question scores a SS score of at least 6 of 9 maximum points.

76. **B)** Pronator syndrome refers to median nerve compression as the nerve passes between the two heads of the pronator teres. It often mimics CTS, as it presents with numbness over the first three digits. Whereas pain in patients with CTS can wake patients from sleep, pain from pronator syndrome usually does not. Weakness is seen in median nerve innervated muscles distal to the pronator teres.

77. **A)** Sixty percent of burns result from fire/flame injuries. Scald, electric, and chemical injuries only make up a minority of burn injuries.

78. **B)** Chronic use of high-dose opioids has been shown to decrease libido in men and women, and to cause amenorrhea and a reduced cortisol response to stress.

79. **B)** The cervical facet joint receives innervation from the same level and one level below. The nerve is blocked at the waist of the articular process in the cervical region. This differs from the lumbar facet joint. The lumbar facet joint is supplied by the medial branches of the dorsal rami, exiting at that same level and one level above. So, as examples, the L4-L5 facet joint receives sensory innervation from the medial branches of the dorsal rami of the L3 and L4 nerve roots, whereas the C3-C4 facet joint receives sensory innervation from the dorsal rami of the C3 and C4 nerve roots. Two special cases in the neck include the C2-C3 facet joint, which receives innervation from the third occipital nerve and the medial branch of the dorsal ramus of the C3 nerve root, and the C7-T1 facet joint, which receives innervation from the C7 and C8 medial branches.

80. **C)** Hypogastric plexus block can be effective for pelvic visceral pain. Celiac plexus blocks can be used for upper abdominal visceral pain. Stellate-ganglion block is used in sympathetically maintained upper extremity pain. Lumbar sympathetic block is effective in sympathetically mediated lower extremity pain.

81. **C)** Consider a trial of pregabalin (Lyrica) in this patient as she most likely has fibromyalgia. A stepwise approach to fibromyalgia management is recommended. After confirming the diagnosis, it is important to explain the condition and treat any comorbid conditions. This may include sleep or mood disturbances. Physical therapy is considered important to help improve fitness function and ultimately decrease pain. This may include educating patients in stretching, gentle strengthening, and a cardiovascular fitness program. Medications may be tried, including agents such as pregabalin (Lyrica), which is started at 50 mg three times daily and increased to 100 mg three times daily over 7 days. Acetaminophen or nonsteroidal anti-inflammatory medications can also be used for pain relief. Opioids should be rarely used in patients with fibromyalgia.

82. **D)** Acetaminophen. Acetaminophen alleviates pain by inhibiting cyclooxygenase in the central nervous system and has analgesic and antipyretic, but **not** anti-inflammatory actions.

83. **B)** The goal of chronic pain management is to help people with pain function better and live rewarding lives. Often the pain can be reduced, but not eliminated.

84. **B)** Phantom pain refers to a painful sensation perceived in a body part that is no longer present following surgical or traumatic removal. This pain most commonly occurs after amputation of a limb (phantom limb pain), but can also occur after surgical removal of breast, rectum, penis, testicles, eye, tooth, tongue, or lesion of the peripheral or central nervous system. Phantom limb pain usually starts within days after amputation, but can also present months to years later. It is less common in congenital amputation and loss of limb in early childhood. Phantom limb pain is not relieved with position, and can be problematic. It can lead to interference with prosthesis training/use and permanent disability in greater than 40% of amputees. Stump pain occurs in the residual limb or stump. Phantom limb sensation is a nonpainful sensation (not pain) of the absent part. Although this patient has a history of lumbar spinal stenosis, the pain does not worsen with walking (neurogenic claudication), thus making this less likely as the pain generator.

85. **A)** Conduction is a method whereby energy is transferred by direct interaction of molecules in a different energy state. Cryotherapy is a method of therapeutic cooling by causing the transfer of energy from warmer to cooler particles.

86. **B)** The most common needle used for lumbar image-guided injection is the 22-gauge, 3.5-inch Quincke (straight) spinal needle. The 22-gauge is an adequate compromise between needle diameter and stiffness. Although, choices (C) and (D) are smaller diameter needles that will produce less pain, they will also bend more easily because they lack stiffness. The curved (Tuohy) needle is an alternative to the straight needle. The use of a curved needle requires a minimum of 22-gauge. Ultimately, the choice of needles depends on operator comfort.

87. **B)** The three major primary headache disorders are migraine, cluster, and tension-type headaches. Prodrome (aura) can occur preceding a migraine headache and may consist of focal neurologic signs or symptoms that will usually fade away within 30 to 60 minutes as the headache begins. Common auras include visual disturbances including field cuts, photophobia, and scintillating scotomata. There have been three gene mutations identified and associated with familial hemiplegic migraine. Migraines are three times more common amongst women, and peak prevalence occurs in midlife. Twenty-five percent of all women may be affected with migraine headache during midlife.

88. **A)** Although elimination of all pain is a noble and desirable goal, it is not a realistic goal in patients with chronic pain. The others are realistic goals and will hopefully lead to normalization of function.

89. **C)** Dysesthesia is an unpleasant abnormal sensation, whether painful or evoked. Allodynia is pain from a stimulus that ordinarily will not provoke pain. Anesthesia is a loss of sensation. Hyperesthesia is an increased sensation or sensitivity. Hyperalgesia is increased pain response from a normally painful stimulus (the degree of pain is disproportionate to the stimulus).

90. **D)** Studies have shown that patients suffering from chronic pain can suffer from sleep disturbances, including longer time to fall asleep, sleep fragmentation, and decreased quality of sleep.

91. **C)** Spondylolisthesis refers to the slippage of one vertebra relative to the one above it. Spondylolisthesis can result from many causes. In older patients who develop spondylolisthesis, most are degenerative in nature (usually caused by disk or facet disease). Spondylolisthesis most commonly affects the L4-L5 level.

92. **A)** Both fluoroscopically guided facet joint injection and fluoroscopically guided medial branch block (not ablation) may be used to confirm the diagnosis of facet joint–mediated pain. After confirmation of the diagnosis, fluoroscopically guided medial branch ablation is usually performed for treatment.

93. **D)** Aspirin. Aspirin alleviates pain by inhibiting prostaglandin synthesis and release and inhibits platelet aggregation. It may take two weeks for a therapeutic response.

94. **A)** Methadone hydrochloride is a relatively potent NMDA receptor antagonist, blocking the activation of NMDA receptors, which are largely responsible for central sensitization. Methadone is cheap, has no active metabolites, and has a half-life varying from 7 hours to 5 days. Methadone is also an opioid and acts as a mu-receptor agonist.

95. **D)** Allodynia is pain from a stimulus that ordinarily will not provoke pain. Anesthesia is a loss of sensation. Hyperesthesia is an increased sensation or sensitivity. Hyperalgesia is increased pain response from a normally painful stimulus (the degree of pain is disproportionate to the stimulus).

96. **B)** The best type of exercises for patients with osteoporosis is progressive resistive spinal extension exercises. Studies have shown that patients with osteoporosis have weaker back extensors than the general population. Spinal flexion exercises should be avoided, as these can aggravate compression fractures in patients with osteoporosis.

97. **A)** Amitriptyline is a tricyclic antidepressant (TCA) that also has a side-effect profile of an anticholinergic and sedative. This TCA can work to help with the patient's neuropathic pain complaints secondary to his spinal cord injury. The side-effect profile of this medication would also serve to help with the patient's urinary leakage and sleep difficulty. Fluoxetine does not have significant anticholinergic effects. Trazodone can help with sleep difficulty, but not pain complaints. Gabapentin would help with neuropathic pain and may cause some drowsiness, but has no anticholinergic effects.

98. **B)** Increased response to a stimulus that is normally painful.
The answer choices are all key definitions. Pain due to a stimulus that does not normally provoke pain is allodynia. Increased sensitivity to stimulation is hyperesthesia. An unpleasant abnormal sensation, whether spontaneous or evoked, is dysesthesia.

Complex regional pain syndrome (CRPS) is classically divided into three stages. These stages are useful for descriptive purposes, but the syndrome does not always follow this stepwise progression. The stages of CRPS are:

Stage 1: Severe pain; pitting edema; redness; warmth; increased hair and nail growth; hyperhidrosis may begin; osteoporosis may begin.

Stage 2: Continued pain; brawny edema; periarticular thickening; cyanosis or pallor; livido reticularis; coolness; hyperhidrosis; increased osteoporosis; rigid nails.

Stage 3: Pallor; dry, cool skin; atrophic soft issue (dystrophy); contracture; extensive osteoporosis.

99. **A)** These two medications affect the sodium channels and help to reduce neuropathic pain, especially trigeminal neuralgia.

100. **A)** Contusions to muscular structures are common after blunt trauma. X-ray will be negative for acute fractures, but will show soft-tissue swelling. Patients will usually present with pain, swelling, and difficulty with range of motion.

101. **C)** Therapeutic ultrasound works by converting electrical energy into high-frequency sound waves, which have the ability to increase tissue temperature and promote tissue healing.

102. **C)** Methadone has a half-life of 13 to 47 hours. Morphine and codeine have a half-life of 2.5 to 3.5 hours. Oxymorphone has a half-life of 7 to 9 hours.

103. **B)** Convection is the act of conveying or transmitting heat in a liquid or gas by bulk movement of heated particles to a cooler area.

104. **B)** Sacroiliac joint (SI) dysfunction or sacroiliitis causes back, buttock, leg, or groin pain with tenderness over the SI joint. This joint is an L-shaped articulation of the sacrum and the ilium. There are many tests that can be utilized to assist in diagnosis of sacroiliitis. Patrick's Test (or flexion, **ab**duction, **e**xternal **r**otation, and **e**xtension [FABERE] test) is positive if pain is elicited with flexion, abduction, external rotation of the hip joint, and extension of the leg. Contralateral pain occurs with this test in a dysfunctional SI joint. Diagnostic SI joint injection under fluoroscopy has a high diagnostic value and can also be therapeutic. The other answer choices are not seen with SI joint pathology.

105. **A)** The initial gate control theory by Melzack and Wall published in *Science* in 1965 indicated that stimulation of large diameter A beta fibers modulated the dorsal horn "gate" and therefore reduced the nociceptive input from periphery.

106. **C)** Postdural-puncture headache (PDPH) is a complication of a punctured dura mater and may occur after a lumbar epidural injection. There is a higher incidence of headache following lumbar puncture (rather than cervical), likely due to a decreasing column of cerebrospinal fluid (CSF) cephalad to the point of dural puncture. PDPH typically occurs hours to days after puncture and presents with symptoms such as bifrontal or occipital headache and nausea, which typically worsen when the patient assumes an upright posture. Some patients only require analgesics, fluids, and bed rest. However, this patient's symptoms have persisted for almost 48 hours without improvement. Epidural blood patch using autologous blood is a safe and effective treatment that will relieve the headache symptoms promptly in this patient. A small amount of autologous blood is injected into the epidural space near the site of the original puncture, and the resulting clotting will "patch" the meningeal leak.

For the following answers (107–126), if necessary, please refer to the following medication conversion table.

**Medication Conversion**

| Medication | Morphine milligram equivalent |
| --- | :---: |
| Morphine | 1 |
| Hydrocodone | 1 |
| Oxycodone | 1.5 |
| Codeine | 0.15 |
| Methadone (1–20 mg/day) | 4 |
| Methadone (21–40 mg/day) | 8 |
| Methadone (41–60 mg/day) | 10 |
| Tapentadol | 0.4 |
| Vicodin | 1 |
| Tramadol | 0.1 |
| Hydromorphone (Dilaudid) | 4 |
| Fentanyl patch | 7.2 |
| Oxymorphone | 3 |

107.  **B)** This is a complicated pain management regimen, and in a live patient would not be appropriate owing to involving two short-acting opioids, but the morphine equivalent dosing for this patient is simple to calculate with the appropriate conversion factors on hand (oxycodone 1.5, and Dilaudid 4). We will solve this problem with the following calculations (see also the medication conversion table):
OxyContin 20 mg × 2 (doses per day) = 40 mg/day
Oxycodone 10 mg × 6 (doses per day) = 60 mg/day
100 × 1.5 = 150 morphine milligram equivalent
Dilaudid 2 mg × 4 (doses per day) = 8 mg/day
8 × 4 = 32 morphine milligram equivalent
150 + 32 = 182 morphine milligram equivalent

108.  **A)** The morphine milligram equivalence factor for codeine is 0.15. The morphine milligram equivalence factor for hydrocodone is 1. The morphine milligram equivalence factor for hydromorphone is 4. The morphine milligram equivalence factor for tapentadol is 0.4 (see also the medication conversion table).

109.  **B)** IV access for pain medications is not always necessary and carries additional risks from the management perspective. Often, the use of PO analgesics is preferred. In this problem the original regimen of Dilaudid (morphine conversion factor 4) IV 2 mg every 4 hours can be converted to the following morphine equivalent:
2 mg × 6 (doses per day) = 12 mg/day
12 × 4 = 48 morphine milligram equivalent
Similarly, we can calculate the same morphine equivalent dosing for oxycodone, the morphine milligram equivalent conversion factor for which is 1.5 (see also the medication conversion table):

5 mg × 6 (doses per day) = 30 mg/day
30 × 1.5 = 45 morphine milligram equivalent

110. **D)** The morphine milligram equivalence factor for methadone is greater than 4. Hydrocodone and morphine are 1. The morphine milligram equivalence factor for tramadol is 0.1 (see also the medication conversion table).

111. **B)** We can easily calculate the morphine equivalence of a medication by noting its appropriate morphine conversion factor. In this case oxycodone has a conversion factor of 1.5. Using this information we calculate (see also the medication conversion table):
Oxycodone 10 mg × 4 (doses per day) = 40 mg/day
40 × 1.5 = 60 morphine milligram equivalents
Tramadol = 50 mg × 6 (doses per day) = 300 mg/day × 0.1 morphine milligram equivalent = 30
Dilaudid = 8 × 4 = 32 morphine milligram equivalents

112. **D)** Due to the wide range of opioids available for analgesic purposes, it is helpful to be able to stratify their effects relative to one another. We can use the drugs' morphine milligram equivalence to speak of the difference in potency between these medications. The morphine milligram equivalent conversion factor for morphine is 1, oxycodone is 1.5, codeine is 0.15. The morphine milligram equivalent conversion factor for methadone varies by dose, but is 4.0 or greater (see also the medication conversion table).

113. **C)** When a patient makes a change to his pain management regimen, it is important to recalculate their morphine milligram equivalence dosing. Also note, the patient would more likely take the 20-mg tablet less often, unless he has scored tablets or you are providing him 20 mg q 6 hours in the form of eight tablets per day. The morphine equivalence factor for oxycodone is 1.5 and we use this information to calculate the change in morphine milligram dosing as follows (see also the medication conversion table):
20 mg × 4 (doses per day) = 80 mg/day
80 × 1.5 = 120 morphine milligram equivalent
10 mg × 4 (doses per day) = 40 mg/day
40 × 1.5 = 60 morphine milligram equivalent
120 − 60 = 60 morphine milligram equivalent

114. **B)** Methadone's morphine equivalent conversion factor is based on its daily dosing. A dose of 1 to 20 mg/day has a factor of 4; 21 to 40 mg/day has a factor of 8; and 41 to 60 mg/day has a factor of 10. We can use this knowledge to calculate morphine conversions by totaling methadone milligram dosages per day and then multiplying that number by the appropriate conversion factor (see also the medication conversion table).

115. **D)** The highest morphine milligram dosage listed is OxyContin 30 mg every 12 hours. We can calculate the appropriate morphine conversions by noting the correct conversion factor for oxycodone (1.5) and calculating as follows (see also the medication conversion table):
OxyContin 30 mg × 2 (doses per day) = 60 mg OxyContin per day
60 × 1.5 = 90 morphine milligram equivalent
Tramadol 100 mg every 4 hours is 100 mg × 6 (doses per day) = 600 mg tramadol
600 mg × 0.1 = 60 morphine milligram equivalents
Of note, this particular regimen would be higher than the maximum safe dose of tramadol due to concerns about serotonin syndrome.
Oxycodone 10 mg every 6 hours is 10 mg × 4 (doses per day) = 40 mg oxycodone

40 mg × 1.5 = 60 morphine milligram equivalents
Dilaudid 4 mg every 8 hours is 4 mg × 3 (doses per day) = 12 mg Dilaudid
12 mg × 4 = 48 morphine milligram equivalents

116. **B)** Tapentadol (also known as Nucynta) is a relatively mild opioid medication used commonly for pain control. In addition to being a relatively weak agonist of the opioid receptors, tapentadol also has some serotonergic properties. Tapentadol is available in both long-acting (Nucynta ER) and short-acting (Nucynta) forms. The maximum total dose of Nucynta ER in a day is 500 mg, the maximum total dose of Nucynta combining both long- and short-acting forms is 600 mg/day. While the regimen in the question stem is acceptable for acute pain in the SICU, if you are transitioning to longer term use of tapentadol, you would want to switch to a regimen using primarily the long-acting Nucynta ER for chronic pain management. One other consideration with tapentadol is that the long-acting formulation has a U.S. Food and Drug Administration (FDA) indication for neuropathic pain, unlike the other opioids. The conversion factor for Nucynta to morphine equivalents is 0.4, the calculation for its morphine equivalents is relatively straightforward, and is determined as follows (see also the medication conversion table):
50 mg × 6 (doses per day) = 300 mg/day
300 × 0.4 = 120 morphine milligram equivalent

117. **B)** Methadone is a typical medication used for opioid maintenance therapy in heroin addicts. The conversion factor for methadone is variable. Based on the dosage of the methadone, in this case the conversion factor is 4 morphine milligram equivalents. Methadone's morphine equivalent conversion factor is based on its daily dosing. A dose of 1 to 20 mg/day has a factor of 4; 21 to 40 mg/day has a factor of 8; 41 to 60 mg/day has a factor of 10. The calculation for its morphine equivalents is relatively straightforward and is determined as follows (see also the medication conversion table):
20 mg × 1 (doses per day) = 20 mg/day
20 × 4 = 80 morphine milligram equivalents

118. **D)** The solution to this problem requires knowledge of morphine milligram equivalents for multiple opioid medications. OxyContin and oxycodone both have a morphine equivalence factor of 1.5. Extended release does not impact the conversion factor for these medications. Morphine has a 1:1 conversion to its milligram equivalence, and tramadol has a conversion factor of 0.1. Using this information we can calculate the morphine equivalent dosing for tramadol, the morphine milligram equivalent conversion factor for which is 0.1 (see also the medication conversion table):
50 mg × 4 (doses per day) = 200 mg/day
200 × 0.1 = 20 morphine milligram equivalent
Similarly, the morphine equivalence for morphine in this problem would be 60, for oxycodone it would be 45, and OxyContin would be 60.

119. **C)** The calculation of morphine milligram equivalents for Dilaudid is a simple matter when using the appropriate conversion factor (4.0). We calculate as follows (see also the medication conversion table):
Dilaudid 2 mg × 3 (doses per day) = 6 mg/day
6 × 4.0 = 24 morphine milligram equivalent

120. **A)** The morphine equivalent conversion for hydrocodone is 1:1 and thus no conversion is necessary to determine the morphine equivalents in this scenario (see also the medication conversion table).

121. **D)** This patient is receiving a typical opioid for pediatric patients. Codeine's morphine equivalent is 0.15, thus to calculate the daily morphine equivalence we proceed as follows (see also the medication conversion table):
60 mg × 4 (doses per day) = 240 mg/day
240 × 0.15 = 36 morphine milligram equivalent

122. **B)** To solve this problem we will have to recall the morphine equivalence factors for each of the named medications: OxyContin is 1.5, tramadol is 0.1, Dilaudid is 4, and morphine is 1. Using this information, we calculate the solution as follows (see also the medication conversion table): Tramadol (morphine milligram equivalent conversion factor is 0.1) is calculated before and after changing the dosage:
100 mg × 6 (doses per day) = 600 mg/day
600 × 0.1 = 60 morphine milligram equivalent
100 mg × 4 (doses per day) = 400 mg/day
400 × 0.1 = 40 morphine milligram equivalent
60 − 40 = 20 morphine milligram equivalent
The other regimen changes would not produce the desired reduction in morphine milligram equivalents. However, please remember that the maximum safe dose of tramadol in a 24-hour period is 400 mg because of concerns about serotonin syndrome.

123. **D)** The morphine milligram equivalence factor for hydrocodone is 1; for morphine is 1; for codeine is 0.15; and for oxycodone is 1.5 (see also the medication conversion table).

124. **B)** This patient is receiving two analgesic pain medications: oxycodone and ibuprofen. It is important to realize that morphine equivalents are calculated only for opioid pain medications, thus ibuprofen will not contribute to the morphine equivalent dosing for this patient's regimen. The conversion for oxycodone to morphine equivalents is 1.5, thus we calculate the morphine equivalents for this patient's regimen as follows (see also the medication conversion table):
10 mg × 3 (doses per day) = 30 mg/day
30 × 1.5 = 45 morphine equivalents

125. **D)** The morphine milligram equivalence conversion factor for both hydrocodone and morphine is 1. Therefore, 1 mg of morphine and 1 mg of hydrocodone can be expected to have an equivalent analgesic effect. Thus, if we calculate the morphine milligram equivalence for hydrocodone and morphine as administered in this scenario, we find that they are each written as 60 morphine milligram equivalents per day (see also the medication conversion table).

126. **C)** Gastrointestinal side effects are the most common adverse reactions associated with opioid therapy. Often times, switching to a different drug will help to reduce these symptoms. In this problem, the original regimen of oxycodone 10 mg every 6 hours can be converted to the following morphine equivalent (see also the medication conversion table):
10 mg × 4 (doses per day) = 40 mg/day
40 × 1.5 = 60 morphine milligram equivalent
Similarly, we can calculate the same morphine equivalent dosing for tramadol whose morphine milligram equivalent conversion factor is 0.1:
100 mg × 6 (doses per day) = 600 mg/day
600 × 0.1 = 60 morphine milligram equivalent
Tramadol is available in both short-acting and long-acting forms. The long-acting formulation is called Ultram ER. If this patient's pain lasts beyond the acute care setting, you should consider a regimen that uses both a long-acting and a short-acting form. A word of caution, however: the maximum safe dose of tramadol, combining long- and short-acting formulations is 400 mg/day.

# 16

# Ultrasound and Regenerative Medicine

## QUESTIONS

1. Characteristic findings of this condition when viewed on musculoskeletal ultrasound include hypoechogenic synovium, increased flow on color or power Doppler imaging in the synovium, and discontinuity of the bone cortex in two orthogonal planes.
   A) Osteoarthritis
   B) Stress fracture
   C) Rheumatoid arthritis
   D) Heterotopic ossification

2. Which of the following is a characteristic of tendinosis (tendinopathy) on ultrasound?
   A) On ultrasound, the tendon will be hypoechoic, with equal echogenicity to the adjacent muscle
   B) On ultrasound, the tendon will have a well-defined focal hypoechoic or anechoic abnormality
   C) In the supraspinatus, associated cortical irregularity of the adjacent greater tuberosity is common
   D) There are active inflammatory cells in this condition

3. Which of the following is **not** a potential cause of ulnar nerve entrapment which can be viewed on ultrasound?
   A) Anconeus epitrochlearis muscle
   B) Triceps brachii tissue within the ulnar groove
   C) Absence of cubital tunnel retinaculum
   D) Transient dislocation of the ulnar nerve

4. While longitudinally tracking a tendon posterior to the lateral malleolus, you follow it distally to find that it inserts on the base of the fifth metatarsal. You are looking at the:
   A) Peroneus longus
   B) Peroneus brevis
   C) Tibialis anterior
   D) Tibialis posterior

5. How are mesenchymal stem cells (MSC) classified?
   A) Hematopoietic
   B) Nonhematopoietic
   C) Epidermal
   D) Embryonic

ANSWERS TO THIS SECTION CAN BE FOUND ON PAGE 469

6. Why are large bore needles, such as 22-gauge needles, recommended for platelet-rich plasma (PRP)?
   A) To promote intentional activation of platelets
   B) To prevent unintentional activation of platelets
   C) To cause endogenous activation of platelets
   D) To ensure enough blood is drawn

7. Mesenchymal stem cells (MSCs) are considered optimal regenerative cells for degenerative musculoskeletal conditions such as osteoarthritis because they:
   A) Slowly proliferate and differentiate to tenocytes
   B) Rapidly proliferate and differentiate to musculoskeletal lineages
   C) Slowly proliferate and differentiate to smooth muscle
   D) Rapidly proliferate and differentiate to mature osteoblasts

8. Your patient with knee osteoarthritis has been advised by his orthopedic surgeon to consider hyaluronic acid versus platelet-rich plasma (PRP) injections prior to surgical intervention. The patient asks you if you have read any literature on whether one is better than the other. You tell him that for his condition:
   A) Hyaluronic acid is the better option
   B) PRP is the better option
   C) The studies have shown PRP does not provide more benefit than hyaluronic acid
   D) Staggered treatment of PRP and hyaluronic injections is best

9. A 60-year-old male who has continuously attempted conservative management for his osteoarthritis asks you to perform his fourth corticosteroid injection of the year for relief. Although he may have temporary relief of pain, you warn him that the medication:
   A) May be toxic to the chondrocytes and the mesenchymal stem cells (MSCs)
   B) Increases the need for surgery
   C) Improves wound healing
   D) Halts the progression of osteoarthritis

10. Which of the following is **not** a property of a chronic tendon injury (tendinosis) when viewed on ultrasound?
    A) Neovascularization
    B) Disruption of tendon fibers
    C) Increased blood flow on power Doppler imaging
    D) Hypoechoic swelling of the involved tendon

11. How is a tear that extends from the articular to bursal surface of the supraspinatus described on an ultrasound report?
    A) Full width
    B) Full thickness
    C) Complete tear
    D) Focal

12. Which key bony landmark is used to identify the attachment sites of the gluteus medius and gluteus minimus when performing lateral hip evaluation?
    A) Tubercle of the lesser trochanter
    B) Ischial tuberosity
    C) Posterior superior iliac spine
    D) Apex of the greater trochanter

13. After months of occupational therapy and compliance with the recommended night splints, your patient states she would like to try an injection for her carpal tunnel syndrome with the goal to postpone the release recommended by her hand surgeon. After visualizing the median nerve with your transducer transversely oriented over the carpal tunnel, you use _____ to separate the median nerve from the flexor retinaculum (deep surface).
   A) Hydroplaning
   B) Hydrodiversion
   C) Hydroinversion
   D) Hydrodissection

14. Which type of stem cells in particular differentiate into bone and cartilage tissue?
   A) Hematopoietic stem cells
   B) Mesenchymal stem cells
   C) Epidermal stem cells
   D) Embryonic stem cells

15. Platelet-rich plasma (PRP) causes regeneration of cartilage or tendons by:
   A) Breakdown of fibrin
   B) Formation of fibrin
   C) Formation of thrombin
   D) Breakdown of thrombin

16. After preparing the platelet-rich plasma (PRP) and letting it stabilize in the anticoagulated state for at least 8 hours, it must be _____ before its use.
   A) Melted
   B) Transduced
   C) Charged
   D) Activated

17. Although open procedure autologous chondrocyte implantation (ACI) is less invasive and patients experience less morbidity, patients need to still perform a practical rehabilitation protocol because of:
   A) The maturing process of the cartilage
   B) Pain control
   C) Monitoring of side effects
   D) Need for reinjection

18. What phase of tissue repair begins with the release of growth factors?
   A) Proliferation
   B) Inflammation
   C) Remodeling
   D) Hemostasis

19. An acute muscle contusion without muscle tear will appear on ultrasound as:
   A) An area of relative hypoechogenicity within the muscle
   B) Areas of hyperechoic hemorrhage within the muscle
   C) Heterogeneous, with mixed echogenicity
   D) Hyperechoic, with posterior acoustic shadowing

20. Which of the following is **not** true about tendon sheath injections?
    A) Placing the needle deep in the tendon when injecting corticosteroids decreases the risk for fat atrophy
    B) The needle should be introduced from lateral to medial over the extremity curvature in order to improve needle visualization
    C) The long axis approach is preferred
    D) An area of fluid distension around the tendon in the tendon sheath is an ideal target for needle placement

21. When evaluating the anterior ankle, which structure is located most medial?
    A) Tibialis anterior
    B) Deep peroneal nerve
    C) Extensor digitorum longus
    D) Extensor hallucis longus

22. A college tennis player comes to your office with progressively worsening elbow pain after repetitively practicing his backhand swing. He has tenderness to palpation over the lateral elbow, and a positive Cozen's sign (pain on resisted wrist extension). You prepare an injection to treat his tennis elbow. Your goal with the ultrasound is to get a proper view of the:
    A) Lateral epicondyle and the common extensor tendon
    B) Lateral epicondyle and the common flexor tendon
    C) Medial epicondyle and the common extensor tendon
    D) Medial epicondyle and the common flexor tendon

23. What is platelet-rich plasma (PRP) composed of?
    A) Highly concentrated platelets
    B) Low concentration of platelets
    C) Highly concentrated red blood cells
    D) None of the above

24. What is an effect of citrate dextrose on plasma pH level when used in platelet-rich plasma preparation?
    A) Lowers pH level
    B) Elevates pH level
    C) Has no effect on pH level
    D) Causes plasma to become neutral

25. Which of the following is used to quantify the level of growth factors released from the platelets upon activation of platelet-rich plasma?
    A) Southern blot
    B) Western blot
    C) Enzyme-linked immunosorbent assay (ELISA)
    D) Sohal assay

26. With regards to autologous chondrocyte implantation, the first-generation cells refers to the:
    A) Periosteum
    B) Collagen membrane
    C) Cell-seeded matrices
    D) Cell-seeded carriers

27. What is an orthopedic indication for platelet-rich plasma (PRP)?
    A) Tendinopathy
    B) Alopecia
    C) (A) and (B)
    D) None of the above

28. Anisotropy occurs in all of the following structures except:
    A) Subcutaneous fat
    B) Ligament
    C) Tendon
    D) Muscle

29. Which of the following statements is **false** about tendon fenestration?
    A) A 20- or 22-gauge needle is recommended
    B) After the procedure, patients should ice the area and take nonsteroidal anti-inflammatory drugs (NSAIDs) for pain relief
    C) Patients are immobilized after the procedure as a precaution
    D) Tenotomy into a partial tear stimulates healing by causing local bleeding that releases growth factors

30. Which bony protuberance, located between the second and third dorsal compartments of the wrist, is used as a landmark to start dorsal compartment sonography?
    A) Gerdy's tubercle
    B) Guyon's tubercle
    C) Lister's tubercle
    D) Radial tuberosity

31. You are going to perform an injection on a patient with bicipital tendonitis. Once positioned properly, you are now ready to administer the medication. You insert the needle _____ to the transducer and are mindful to not inject into the _____ artery.
    A) Out-of-plane; humeral circumflex
    B) In-plane; humeral circumflex
    C) Out-of-plane; brachial
    D) In-plane; brachial

32. Which type of collagen (COL) is found in injured tendons?
    A) COL1
    B) COL2
    C) COL3
    D) COL4

33. Citrate dextrose is used in platelet-rich plasma (PRP) preparation. How does citrate dextrose cause anticoagulation?
    A) Binds calcium thereby preventing the clotting cascade
    B) Releases calcium thereby preventing the clotting cascade
    C) Binds calcium to allow the clotting cascade
    D) Binds sodium thereby initiating the clotting cascade

34. The healing of both soft and hard tissue is mediated by a complex array of intracellular and extra-cellular events regulated by:
    A) Vascular endothelial growth factor
    B) Signaling proteins
    C) Target cells
    D) Allogenic fibrin glue

35. Lesions to the articular cartilage have a poor ability for self-repair and therefore have become an important area of study for engineering tissues. It is an ideal tissue to engineer as it only requires one type of cell to regenerate, the:
    A) Osteoblast
    B) Osteoclast
    C) Chondrocyte
    D) Tenocyte

36. A female patient has recently started preparing for a marathon, and has pain on the bottom of her foot which is worse with the first few steps of the day. She states it has progressively worsened and her coach told her to rest for a few days and apply ice to decrease inflammation. Which of the following, upon ultrasound examination of the plantar fascia, would be considered abnormal and indicative of plantar fasciitis?
    A) Hyperechoic thinning of less than 2 mm
    B) Hyperechoic thickening of more than 4 mm
    C) Hypoechoic thickening of more than 4 mm
    D) Hypoechoic thinning of less than 2mm

37. On short-axis ultrasound imaging, this structure has a speckled or honeycomb appearance:
    A) Ligament
    B) Peripheral nerve
    C) Artery
    D) Tendon

38. Which of the following statements is **true**?
    A) Eighty percent of Baker's cysts communicate to the knee joint
    B) A Baker's cyst is an accumulation of joint fluid between the semitendinosus and the lateral gastrocnemius
    C) Baker's cysts do not communicate with the knee joint
    D) The knee joint should be aspirated prior to aspiration of a Baker's cyst

39. Which bursa is located between the patellar tendon and the tibia?
    A) Superficial infrapatellar bursa
    B) Deep infrapatellar bursa
    C) Suprapatellar bursa
    D) Prepatellar bursa

40. A 50-year-old woman presents to your office with anterior shoulder pain secondary to bicipital tendonitis. After 2 years of performing blind injections to the biceps tendon, you decide to use the new ultrasound machine in your office. For the best visualization of the biceps tendon, you ask the patient to sit with:
    A) Elbow flexed and forearm supinated
    B) Elbow extended and forearm supinated
    C) Elbow flexed and forearm pronated
    D) Elbow extended and forearm pronated

41. Which type of collagen (COL) is found in healthy tendons?
    A) COL1
    B) COL2
    C) COL3
    D) COL4

42. As per International Cellular Medicine Society (ICMS) guidelines, what is commonly used to anticoagulate blood in preparation for platelet-rich plasma injections?
    A) Citrate dextrose
    B) Coumadin
    C) Heparin
    D) Lovenox

43. In healthy individuals approximately how long does the remodeling phase of tissue repair take?
    A) 1 day
    B) 3 days
    C) Several weeks
    D) 6 months

44. With regards to self-reported pain levels in patients, mesenchymal stem cells (MSCs) injection can:
    A) Improve pain
    B) Have no effect on pain
    C) Increase pain
    D) Be inconclusive

45. Which one of the following structures appears hyperechoic under ultrasound?
    A) Blood vessels
    B) Fluid collection
    C) Tendinosis
    D) Tendons

46. Under musculoskeletal ultrasound guidance, normal muscle appears:
    A) Hyperechoic with posterior acoustic shadowing
    B) Hyperechoic, with fibrillar echotexture
    C) Hypoechoic, with hyperechoic septa
    D) Uniformly hypoechoic

47. Which of the following adjustments can be made to visualize a deep structure such as the hip on ultrasound?
    A) Use a higher frequency transducer
    B) Use a curvilinear probe
    C) Use a linear probe
    D) Adjust the gain

48. Which of the following structures is easiest to visualize on ultrasonography?
    A) Popliteofibular ligament
    B) Medial collateral ligament
    C) Anterior cruciate ligament
    D) Posterior cruciate ligament

49. The best way to improve the visualization of the needle under the transducer while performing an ultrasound guided injection is to:
    A) Use a lower gauge needle
    B) Increase the amount of gel
    C) Keep the needle parallel to the transducer
    D) Have a steeper approach

50. What is true about how platelet-rich plasma (PRP) must be prepared?
    A) Must be clotted
    B) Must be anticoagulated
    C) Must be dehydrated
    D) Must be hydrated

51. How soon should a patient be followed up (as recommended by the International Cellular Medicine Society [ICMS]) after injection of platelet-rich plasma (PRP)?
    A) 2 to 6 days
    B) 2 to 6 weeks
    C) 2 to 6 months
    D) 12 months

52. In healthy individuals, approximately how long does the proliferative phase of tissue repair take?
    A) 1 day
    B) 3 days
    C) Several weeks
    D) 6 months

53. Mesenchymal stem cells (MSCs) are the best source for seeding scaffolds in tissue engineering due to their ability to differentiate. They are:
    A) Hematopoietic stromal stem cells
    B) Nonhematopoietic stromal stem cells
    C) Hematopoietic adipose stem cells
    D) Non-hematopoietic adipose stem cells

54. Which condition is likely if a patient has limited external shoulder rotation when evaluating the subscapularis at sonography?
    A) Impingement syndrome
    B) Subscapularis tear
    C) Supraspinatus tendinosis
    D) Adhesive capsulitis

55. Which of the following injection techniques has been shown to be the most accurate way to perform a piriformis injection?
    A) Use of anatomical landmarks (ie, "blind" technique)
    B) Fluoroscopy with contrast dye
    C) Ultrasound guidance
    D) Electrodiagnosis (EMG) guidance

56. All of the following are signs of peripheral nerve entrapment on ultrasound **except**:
    A) Muscle atrophy noted in muscles supplied by the affected nerve
    B) Hypoechoic swelling of the involved nerve at the compression site

    C) Symptoms of numbness and tingling with transducer pressure over the nerve
    D) Cystic areas and calcification within the entrapped nerve

57. A patient is thought to have a medial collateral ligament tear. On sonography, valgus stress is applied to the knee and it widens by 8 mm. What is the diagnosis?
    A) Intact medial collateral ligament
    B) Grade 1 injury
    C) Grade 2 injury
    D) Grade 3 injury

58. When performing an ultrasound-guided injection, if the needle is introduced perpendicularly to the transducer, it is considered:
    A) In plane
    B) Out of plane
    C) Cross plane
    D) Linear plane

59. What is the sequence in which cellular response to injury occurs?
    A) Inflammation, remodeling, hemostasis, proliferation
    B) Proliferation, inflammation, remodeling, hemostasis
    C) Hemostasis, proliferation, inflammation, remodeling
    D) Hemostasis, inflammation, proliferation, remodeling

60. According to the International Cellular Medicine Society (ICMS) what is recommended about nonsteroidal anti-inflammatory drug (NSAID) use post–platelet-rich plasma (PRP) injection?
    A) Take every 4 to 6 hours
    B) Take every 12 hours
    C) Take every 24 hours
    D) Avoid use

61. In healthy individuals, approximately how long does the inflammatory phase of tissue repair take?
    A) 1 day
    B) 3 days
    C) Several weeks
    D) 6 months

62. When explaining to a patient the benefit of stem cell therapy, they ask if there is any anti-inflammatory effect of the treatment. You remember reading a recent study which proves mesenchymal stem cells (MSCs) can modulate the functions of the adaptive immune system cells including:
    A) B-cells only
    B) T-cells only
    C) Both B-cells and T-cells
    D) Red blood cells

63. Which of the following is a finding on ultrasound that is characteristic of osteoarthritis?
    A) Well-defined bony protrusions at the margins of an involved joint
    B) Synovial hypertrophy with increased flow on color or power Doppler
    C) The double contour sign
    D) Hyperechoic soft tissue deposits with a hypoechoic rim in affected joints

64. Which of the following is an advantage to using ultrasound to perform an injection as opposed to performing an injection "blindly"?
    A) Avoidance of neurovascular structures
    B) Reduction in pain/discomfort
    C) Reduced rate of infection
    D) Decrease in time required for each procedure

65. Which of the following is **true** regarding ultrasound-guided percutaneous joint procedures?
    A) The needle should always be aimed directly at joint articulations
    B) Joint recesses that are filled with fluid should be avoided
    C) For proper visualization, it is recommended to use a needle that is 18-gauge
    D) Accuracy of ultrasound-guided joint procedures is improved if the needle tip is directly visualized within the target

66. What is the sensitivity of ultrasound for diagnosing meniscal tears?
    A) 45%
    B) 65%
    C) 75%
    D) 85%

67. When considering the resolution quality of an ultrasound transducer, which of the following frequencies leads to the highest resolution?
    A) High frequency
    B) Medium frequency
    C) Low frequency
    D) Cross frequency

68. A patient who recently performed daily prolonged walking on vacation presents to your clinic complaining of pain distal to the medial aspect of the knee. After evaluating the medial collateral ligament, you notice three tendons inserting into the anteromedial proximal tibia. She complains of pain as the transducer is pressed to improve the visualization of these tendons. What is her most likely diagnosis?
    A) Medial meniscal tear
    B) Baker's cyst
    C) Pes anserine bursitis
    D) Saphenous nerve compression

69. Which of the following is a relative contraindication to platelet-rich plasma (PRP) according to the International Cellular Medicine Society (ICMS)?
    A) Cancer, especially hematopoietic, or of the bone
    B) Sepsis
    C) Patient not willing to accept the risk
    D) Platelet dysfunction syndrome

70. What phase of tissue repair leads to the formation of new tissue?
    A) Inflammation
    B) Proliferation
    C) Remodeling
    D) Hemostasis

71. An elderly patient arrives in the office asking for alternative options for his knee osteoarthritis (OA) as conservative management as corticosteroid injections did not provide any relief. You recommend adipose-derived stem cell therapy because it is effective in:
    A) Cartilage healing
    B) Reducing pain
    C) Improving function
    D) All of the above

72. Which of the following techniques is the most accurate way to diagnose carpal tunnel syndrome (CTS) via ultrasound?
    A) Measure the cross-sectional area (CSA) of the median nerve at the carpal tunnel and diagnose CTS if the CSA is greater than 9 mm$^2$
    B) Measure the diameter of the median nerve at the carpal tunnel and if it is greater than 12 mm, the patient has CTS
    C) Do a side-to-side comparison of the cross-sectional area of the median nerve at the carpal tunnel, and if it is 20% larger than the unaffected side, the patient has carpal tunnel syndrome
    D) Measure the difference between the CSA of the median nerve at two levels—the carpal tunnel and the pronator quadratus—and diagnose CTS if the difference in the CSA is more than 2 mm

73. Ultrasound findings of trigger finger may include all of the following **except:**
    A) Accumulation of granular, hyperechoic material in the synovial sheath
    B) Diffuse hypoechoic thickening of the A1 pulley
    C) Synovial sheath effusion
    D) Swelling of the flexor digitorum superficialis (FDS) and profundus (FDP) tendons

74. Techniques to improve needle visualization include all of the following except:
    A) Positioning the needle so that the ultrasound beam is perpendicular to the needle's surface
    B) "Jiggling" the needle while moving the transducer over the needle path, which moves the adjacent soft tissue
    C) Rotating the bevel downward
    D) Using a lower gauge needle

75. How should the shoulder be positioned to best visualize the supraspinatus tendon?
    A) Neutral position
    B) Internally rotated
    C) Hyperextended
    D) Externally rotated

76. When the ultrasound probe is looking at a cross-sectional view of a structure it is considered to be:
    A) Long axis
    B) Short axis
    C) Cross axis
    D) Sagittal

77. While preparing to perform an aspiration of a patient's olecranon bursitis, you note that he has significant limitation of range of motion during exam secondary to pain, severe tenderness to palpation, and hyperechoic particles on ultrasound exam. He denies any numbness/tingling or weakness. At this point you should:
    A) Perform the aspiration and steroid injection as planned
    B) Not give steroids at this point and consider further workup for possible septic joint
    C) Refer for surgical bursectomy
    D) Recommend electrodiagnosis (EMG) to rule out ulnar neuropathy

78. Which of the following is not an absolute contraindication for platelet-rich plasma (PRP) as listed in the International Cellular Medicine Society (ICMS)?
    A) Platelet dysfunction syndrome
    B) Tobacco use
    C) Septicemia
    D) Local infection at site of injection

79. Fibroblasts initiate what phase of tissue repair?
    A) Inflammation
    B) Proliferation
    C) Remodeling
    D) Hemostasis

80. It is understood that mesenchymal stem cells (MSCs) have the ability to differentiate to all tissues within a joint and modulate a local inflammatory response, making injection thereof a potential regenerative solution, providing building blocks to restore damaged joints. Evidence also suggests they stimulate native tissue through _____ stimulation.
    A) Exocrine
    B) Paracrine
    C) Endocrine
    D) Autocrine

81. The repairing of cartilage by mesenchymal stem cell (MSCs) implantation can best be evidenced by which imaging modality?
    A) X-ray
    B) MRI
    C) Bone scan
    D) Ultrasound

82. During the late stage of osteoarthritis, the repaired tissue from human articular cartilage has a unique progenitor cell population known as *chondrogenic progenitor cells* (CPCs). They exhibit:
    A) Multipotent differentiation capacity toward the adipose lineage
    B) Unipotent differentiation capacity toward the chondrocytic lineage
    C) Pluripotent differentiation capacity toward the adipose lineage
    D) Multipotent differentiation capacity toward the chondrocytic lineage

# Ultrasound and Regenerative Medicine

## ANSWERS

1. **C)** The characteristic appearance of rheumatoid arthritis on musculoskeletal ultrasound includes hypoechoic synovium (due to synovial hypertrophy), hyperemia (increased color or power Doppler flow) in joints with active synovitis, and discontinuity of the bony cortex in two orthogonal planes (erosions). Stress fractures may initially appear on ultrasound as a focal hypoechoic area adjacent to bone that may later progress to fracture step-off deformity. Heterotopic ossification appears hyperechoic, with posterior acoustic shadowing. Osteoarthritis is characterized by cartilage loss and osteophyte formation in affected joints. Osteophytes appear as well-defined bony outgrowths at the margin of the involved joint.

2. **A)** Tendinosis (tendinopathy) is characterized by a lack of active inflammation. On ultrasound, the tendon will typically have an ill-defined heterogeneous and hypoechoic area with no well-defined defect. The tendon may be similarly hypoechoic to the adjacent muscle. Cortical irregularity of the greater tuberosity is associated with supraspinatus tears.

3. **B)** During elbow flexion, it is normal for the triceps brachii to be located between the medial epicondyle and the olecranon (the ulnar groove). However, during extension, no muscle should be present in the ulnar groove. The anconeus epitrochlearis can be found by bringing the elbow into extension and looking for muscle tissue in the ulnar groove. Absence of the cubital tunnel retinaculum can predispose individuals to transient dislocation of the ulnar nerve. Transient dislocation generally occurs anteromedial to the medial epicondyle with elbow flexion and can irritate the ulnar nerve.

4. **B)** Both the peroneus brevis and peroneus longus can be visualized posterior to the lateral malleolus. The peroneus brevis inserts onto the base of the fifth metatarsal and the peroneus longus inserts on the first metatarsal. The tibialis anterior inserts on the medial cuneiform. The tibialis posterior inserts on the navicular.

5. **B)** MSCs are nonhematopoietic stromal stem cells that originate from bone marrow, periosteum, blood vessel walls, adipose tissue, muscle, tendon, umbilical cord blood, skin, and dental tissues. They are able to self-replicate and differentiate into mesenchymal tissues, such as bone, cartilage, ligament, tendon, muscle, and adipose tissue.

6. **B)** Large bore needles are used to draw up and to inject PRP to prevent unintentional activation of platelets.

7. **B)** MSCs are found in a variety of tissues. They have the ability to rapidly proliferate and differentiate into musculoskeletal lineages. This includes bone and cartilage. MSCs do not slowly proliferate. MSCs can also differentiate into tenocytes (tendons), osteoblasts (bone), and smooth muscle; however, the bone and cartilage musculoskeletal lineage is of most importance for osteoarthritis.

8. **C)** According to evidence-based orthopedics in the *Journal of Bone and Joint Surgery*, studies have shown that in patients with knee-joint degeneration, PRP did not provide more benefit than injections of hyaluronic acid (HA). These patients were given three weekly intra-articular injections of PRP or HA.

9. **A)** A known side effect of injected corticosteroids is toxicity to the chondrocytes and the MSCs. Despite giving temporary pain relief, injected corticosteroids impair wound healing for 8 to 12 weeks, may postpone the need for surgical intervention temporarily, and will not halt the progression of osteoarthritis. Joint replacement is the ultimate solution.

10. **B)** Tendon fibers should remain undisrupted in tendinosis. Neovascularization refers to the growth of new blood vessels into chronically damaged areas of tendon and can be viewed on ultrasound using color Doppler imaging. Neovascularization and the accompanying nerve fibers that coincide with vessel growth is hypothesized to be the source of pain in chronic tendinopathy. Tendinosis appears as hypoechoic swelling of the involved tendon.

11. **B)** A full-thickness tear of the supraspinatus extends from the articular to the bursal side. It can be focal or incomplete, or it may involve the entire width of a tendon. A full-width or complete tear involves the entire width of the tendon.

12. **D)** The apex of the greater trochanter is a key landmark between the anterior and lateral facets of the greater trochanter. The gluteus minimus tendon is identified over the anterior facet and the distal gluteus medius is over the lateral facet. The gluteus maximus courses over the posterior facet.

13. **D)** The carpal tunnel is surrounded by the carpal bones inferiorly and the flexor retinaculum superiorly. A total of nine tendons and one nerve run through the carpal tunnel—four tendons of the flexor digitorum profundus, four tendons of the flexor digitorum superficialis, one tendon of the flexor pollicis longus, and the median nerve. By hydrodissecting the median nerve away from the flexor retinaculum using ultrasound guidance, patients may have prolonged relief of symptoms. This serves as a way to delay or end the impending need for surgical intervention.

14. **B)** Embryonic stem cells are pluripotent, meaning they can differentiate into any cell type except for the placenta and umbilical cord. Mesenchymal stem cells are nonhematopoietic stromal stem cells that originate from bone marrow, periosteum, blood vessel walls, adipose tissue, muscle, tendon, umbilical cord blood, skin, and dental tissues. They are able to self-replicate and differentiate into mesenchymal tissues, such as bone, cartilage, ligament, tendon, muscle, and adipose tissue. Epidermal stem cells regenerate layers of the epidermis found in the basal layer. Hematopoietic stem cells differentiate into blood and immune cells.

15. **B)** Fibrin needs to be laid down to allow membrane formation. Platelet-rich plasma stimulates the proliferation of stem cells and fibroblasts.

16. **D)** Activating the PRP allows for the release of the contents of their alpha granules from the platelets. The clot contains the secreted proteins and maintains their presence at the application site. It is usually done by adding a solution of 1,000 units of topical bovine thrombin per milliliter of 10% calcium chloride to the PRP. It is neither melted (as it is already in liquid form), nor charged (as there is no electric gradient used for PRP), nor transduced (as it does not change form).

17. **A)** The maturing process of the cartilage requires a rehabilitation protocol including possibly immobilizing the joint with a brace (eg, knee in extension with full weight bearing while in the brace). Return to running usually occurs between 7 and 9 months, and return to sports usually occurs in 12 months. Pain control, monitoring of side effects, and need for reinjection are important things to monitor. However, they are not the most important in the postprocedural rehabilitation protocol.

18. **B)** Prior to the inflammation phase, the clotting cascade takes place to stop blood loss, that is, hemostasis. During the inflammatory phase chemokines, cytokines, growth factors, histamine, prostaglandins, and prostacyclins are released. Fibroblasts enter about 2 to 3 days after the injury, initiating the proliferative phase. The proliferative phase includes angiogenesis, granulation tissue formation, epithelialization, and contraction. The next phase is maturation and remodeling. During this phase, type I collagen replaces type III collagen that was laid down in the proliferative phase. Remodeling begins 21 days from the injury or when the collagen content of the wound is stable.

19. **B)** Acute muscle injury appears hyperechoic on sonography due to areas of hemorrhage. In fact, excessive exercise can even cause diffuse muscle hyperechogenicity due to transient muscle edema. Hemorrhage will appear more hypoechoic later in the course of injury, or may look heterogeneous with mixed echogenicity. Heterotopic ossification is hyperechoic with posterior acoustic shadowing.

20. **C)** The short axis view is preferred for tendon sheath procedures because it enables flexibility in targeting the needle either above, next to, or deep to the tendon. In contrast, when using the long axis approach, the needle can only be placed superficial to the tendon. Superficial placement of the needle relative to the tendon when using corticosteroids increases the risk of subcutaneous fat atrophy or depigmentation.

21. **A)** Tibialis anterior is the largest and most medial tendon in the transverse plane of the anterior ankle. The next structures, from medial to lateral, are the extensor hallucis longus, the anterior tibial artery, the deep peroneal nerve, and the extensor digitorum longus.

22. **A)** The patient with tennis elbow (lateral epicondylitis) may either be positioned supine with the arm internally rotated and elbow flexed, or sitting upright with the elbow flexed in order to get proper visualization of both the lateral epicondyle and the common extensor tendon for the injection. The common extensor tendon includes the extensor carpi radialis brevis, extensor digitorum, extensor digiti minimi, and extensor carpi ulnaris. Alternatively, golfer's elbow (medial epicondylitis) would warrant visualization of the medial epicondyle and the common flexor tendon.

23. **A)** PRP is prepared by centrifugation to obtain a high concentration of platelets. Platelets then degranulate and release growth factors that have healing properties.

24. **A)** Citrate dextrose lowers pH levels and therefore must be buffered prior to the injection, as some growth factors are dependent on pH levels. Citrate-based anticoagulants bind to calcium, which is required for the thrombin cascade.

25. **C)** Levels of growth factors released can be quantified using ELISA. The northern blot is used to identify particular mRNA sequences and the western blot is used to identify specific amino acid sequences in proteins. The Sohal assay does not exist.

26. **A)** With regards to autologous chondrocyte implantation, the cell suspension to be injected is split into three generations. The first is periosteum, second is collagen membrane, and the third is split into two categories: cell-seeded matrices, and cell-seeded carriers.

27. **A)** Indications for PRP include the following: tendinopathies, ligament sprains, muscle strains, joints, intervertebral disks, and fractures.

28. **A)** Anisotropy refers to a variation in the ultrasound appearance of fibrillar tissues whereby the hyperechoic fibrillar appearance is lost when the ultrasound beam is not perpendicular to the visualized structure. Tendons and ligaments are especially subject to anisotropy, and muscle's appearance is affected to a lesser extent. Fat is hyperechoic on ultrasound and is not subject to anisotropy.

29. **B)** Patients should not take NSAIDs after needle tenotomy so the release of growth factors will not be inhibited. They are instructed to immobilize the area after treatment as a precaution. The procedure is typically done with a 20- or 22-gauge needle, which is inserted into the abnormal segment approximately 20 to 30 times. This is thought to stimulate local bleeding and subsequent release of growth factors, which will promote healing of a partially torn tendon.

30. **C)** Lister's tubercle is a pronounced bony prominence on the distal radius located between the second and third dorsal compartments of the wrist. It is typically the starting point for evaluation of the dorsal wrist.

31. **A)** The long head of the biceps tendon runs through the intertubercular groove. The best approach to inject into the tendon sheath is in-plane from the lateral side. Care should be taken to avoid the humeral circumflex artery, which crosses almost perpendicularly posterior to the tendon.

32. **C)** COL3 has less cross-links and is seen within tropocollagen. There are five types of collagen. Collagen type I is found in skin, tendon, vessels, organs, and bone. Collagen type II is found in cartilage. Collagen type III is found in reticular fibers. Collagen IV forms basal lamina and collagen type V is found on cell surfaces, hair, and placenta.

33. **A)** Citrate dextrose binds calcium, preventing the clotting cascade.

34. **B)** Although not completely understood, signaling proteins aid in healing both soft and hard tissues by inducing an interaction between growth factors and surface receptors on the target cells, which activate pathways that induce the production of proteins needed for the regenerative process. Vascular endothelial growth factor (VEGF) is one of the many growth factors necessary for this pathway. Target cells contain the surface receptors mentioned. Allogenic fibrin glue was described in 1970 and is formed by polymerizing fibrinogen with thrombin and calcium.

35. **C)** Chondrocytes are the building blocks of articular cartilage, and have limited cell regeneration. This makes them ideal tissue to engineer. Osteoblasts build bone, osteoclasts break down bone, and tenocytes are the building blocks of tendons.

36. **C)** In plantar fasciitis, the fascia is thickened and is hypoechoic, as compared to the normal fascia, which is echogenic. This is best seen at the calcaneal insertion of the plantar fascia.

37. **B)** Normal peripheral nerves have a honeycomb or speckled appearance on short axis, and look fascicular on long axis. The individual nerve fascicles are hypoechoic and are surrounded by hyperechoic connective tissue (epineurium). Ligaments are hyperechoic, with a striated appearance that is more compact than tendons. Ligaments also can be distinguished from tendon because they connect two bony structures. Arteries can be seen pulsating and are hypoechoic circles surrounded by hyperechoic connective tissue. Tendons are hyperechoic with a fibrillar echotexture, which represents the endotendineum septa.

38. **D)** Baker's cysts communicate with the knee joint in 50% of patients over 50 years old. A Baker's cyst is a distended bursa between the semimembranosus and the medial gastrocnemius. Prior to aspirating a Baker's cyst, the knee should be aspirated for fluid. If there is a communication and the knee contains fluid, failure to do this step will result in immediate reaccumulation of joint fluid within the Baker's cyst.

39. **B)** The deep infrapatellar bursa is between the distal patellar tendon and the proximal tibia. The superficial infrapatellar bursa is anterior to the distal patellar tendon. The prepatellar bursa is located anterior to the patella. The suprapatellar bursa extends superiorly from the knee joint between the patella and femur and is bordered anteriorly by the quadriceps fat pad.

40. **A)** In order to best visualize the biceps tendon, the transducer is held over the proximal humerus in the axial plane, the elbow is flexed, and the hand is supinated. The biceps is best visualized in this position. Elbow extension and hand pronation does not improve visualization.

41. **A)** There are five types of collagen. Collagen type I is found in skin, tendon, vessels, organs, and bone. Collagen type II is found in cartilage. Collagen type III is found in reticular fibers. Collagen IV forms basal lamina, and collagen type V is found on cell surfaces, hair, and placenta.

42. **A)** Citrate dextrose is a solution of citric acid, sodium citrate, and dextrose in water. It is used to anticoagulate blood, but preserve the blood contents.

43. **D)** The remodeling phase of tissue repair takes about 6 months or longer depending on the type of wound.

44. **D)** Many studies have been done showing improved levels of self-reported pain when compared to controls. However, most of the studies have been deemed of poor quality and, at the time of writing, the effect of MSCs injection on pain is inconclusive.

45. **D)** Tendons, ligaments, bone, and calcifications appear as hyperechoic structures. Tendons distinctly have a fibrillar pattern under ultrasound. Blood vessels and fluid collections are anechoic, and tendinosis is hypoechoic.

46. **C)** Using musculoskeletal ultrasound, various soft tissue structures can be distinguished from one another by their characteristic appearance. Normal muscle is hypoechoic (dark) and has hyperechoic septa. Bone is hyperechoic (bright) at its surface, with posterior acoustic shadowing (darkness) deep to the bone's surface. Normal tendons are hyperechoic with a fibrillar pattern. Hyaline cartilage is uniformly hypoechoic.

47. **B)** Linear transducers with high-frequency (10 MHz or greater) are typically used to view musculoskeletal structures, which are mostly superficial. In order to visualize a deeper structure, such as the hip, a lower-frequency transducer with a curvilinear probe should be used. The gain refers to the overall brightness of the screen, and should be adjusted until the ultrasound characteristics of normal soft tissues can best be visualized.

48. **B)** Superficial ligaments, such as the medial and lateral collateral ligaments, can be effectively evaluated by ultrasound. However, deeper structures like the anterior and posterior cruciate ligaments can only be partially visualized on sonography. MRI should be utilized if damage to these ligaments is suspected. The popliteofibular ligament is also difficult to evaluate, but injury to it often coincides with a lateral collateral ligament tear or abnormal widening of the lateral joint space with varus stress.

49. **C)** Improving the visualization of the needle is best done by keeping the needle as parallel to the transducer as possible, possibly by using a gel standoff. A lower gauge needle (larger size) does not always improve visualization if it is not parallel to the transducer. Excess gel may help to create a gel standoff; however, the positioning is the most important aspect to improving visualization. A steeper approach actually makes it more difficult to see the needle as it is introduced.

50. **B)** PRP must be made from anticoagulated blood to ensure platelets do not clot.

51. **B)** As per the ICMS recommendations, patients should be followed up in 2 to 6 weeks after injection of PRP for assessment of range of motion, pain, and function.

52. **C)** The proliferative phase of tissue repair initiated approximately 3 to 5 days from the initial injury and overlaps with the inflammatory phase.

53. **B)** As nonhematopoietic stromal stem cells, MSCs have many sources and are capable of self-replication and differentiating into and contributing to the regeneration of mesenchymal tissues. These include cartilage, bone, ligament, muscle, tendon, and adipose tissue. Hematopoietic stem cells give rise to all types of blood cells and derived from mesoderm.

54. **D)** Adhesive capsulitis is suggested on sonography when a patient has limited external rotation while evaluating the subscapularis. Sonography can suggest subacromial impingement when there is gradual pooling of subacromial-subdeltoid bursal fluid at the acromion tip during active arm elevation. Subscapularis tears are rarely isolated, and are characterized on sonography by the abnormal appearance of the tendon, which may be retracted or have an area of focal hypoechogenicity.

55. **C)** A cadaver study comparing fluoroscopically guided injection of the piriformis to ultrasound-guided injections found a statistically significant difference in accuracy in favor of the ultrasound-guided technique. The "blind" anatomical technique is not favored due to the small size of the piriformis muscle, its deep location, and its proximity to neurovascular structures. EMG guidance is not usually used for piriformis injections.

56. **D)** Cystic areas and calcifications within peripheral nerves can occur in longstanding peripheral nerve sheath tumors, such as schwannomas. Muscle atrophy can be noted in muscles supplied by the affected nerve. Hypoechoic swelling of the involved nerve at the compression site is characteristic of peripheral nerve entrapment. The patient may experience numbness and tingling with transducer pressure over the nerve.

57. **C)** The medial collateral ligament can be evaluated dynamically by applying valgus stress and observing for medial joint space widening. Medial joint space widening less than 5 mm is a grade 1 injury. Widening of 5 to 10 mm is a grade 2 injury, and more than 10 mm of widening is considered a grade 3 injury.

58. **B)** Out-of-plane injections are performed with the needle inserted perpendicularly to the transducer. In-plane injections are parallel. Cross-plane and linear-plane are not formally used ultrasound terms to describe needle insertion with respect to the transducer.

59. **C)** Hemostasis is the first stage of wound healing and involves blood plasma and platelets for coagulation. Inflammation is mediated by granulocytes, especially leukocytes, and platelets. Tissue regeneration involves growth factors that are found in alpha granules.

60. **D)** According to the guidelines/recommendations listed in the ICMS, NSAIDs should be avoided until the patient has healed, is pain free, has full function, or has reached a plateau.

61. **B)** The inflammatory phase of tissue repair takes about 3 days.

62. **C)** Several studies show the effect on the adaptive immune system cells such as B- and T-cells. It has been shown that these cells also induce expression of anti-inflammatory mediators in macrophages.

63. **A)** Characteristics of osteoarthritis on ultrasound include osteophytes and cartilage loss of affected joints. Osteophytes appear as well-defined bony protrusions at the margins of an involved joint. Hallmarks of gout include the "double contour sign" and tophi. The double contour sign refers to a double layer of hyperechogenicity, which is due to urate crystal deposition on the surface of cartilage and the normally hyperechoic bony surface. Tophi appear as hyperechoic soft tissue deposits with a hypoechoic rim in affected joint.

64. **A)** Ultrasound image guidance assures avoidance of neurovascular structures, which can be visualized and avoided by the sonographer. However, injections may be equally painful. The rate of infection has not been shown to be lower with the use of ultrasound guidance. Each procedure may take longer due to the added step of ultrasound visualization, depending on the experience of the sonographer.

65. **D)** The needle should not be aimed directly into joint articulations, as this can potentially damage the cartilage lining the joint. Instead, the target should be the joint recess that directly communicates with the joint articulation. Fluid-filled joint recesses are ideal targets for therapeutic injections. Any needle gauge can be used for an ultrasound-guided procedure, but if aspiration is considered, the needle should be at least 22-gauge (18-gauge if the fluid is heterogeneous). Direct visualization of the needle tip is the best way to ensure procedure accuracy.

66. **D)** Ultrasound has a sensitivity of 85% and a specificity of 86% in the diagnosis of meniscal tears. MRI is the imaging method of choice owing to its higher sensitivity. Ultrasound is limited due to incomplete or poor visualization of the entire menisci but can often identify pathology in the posterior horn of the medial meniscus, which is the most common site for tears. Therefore, evaluation is still recommended during sonography of the knee.

67. **A)** Although high-frequency transducers offer a higher resolution, they also offer less depth. Low-frequency transducers, on the other hand, offer poorer resolution, but better depth.

68. **C)** The sartorius, gracilis, and semitendinosus (from anterior to posterior) join to form the pes anserine. Repetitive stress to this area (including prolonged walking) can predispose a patient to pes anserine bursitis, especially in those with knee osteoarthritis. This can be visualized with the technique noted using an oblique orientation of the transducer.

69. **A)** Absolute contraindications include platelets dysfunction syndrome, septicemia, local infection at site of injection, critical thrombocytopenia, and the patient not willing to accept the risks, as listed in the ICMS. Cancer is a relative contraindication.

70. **C)** Prior to the inflammation phase, the clotting cascade takes place to stop blood loss, that is, hemostasis. During the inflammatory phase, chemokines, cytokines, growth factors, histamine, prostaglandins, and prostacyclins are released. Fibroblasts enter about 2 to 3 days after the injury, initiating the proliferative phase. The proliferative phase includes angiogenesis, granulation tissue formation, epithelialization, and contraction. The next phase is maturation and remodeling. During this phase, type I collagen replaces type III collagen that was laid down in the proliferative phase. Remodeling begins 21 days from the injury or when the collagen content of the wound is stable.

71. **D)** Adipose-derived stem cell therapy has been proven to be effective in cartilage healing, pain reduction, and improvement in function, and therefore, appears to be a good option for OA treatment in elderly patients who do not want joint replacement.

72. **D)** Using the difference in the CSA of the median nerve at the carpal tunnel and the pronator quadratus improves the sensitivity and specificity of ultrasound nerve measurements for the diagnosis of carpal tunnel syndrome to 99% and 100%, respectively. Prior studies used the CSA of the median nerve at the carpal tunnel alone and made the diagnosis based upon a 10 to 12 mm$^2$ threshold, which yielded lower sensitivity and specificity. The use of an internal control (the cross-sectional area at the pronator quadratus) compensates for interindividual variability in the CSA of the median nerve.

73. **A)** The A1 pulley is contiguous with the flexor tendon sheath, and is composed of annular bands of connective tissue. It is located at and proximal to the metacarpophalangeal (MCP) joint. A patient with trigger finger will have ultrasound findings that include diffuse hypoechoic thickening of the A1 pulley, swelling of the FDP and FDS tendons, synovial sheath effusion, and dynamic changes in the shape of the synovial sheath during flexion and extension.

74. **C)** Rotating the bevel upward so it is facing toward the ultrasound beam produces a more echogenic appearance. A lower gauge needle is more conspicuous under ultrasound, but should not necessarily be used for this reason alone. Some manufacturers produce coated or etched needles that are more echogenic. "Jiggling" the needle (ie, moving it minimally forward and backward) moves the surrounding soft tissue and can help localize the needle. Positioning the soundbeam perpendicular to the needle increases the echogenicity of the needle; this alignment can be accomplished by moving the puncture site farther from the transducer.

75. **C)** In order to expose the supraspinatus, which is hidden behind the acromion when the shoulder is in a neutral position, the shoulder should be hyperextended. Two common positions used are the Crass position and the modified Crass position.

76. **B)** Short axis gives a cross-sectional view of the structure being examined. Long axis refers to a sagittal view of the structure being examined.

77. **B)** As per the patient's exam and ultrasound evidence of hyperechoic particles, there may be a septic etiology for the patient's pain. Steroids are contraindicated at this time, and the patient needs a more comprehensive workup.

78. **B)** Absolute contraindications include platelets dysfunction syndrome, septicemia, local infection at site of injection, critical thrombocytopenia, and the patient not willing to accept the risks.

79. **B)** Prior to the inflammation phase, the clotting cascade takes place to stop blood loss, that is, hemostasis. During the inflammatory phase, chemokines, cytokines, growth factors, histamine, prostaglandins, and prostacyclins are released. Fibroblasts enter about 2 to 3 days after the injury, initiating the proliferative phase. The proliferative phase includes angiogenesis, granulation tissue formation, epithelialization, and contraction. The next phase is maturation and remodeling. During this phase, type I collagen replaces type III collagen that was laid down in the proliferative phase. Remodeling begins 21 days from the injury or when the collagen content of the wound is stable.

80. **B)** Paracrine stimulation works by local hormones diffusing a short distance to other cells. Exocrine stimulation works by nonhormone secretion into the external environment via ducts. Endocrine stimulation works by hormones being secreted into the blood acting at a distance without ducts. Autocrine stimulation works by hormones that act on the cells producing them.

81. **B)** After MSC implantation with fibrin glue as a scaffold in osteoarthrtitic knees, the regeneration of cartilage is best evidenced via MRI evaluation. X-ray, bone scan, and ultrasound would not be the best imaging modalities to show cartilage regeneration.

82. **D)** As they have a multipotent differentiation capacity toward the chondrocytic lineage, CPCs provide a potential starting point for the development of cell-based therapy for osteoarthritis (OA). They repair and may even be more effective than cells derived from a different source, especially in late OA.

# Index

*Italic page numbers indicate a Question.*